Seafood: Resources, Nutritional Composition, and Preservation

Editor

Zdzisław E. Sikorski, Ph.D., D.Sc.
Head
Department of Food Preservation and Technical Microbiology
Technical University Politechnika Gdańska
Gdansk, Poland

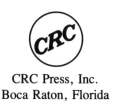

CRC Press, Inc.
Boca Raton, Florida

Library of Congress Cataloging-in-Publication Data

Seafood—resources, nutritional composition, and preservation
  editor, Zdzisław E. Sikorski.
    p. cm.
  Includes bibliographical references.
  ISBN 0-8493-5985-6
  1. Fishery products—Preservation. 2. Fishery products—
Composition. 3. Seafood—Preservation. 4. Seafood—Composition.
5. Fishery resources. I. Sikorski, Zdzisław E.
  SH337.S43 1990
  664'.94—dc20   89-25331
                                                               CIP

This book represents information obtained from authentic and highly regarded sources. Reprinted material is quoted with permission, and sources are indicated. A wide variety of references are listed. Every reasonable effort has been made to give reliable data and information, but the author and the publisher cannot assume responsibility for the validity of all materials or for the consequences of their use.

All rights reserved. This book, or any parts thereof, may not be reproduced in any form without written consent from the publisher.

Direct all inquiries to CRC Press, Inc., 2000 Corporate Blvd., N.W., Boca Raton, Florida 33431.

© 1990 by CRC Press, Inc.

International Standard Book Number 0-8493-5985-6

Library of Congress Number 89-25331
Printed in the United States

FOREWORD

Seafood technology is a very broad field. Its characteristic feature is the application of biochemical, microbiological, chemical, and engineering principles for the preservation and processing of a very large number of species of marine organisms, differing in their composition and properties, to produce safe foods, satisfying the human nutritional requirements and diversified eating habits. There has been a large impact of locally prevailing conditions and of the characteristics of available raw materials on the traditionally developed procedures of fish processing. On the other hand, limitations in availability of conventional resources and the progress in food chemistry and engineering brought about very dramatic changes in the methods of handling, processing, and utilization of seafoods. These broad aspects of seafood technology can be best treated by an international group of specialists.

As the editor of this book, many opportunities to widen my knowledge of various aspects of fish technology had been offered to me by Dr. June Olley from the Commonwealth Scientific and Industrial Research Organization (CSIRO) in Hobart, Tasmania, and by Nick Jarman, the General Manager of the New Zealand Fishing Industry Board. The observations made in Australia and New Zealand added to my European experience. Furthermore, I could count on the cooperation of many internationally recognized specialists in preparing a book on seafood technology.

I would like to extend my gratitude to all colleagues who contributed to this volume and to all persons who gave the permission to use previously published material. A large part of the book was prepared on time, thanks to Mrs. Anna Wilk, who provided the necessary contact with the coauthors and expertly typed many chapters. I would also like to acknowledge the help of Miss Joanna Stroińska and Miss Joanna Chudoba in preparing a large part of the figures. I am also pleased to acknowledge the Politechnika Gdańska in permitting to pursue of the undertaking involving such international cooperation of specialists.

I thank my wife Krystyna for her assuming the responsibilities for the family during the years of my peregrinations abroad.

Zdzisław E. Sikorski
Gdansk, March, 1989.

THE EDITOR

Zdzisław E. Sikorski, Ph.D., is Head of the Department of Food Preservation and Technical Microbiology of the Technical University Politechnika Gdańska.

Dr. Sikorski obtained his training in the Faculty of Chemistry, Technical University Politechnika Gdańska, receiving the B.S. degree in 1954, M.S. in 1956, and Ph.D. in 1960. He gained industrial experience working for short periods from 1956 to 1958 in food processing plants in West Germany and on a deep-sea fishing trawler. In 1964 and 1965, while doing postdoctoral work in the Department of Agricultural Biochemistry at Ohio State University, Columbus, he also served as a Visiting Assistant Professor. In 1965 he earned the degree of Doctor Habilitatus (equivalent to D.Sc.) and in 1966 was appointed Assistant Professor and Head of the Chair of Fish Technology in the Politechnika Gdańska. He became an Associate Professor of Food Science in 1973 and Professor in 1980. He served for 5 years as the Dean of the Faculty of Chemistry. In 1975 and 1976 he was Senior Research Fellow in CSIRO, in Hobart, Tasmania, and in 1981 and 1982 was a Scientist in DSIR in Auckland, New Zealand.

Dr. Sikorski presently is a member of the Committee of Food Technology and Chemistry of the Polish Academy of Sciences, is serving on the Scientific Board of three food research institutions, and has been Chairman of the Scientific Board of the Sea Fisheries Institute in Gdynia. From 1977 to 1988 he was a member of the Main Council of Science and Tertiary Education in Poland. He has received several awards from the Minister of Science and Tertiary Education and from the Secretary of the Division of Agricultural Sciences of the Polish Academy of Sciences.

Dr. Sikorski has published more than 100 papers and 8 books and has obtained 8 patents. His current major research interests relate to changes in muscle proteins due to storage and processing of foods.

CONTRIBUTORS

A. S. Artyukhova, Ph.D.
Senior Scientist
Atlantic Ocean Research Institute of Fish
  Industry and Oceanography
Kaliningrad, Soviet Union

James R. Burt, Ph.D.
Assistant Director
Torry Research Station
Aberdeen, Scotland

Piotr J. Bykowski, Ph.D., D.Sc.
Head
Department of Fish Processing and
  Equipment
Sea Fisheries Institute
Gdynia, Poland

Peter E. Doe, Ph.D.
Senior Lecturer
Department of Civil and Mechanical
  Engineering
University of Tasmania
Hobart, Tasmania, Australia

Zenon M. Ganowiak, Ph.D., D.V.M.
Professor
Department of Food Science
Medical Academy
Gdansk, Poland

Zbigniew Karnicki, Ph.D.
Director
Sea Fisheries Institute
Gdynia, Poland

Anna Kolakowska, Ph.D., D.Sc.
Agricultural Academy of Szczecin
Szczecin, Poland

K. M. B. Miler, Ph.D.
Agricultural Academy of Szczecin
Szczecin, Poland

Marian Naczk
Assistant Professor
Department of Nutrition and Consumer
  Studies
St. Francis Xavier University
Antigonish, Nova Scotia, Canada

June Olley, D.Sc., Ph.D.
Agricultural Science Department
University of Tasmania
Hobart, Tasmania, Australia

Bonnie Sun Pan, Ph.D.
Professor and Dean
College of Fisheries Science
National Taiwan Ocean University
Keelung, Taiwan, ROC

Vladimir I. Shenderyuk, Ph.D.
Laboratory Chief
Department of Semi-Canned Fish
  Technology
Atlantic Ocean Research Institute of Fish
  Industry and Oceanography
Kaliningrad, Soviet Union

Zdzisław E. Sikorski, Ph.D., D.Sc.
Professor and Head
Department of Food Preservation and
  Technical Microbiology
Technical University Politechnika
  Gdańska
Gdansk, Poland

Damazy J. Tilgner, Ph.D., D.Sc.
Professor Emeritus
Technical University Politechnika
  Gdańska
Gdansk, Poland

TABLE OF CONTENTS

Preface 1
Damazy J. Tilgner

Chapter 1
Introduction 5
Zdzisław E. Sikorski

Chapter 2
Resources and Their Availability 9
Zdzisław E. Sikorski and Zbigniew Karnicki

Chapter 3
The Nutritive Composition of the Major Groups of Marine Food Organisms 29
Zdzisław E. Sikorski, Anna Kołakowska, and Bonnie Sun Pan

Chapter 4
Postharvest Biochemical and Microbial Changes 55
Zdzisław E. Sikorski, Anna Kołakowska, and James R. Burt

Chapter 5
The Preparation of the Catch for Preservation and Marketing 77
Piotr J. Bykowski

Chapter 6
Chilling of Fresh Fish 93
Zdzisław E. Sikorski

Chapter 7
Freezing of Marine Foods 111
Zdzisław E. Sikorski and Anna Kołakowska

Chapter 8
Drying and Dried Fish Products 125
Peter E. Doe and June Olley

Chapter 9
Salting and Marinating of Fish 147
Vladimir I. Shenderyuk and Piotr J. Bykowski

Chapter 10
Smoking 163
K. M. B. Miler and Zdzisław E. Sikorski

Chapter 11
Canning of Marine Foods 181
Marian Naczk and A. S. Artyukhova

Chapter 12
Minced Fish Technology 199
Bonnie Sun Pan

Chapter 13
Sanitation in Marine Food Industry..211
Zenon M. Ganowiak

Index 231

PREFACE

Damazy J. Tilgner

TABLE OF CONTENTS

I.	The Resources	2
II.	Wholesomeness	2
III.	Preservation	2
IV.	Nutritive Quality	2
V.	Palatability	3
VI.	Interscience Cooperation	3

I. THE RESOURCES

Around five sixths of the surface of our planet is covered with water. This vast area represents a giant volume in which around 20,000 species live and multiply. Since antiquity fishing and seafood consumption has played an important role in coastal regions. In contrast to other maritime deep water resources seafood undergoes a continuous biological renewal and recycling. Only human interference by overfishing or pollution of the environment can put an end to this eternal biological cycle.

Under the pressure of high demand many valuable species of marine fish and invertebrates are now being produced under controlled conditions in aquaculture. Fish are highly efficient in converting food into animal proteins. For every 1.5 kg of feed they gain 1 kg of body weight. This equals poultry in converting feed protein into body protein. Generally this conversion rate is higher than in slaughter animals. The labor productivity is high since a well-managed catfish farm can yield about 5 ton of fish per man year of labor from 1 acre of earthen ponds. This compares favorably with industrial beef or pork farming.

The steady increase of industrial fish farming shows in some countries great potentials. Catfish, carp, trout, tuna, and salmon are harvested in aquacultures. Fish species with fer bones, white meat, and a mild flavor are attractive to the consumer.

It may be asumed that industrial fish farming will gain further progress and development through organized research including genetic engineering.

II. WHOLESOMENESS

The food industry has to provide wholesome food products without health hazards. It has to guarantee freedom from carriers of disease in its products.

Maritime products, fresh or frozen, should be sampled, inspected, and certified fit for human consumption. In some countries the inspection service and tonnage of consignments is growing. The causes and prevention of quality deterioration are now better known. Rapid microbiological analysis has progressed in recent years and facilitates improved production control.

III. PRESERVATION

The second principal task of the food industry is preservation of the original quality. Fish is very liable to microbiological and biochemical spoilage. Progress has been stimulated by the desire to obtain greater efficiency at lower cost and improved acceptability. Rational packaging techniques based upon considerable scientific findings are interlinked with improved storage and display. Many species in the retail market are now closely trimmed, packaged in transparent wrappers, and always kept under refrigeration. Structural and compositional determinants of sensory properties influence acceptability of food fish.

IV. NUTRITIVE QUALITY

The third task of the food industry is providing products with a high, specified nutritional value. The nutritive quality may be lowered by inadequate care, low speed of delivery, and improper processing, storage, and marketing.

There is a close interdependence between nutrition and health. The general public knows too little about proper diets. Extravagant claims for health food are made, e.g., that fish is good for the brain. This is probably an old wives' tale since there is no food which would improve the memory. However, eating fish and shellfish contributes greatly to good health by reducing the risk of heart disease, strokes, some cancer, and other serious ailments.

V. PALATABILITY

Wholesomeness, stability, and high nutritional value of food are not enough. Neither is convenience in use, since the sensory appeal and pleasing savor are of paramount importance.

The main factor in the success of fish and fish products in the diet is flavor. Since the Second International Congress of Food Science and Technology in Warsaw, 1966, flavorology has developed into detailed sensory and chemical evaluations. Flavor identity, stability, and enhancement are investigated for a better understanding of fish as food. A new seafood nomenclature system to be based on the sensory or edibility characteristics of fish is under development by the National Marine Fisheries Service of the U.S. Department of Commerce. The goal is to enable consumers to make educated choices among fish species. A modified flavor profile method provides comparative sensory data to select a desired flavor and texture of fish. Aroma and flavor characteristics of many species of North Atlantic fish have been evaluated.

The art of fish cookery requires knowledge and imagination. One paramount rule shoud be observed, i.e., do not overcook to obtain a most appreciated savory product. The delicate flavor of most boiled fish is enhanced with butter and good white table wine, preferably chablis, as a seasoning and a pinch of zest.

VI. INTERSCIENCE COOPERATION

Huge marine resources require high international professionalism and cooperation. Closely linked with human needs, marine science has joined forces with food science and technology and with nutrition science. Improving these contacts marine science can contribute best in the area of education and scientific activities. By initiating and sponsoring symposia and courses an international approach can be a real asset. Different systems can learn from each other. Thus, development of marine science and education can be promoted. Human intelligence has changed antique images about sea and fish. International consultancy rectifies errors in adjustments.

The first Consultation of the Fisherics Industry sponsored by UNIDO and FAO was hosted by the Government of Poland and held in Gdańsk in 1987. Two issues have been thoroughly discussed, i.e., the progress in fishing equipment to increase efficiency and the improvement in the processing and marketing chains of fish. The recommendations of the consultation will certainly have a positive impact on the fishery industry.

In comparison with agricultural sciences the size and scope of fishery science requires a substantial increase. It is laudable that this volume informs about the status of marine foods. It must be stressed that seafood products technology requires a solid food science background as the important requisite for positions in the seafood industry.

Chapter 1

INTRODUCTION

Zdzisław E. Sikorski

TABLE OF CONTENTS

I.	Demand for Fish as Food	6
II.	Resources and Availability	6
III.	Developments in Fishing Boats and Gear	6
IV.	Utilization of the Catch	7
V.	The Nutritional Value	7
VI.	Better Sanitary Management	7

I. DEMAND FOR FISH AS FOOD

Marine fish and invertebrates form a substantial part of the human diet, both of the poor and of the wealthy. Their contribution to the world food resources is usually evaluated in terms of protein value. The ratio of the daily fish protein intake per capita to the total animal protein consumption ranged in the 1970s from about 6 in West Germany through 45 in Japan to about 70 in South Korea. In many developing countries, fish, in very simple forms of preparation and artisan preservation, mainly by drying, fermenting, and salting, supply most of the animal protein in the poor man's diet based on staple cereals. On the other hand, many species of fish and marine invertebrates are highly valued because of their superior sensory quality. Therefore, the well-to-do select for their cuisine rare, expensive species of fish, crustaceans, and esoteric mollusks. These seafoods provide the gourmet with exquisite sensory delight. Thus, there is a large and growing demand for fish and marine shellfish as a cheap source of valuable protein, lipids, and other nutrients for the people in need, as well as for the expensive species for the people who can afford. Actually the world catches lag substantially behind the demand in both groups.

II. RESOURCES AND AVAILABILITY

During the last 2 decades, a significant change in the world resources and availability of marine fish and shellfish has taken place. The resources of many traditional species, which formed in the past the basis for large industrial international fisheries, e.g., the herring, pilchard, cod, and some tunas, have been largely overfished. Furthermore, the introduction of the economic zones by the coastal states has restricted the accessibility of many shelf areas for international exploitation. These changes in the availability of resources have led to discoveries of several new rich fishing grounds, both in the shelf seas and in the open oceans. Many of these areas were initially abundant in valuable species; others were quickly recognized as large sources of swarm fish of considerable industrial value. Unfortunately, some of the new resources discovered have also already been overfished because of initial lack of proper international management. There are also resources of species for which there is less demand on the world market, e.g., the capelin and the Antarctic krill. Some of these fish and invertebrates are being caught by a growing number of vessels. The industrial exploitation of other abundant populations, especially of small midwater species in the open oceans, awaits further improvement in the technology of fishing operations and processing. The actual resources available annually for commercial fisheries by contemporary technology are estimated to be about 200 million tons.

The decrease in availability of valuable species, accompanied by a growing demand for top quality seafoods, has brought about rapid developments in sea farming. The quantity of organic material produced in the uncultivated seas, represented by a unit square, is roughly equal to the average in agriculture. The crop taken by the fisheries from the seas, however, is not higher than about 1% of the total production.

III. DEVELOPMENTS IN FISHING BOATS AND GEAR

The changes in worldwide fisheries policy, as well as general technological progress, caused significant alterations in the development trends in fishing boats and gear, as well as in fishing operations. Although the major part of the world catch is now being harvested as before in coastal areas by the crews of small fishing craft, of about 10 m in length, these boats are now better equipped in navigational and communication aids, have more efficient catching gear on board, and many of them have the facilities for chilling the catch in ice of sea water. At the same time, however, very large factory ships are being built, designed for cooperation with fleets of catchers in the Pacific waters and for processing on board, like the new generation floating fish factories for the U.S.S.R., 179 m long, with a crew of 520, equipped for producing frozen fish blocks, canned fish, and crabs, as well as fodder meals.

IV. UTILIZATION OF THE CATCH

The need for better management and utilization of the world resources which are available only at a growing cost for the necessary equipment and energy has encouraged more careful and sophisticated handling and preservation of the catch on board to keep the fish longer in the state of prime freshness, to extend the shelf life, and to reduce losses due to spoilage. In many specialized fisheries, it also proved justifiable to utilize the by-products, which until recently had been discarded overboard. On the other hand, very high prices, paid for top quality fish of prime freshness, have made it possible to apply individual treatment of such resources and air freight the catch to distant quality markets.

The depletion of many species, traditionally used for making worldwide or locally popular fish products, has encouraged efforts to produce the traditional commodities from other, less suitable but abundant raw materials, by properly modifying the technology. Some resources, which were in the past regarded as raw material for fodder meal, are now being used for human consumption. In the wake of the breakthrough made by the American invention of the fish fingers in the 1950s, many fish species of rather low traditional commercial value have made a name as raw material for various products composed of minced fish flesh. Furthermore, the fish minces in form of bland preparations, known as surimi, have been used not only in the seafood industry, but are also being regarded as suitable for blending with other material in non-fish foods. Although much effort was spent in research on dry fish protein concentrates, the commercial application of results has not met high expectations.

V. THE NUTRITIONAL VALUE

There is a growing awareness of the beneficial role of fish and other marine foods in human nutrition. After the discoveries of the first 2 decades of the 20th century, when cod liver oil was found to exhibit preventive and therapeutic effectiveness in vitamin A and D deficiencies, fish liver oils or concentrates were administered to infants and children. Later, due to competition of synthetic vitamins, fish oils lost their important position. They have been, however, again recognized as very beneficial for human health, being the richest source of n-3 fatty acids, which cooperate in preventing both heart disease and heart attack. Fish in the human diet is very important also because it supplies protein of high biological value, as well as a large variety of minerals and microelements. Thus, fish can help to fulfill at least three out of the popular ten suggestions for rational nutrition.

VI. BETTER SANITARY MANAGEMENT

Increasing pollution of many coastal waters brings about serious risks of contamination of the catch, mainly of valuable shellfish. To effectively prevent most of the dangers to human health caused by environmental contaminants, toxins, pathogenic microorganisms, and parasites associated with marine foods from polluted areas, improved sanitary management in the fish industry has been introduced. This is aided by new developments in handling equipment and processing machinery, application of effective refrigeration starting on board the vessel, rationalized parameters of processing, modern protective packaging of the products, good manufacturing practice and sanitary supervision of all operations, and very stringent regulations enforced by various health authorities, especially regarding export licences. Better understanding of the nature of fish and marine invertebrates and of the operations involved in the handling, processing, and preservation of the catch may also help improve the utilization of these resources as human food.

Chapter 2

RESOURCES AND THEIR AVAILABILITY

Zdzisław E. Sikorski and Zbigniew Karnicki

TABLE OF CONTENTS

I. The Marine Habitat 10
    A. The Physical and Chemical Factors 10
        1. Introduction 10
        2. The Depth and the Bottom Deposits 10
        3. The Light 10
        4. The Temperature 11
        5. The Salinity 12
        6. Oxygen, Carbon Dioxide, and Hydrogen Sulfide 12
    B. The Food Chain in the Seas 12

II. The Main Groups of Organisms Exploited for Food 13
    A. Marine Plants 13
        B. Mollusks 14
        C. Crustaceans 15
        D. Fish 17
            1. General Biological Characteristics 17
            2. Fish Families of Commercial Importance 19
                a. Clupeidae and Engraulidae 19
                b. Gadidae 19
                c. Serranidae 19
                d. Carangidae 19
                e. Lutianidae 19
                f. Sparidae 19
                g. Scienidae 19
                h. Nototheniidae 20
                i. Scombridae 20
                k. Scorpenidae 20
                l. Bothidae, Pleuronectidae, and Soleidae 20
                m. Salmonidae 20
                n. Selachii 20

III. Fishing Gear and Boats 21
    A. Fishing Gear 21
        1. Development 21
        2. Wounding Gear and Fishing Lines 21
        3. Fish Traps 22
        4. Nets 22
    B. Fishing Boats 22
        1. Introduction 22
        2. Coastal Fishing Boats 22
        3. Tuna Clippers and Long Liners 24
        4. Trawlers 25
        5. Other Vessels Employed in Fisheries 25

IV.	Accessibility and Limitations of Resources	26
	A. Biological Factors	26
	B. Technical Factors	26

References ... 27

I. THE MARINE HABITAT

A. THE PHYSICAL AND CHEMICAL FACTORS

1. Introduction

The living conditions for marine organisms in oceans and seas depend on a large number of physical and chemical factors of the habitat. These vary extensively under the influence of the geographic location, the seasonal climatic conditions, and in many cases also on the activities of man.[1]

2. The Depth and the Bottom Deposits

Along the coasts of continents the seas are generally shallow, as the land forms there a plateau descends gradually to about 200 m, known as the continental shelf (Figure 1). The shelves account for about 8% of the total ocean area. Their width depends upon the configuration of the coastal zone of the land. Further down, to about 100 m, runs the much steeper continental slope, and beneath, to about 6000 m, extends the deep ocean bottom over some 77% of the ocean area. The bed of the ocean is not quite flat. In many places it forms high underwater ridges and mountain ranges. There are also deep clefts and canyons, some of them reaching down to 10,000 m.

The pressure in the ocean waters, increasing with the depth, is one of the factors that influences the distribution of organic life in the seas. Most of the species of fish and marine invertebrates exploited for commercial purposes are not adapted to live at very great depths. However, even at the extreme high pressures prevailing at the deep ocean bottom, there exist different forms of animal life.

The bottom deposits on the shelves and on the continental slopes are formed by material brought down from the land. Thus, the bottom can be covered with gravel, sand, marls, and muds. There are also deposits of marine origin, i.e., banks of shells or finely ground coral. The vast areas of the deep bed of the ocean are covered with deposits of volcanic nature and remnants of various forms of organic life, composed of tiny calcareous shells, sediments containing skeletons of silica, or so-called red clay, made of volcanic or cosmic dust, and of deposits of animal or plant origin.

3. The Light

Biological life in the seas depends primarily on factors that are necessary for the development of various plant organisms. Most important is the light, the driving force of photosynthesis. Depending on the intensity of light penetration, the sea waters are classified as the translucent zone down to about 80 m, followed by dim waters which extend to 350 m. Further down are dark waters. These zone limits are only approximate, as they are effected significantly by factors influencing light penetration. Sea waters deficient in nutrients, and thus also in unicellular organisms, are more transparent than the more fertile seas.

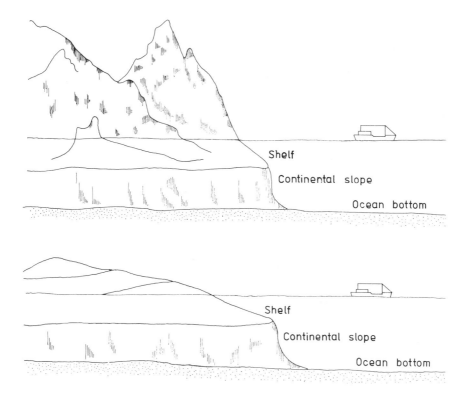

FIGURE 1. The continental shelf and slope.

The irradiation of the seas varies in daily and in seasonal cycles. During the day the phytoplankton, i.e., the drifting, small, unicellular photosynthetizing organisms, can find enough light in the deeper waters rich in nutrients, while during the night they move towards the less dark surface waters. The seasonal cycles of light intensity have a large impact on the biological production in the fertile waters of the temperate and cold zones.

4. The Temperature

The seas and oceans have a very large heat capacity; hence, they are not very susceptible to rapid temperature changes. Usually the surface temperatures of sea waters range from about 28 to $-2.5°C$. Areas of exceptionally high temperature, such as the Persian Gulf, 36°C, are rather rare. The temperature of the sea waters depends on the latitude, water currents, the season, and the depth. Only in the surface layers, influenced by the weather conditions, do the changes in temperature take place within a few hours. In deeper waters, seasonal cycles of temperature are noticeable, while at great depths no fluctuations in temperature take place.

The influence of temperature on the biological life in the seas is both direct and indirect. The temperature affects the solubility of oxygen in the sea water and the intensity of the metabolism of the organisms. Many marine organisms are very well adapted to fluctuating environmental conditions, while others can live only within a very limited range of temperatures. The stenothermic drifting plankton organisms perish instantaneously on being brought with the sea currents into areas of very different temperature. Such zones of convergence of warm and cold waters usually abound in nutrients, originating from mineralization of dead animals or plants.

The water temperature is one of the most essential factors affecting the distribution of fish in the seas. Favorable thermal conditions are especially important for the development of the fertilized eggs. The density of the sea water depends on the salinity and temperature, influencing in turn the vertical distribution of the eggs. Cold waters are generally more fertile than warm seas and are inhabited by a comparatively small number of species, reaching vast populations in years of favorable hatching and feeding conditions. On the other hand, warm seas are generally the habitat of many species competing for food. These species usually do not form large populations.

5. The Salinity

The primary chemical property of sea waters is salinity. Ocean waters contain on the average 35 g salts in 1 dm^3. The salinity of shelf seas of the temperate zones, with a large inflow of fresh water and rather limited connection with the ocean, is much lower — e.g., in the Baltic Sea about 10 g/dm^3. Very salty seas in hot regions contain salt in quantities of about 45 g/dm^3. The quantitative composition of salts from various seas is almost identical: 77.5% NaCl, 10.9% $MgCl_2$, 4.7% $MgSO_4$, 3.6% $CaSO_4$, 2.4% KCl, 0.3% $CaCO_3$, and 0.2% $MgBr_2$. Sea water also contains mineral biogenic compounds, mainly of nitrogen and phosphorus, that are indispensable for organic life. Their concentration is generally very small, about 1 g in 1 m^3 of water. The surface waters in the continental shelf zones, which are heavily supplied by rivers carrying large quantities of inorganic and organic materials, and coastal areas polluted with sewage are much richer in biogenic substances. An excessive accumulation of these compounds at times may cause too massive growth of phytoplankton. This can result in impaired light penetration into the water and depletion of oxygen by the decaying organisms.

In order to be utilized, the biogenic substances must reach the upper water layers where the photosynthetizing organisms can use them. All movements of the sea waters due to drift, currents, tides, and storms bring about a desirable mixing of the pelagic waters and favor the development of all forms of orgnanic life.

6. Oxygen, Carbon Dioxide, and Hydrogen Sulfide

Oxygen accumulates in sea waters mainly in the surface layers due to aeration and the metabolism of plants. The concentration of dissolved oxygen decreases with the increase in temperature, being in 1 dm^3 of water about 8 cm^3 at 0°C and 5.4 cm^3 at 30°C.

Carbon dioxide and hydrogen sulfide accumulate mainly in deeper waters due to decomposition of organic material. Lack of circulation of water in some areas may cause unfavorable conditions for organic life because of too high concentration of these gases and insufficient transport of oxygen to the deeper layers.

B. THE FOOD CHAIN IN THE SEAS

Marine plants are the primary producers of organic material. They utilize the biogenic substances dissolved in the water and assimilate carbon dixoide. They are mainly represented by phytoplankton. These unicellular organisms are abundant in all surface waters. Their growth, however, is especially exuberant in shelf areas, rich in biogenic material and well supplied with light. Shallow coastal belts also form a favorable habitat for many varieties of sea grass and sedentary algae. Many species of algae also inhabit deeper seas. The plant organisms, both unicellular and higher developed plants, provide the necessary food for zooplankton and animal organisms. Furthermore, large colonies of seaweeds thriving off many coasts, form a kind of submarine forest, giving refuge for a vast number of fish and invertebrates of the seas.

The largest biomass of the marine animal kingdom is made up of zooplankton, feeding on the unicellular plant organisms (Figure 2). Most forms of zooplankton can be utilized as food by the plankton-feeding fish and sea mammals. Small benthonic fauna, mainly worms, crustaceans, mollusks, and echinoderms, feed on the seaweeds and they constitute the food of predatory benthos species. Predatory fish prey on all suitable forms of sea animals.

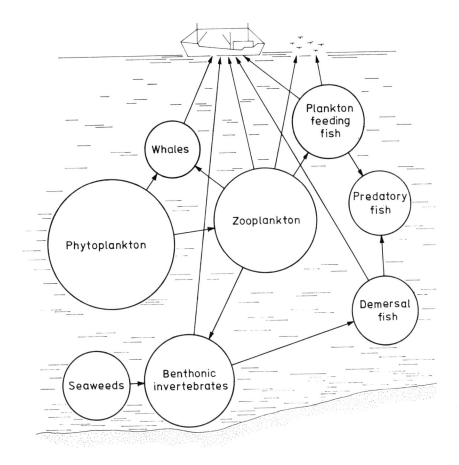

FIGURE 2. The food chain in the seas.

Dead organisms, not utilized by the benthonic fauna, undergo decomposition by microorganisms and mineralization. The mineral products can be thus recycled into the food chain through plants.

II. THE MAIN GROUPS OF ORGANISMS EXPLOITED FOR FOOD

A. MARINE PLANTS

Marine plants or seaweeds occur in an incredibly large variety of life forms, but relatively few are of direct commercial value. Of all marine plants, algae are the most important. They are usually classified into four main groups, taking into consideration their pigmentation, i.e., red Rhodophyceae, brown Phaeophyceae, green Chlorophyceae, and blue-green algae Cyanophyceae.

Red and brown algae appear mainly in the marine environment in cold waters below 20°C and they have the largest commercial importance.

Seaweeds are mainly used for the manufacture of hydrocolloids such as agar, alginates, and carrageenan for direct human consumption and as animal feed and fertilizer. The total world harvest of marine algae in 1986 was 3.5 million metric tons, the three largest producers being China, Japan, and the Republic of Korea.[2]

In the last decade important progress in algae culture technique has been observed, particularly in Asia, especially for species used for colloids production like *Laminaria, Graeilaria, Undaria,* and *Gelidium.*

In the 1960s, attempts have also been made to culture the single cell algae of *Chlorella* spp. and *Spirulina maxima*. However, these attempts never reached a large commercial level.

B. MOLLUSKS

There are over 130,000 species of mollusks, varying in size from a few millimeters to over 20 m. However, only rather small groups of this vast phyla are commercially important. The edible mollusks can be divided into three main groups: univalves having a single shell, bivalves which have two shells, and cephalopods. The first group consists of snails, winkles, whelks, and abalones, the second of oysters, mussels, and clams, and the third of squid, cuttlefish, and octopus. Mollusks form about 7% of the total world catch and play an important role in international trade.

Oysters are considered a delicacy all over the world and over 1 million tons are consumed annually, fresh or processed. Clams, mussels, and scallops are also of considerable importance, forming a base for specialized industry, including not only harvesting and processing sectors but also farming in coastal waters, for example, in Italy, Japan, and China.

The majority of uni- or bivalves are commonly consumed fresh, sold on the market with the shell on. However, freezing as well as canning of shelled meat plays an increasingly important role.

Clams are the most important group of bivalves, with total world catch in 1986 exceeding 1.8 million tons and China, Japan, and the U.S. as the biggest producers and consumers.

The most important of all groups of mollusks are the cephalopods.[3] Their catches have increased threefold in the last 3 decades, reaching in 1986 close to 1.6 million tons. The largest catches are taken by the fisheries of Japan, Korea, Poland, Spain, China, and Thailand.

Cephalopods exist practically in all waters, exhibiting considerable variety of form and eating characteristics. Texture is of particular concern. Of the almost 1000 species of cephalopods, only a few are commercially caught today, mainly for food, but also for bait for other types of fisheries.

Cephalopods are marketed in many forms mainly as fresh, frozen, canned, dried, salted, and smoked. The most important of all cephalopods are squids. Most commercially exploited squids belong to two main families: Ommastrephidae and Loliginidae. About 75% of the world squid catch is composed of the Ommastrephidae.

The most important single species are *Todarodes pacificus* (Figure 3) and *Ommastrephes bartrami*. They compose about 35% of the world squid catch. Other important species of this family are those of genus *Illex*, particularly *I. illecebrosus*, *I. coindetti*, and *I. argentinus*.

The mantle size of the commercially exploited squids from the family Ommastrephidae usually do not exceed 50 cm in length and the weight is below 0.5 kg. Most of these species are taken by highly specialized vessels, using jigging, i.e., light attraction and fishing with hooks. The trawling technique, on the other hand, is commonly used for catching squids of the family Loliginidae. These species have worldwide distribution in both tropical and temperate zones. Of all the species, *Loligo vulgaris* which occurs in the Eastern Atlantic down to South Africa is one of the most important. Generally squids belonging to this family are slightly smaller than Ommastrephidae, with mantle size of 20 to 40 cm.

There are about 130 species of cuttlefish, grouped into two main families, Sepiidae and Sepiolidae. Cuttlefish live in shallow waters of the continental shelf and therefore their resources are very much smaller than those of squid. Cuttlefish are also widely distributed, but are not found eastward of the Japan-Philippines-Australia line and do not occur in the Pacific waters of North and South America.

Though the mantle size of the cuttlefish is very similar to that of most squids, reaching a maximum size of about 45 cm, the weight due to different body shape is much higher, reaching up to 4 kg.

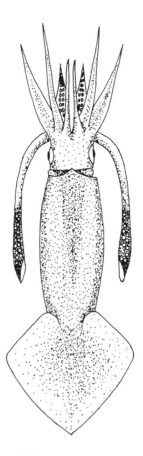

FIGURE 3. Squid *Illex* spp.

Cuttlefish is marketed mainly as fresh or frozen. In Japan and some Far East countries, cuttlefish is served raw or cured in many different ways.

Similar to cuttlefish, octopus inhabit only waters of the continental shelf and usually require some refuge to protect their soft bodies. The most important species is *Octopus vulgaris*, reaching maximum mantle size of up to 1.4 m and about 10 kg weight. The main market for octopus is Japan, Italy, Spain, and Greece.

C. CRUSTACEANS

Crustaceans are the most valuable group of marine organisms. They form about 4% of the total world catch. Almost all species in this group are considered on the world market as high-value commodities.

The most important group are shrimps or prawns (Figure 4). The two names refer to the same group — which one is used depends upon local preferences. The total world catch of shrimp in 1986 reached 1.9 million tons. Shrimp are distributed all over the world. From the commercial point of view, they can be divided into cold-, warm-, and freshwater species.

Coldwater species, e.g., *Pandalus borealis* and *Crangon crangon*, grow slowly and are small in size, compared to warmwater species, mainly of the Penaeus family which grow quickly, reaching a large size. Freshwater species, mainly *Macrobranchium rosenbergii*, inhabit tropical lakes and rivers, growing very fast and reaching a very large size, up to 0.3 kg. For that reason shrimps of Penaeus and Macrobranchium families are now successfully cultured.

Tropical marine species are the most important part of world trade in crustaceans, with

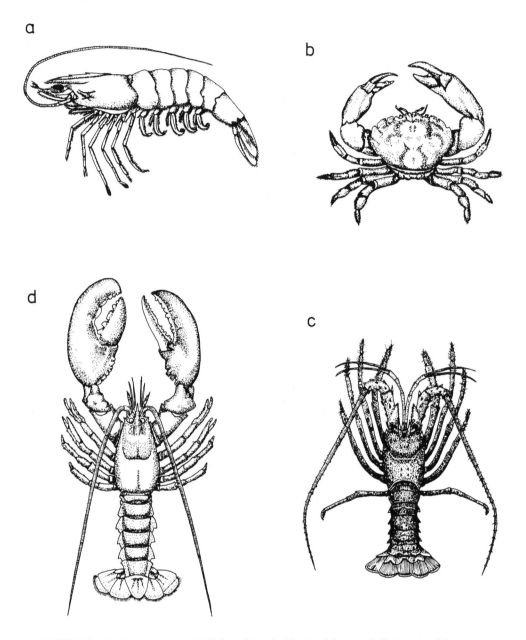

FIGURE 4. Marine crustaceans. (a) Shrimp, (b) crab, (c) spiny lobster, and (d) American lobster.

main markets in the U.S. and Japan. Coldwater species are preferred in Europe. Due to high commercial value, processing and trading of shrimp are highly specialized. Shrimp are sold alive, fresh, frozen, canned, dried, and in a number of different forms, e.g., whole, headless, shell-on, peeled, peeled and deveined, etc. There is precise grading by size systems, i.e., numbers per 1 kg or 1 lb, different in the U.S. and Japan. The main producers of shrimp are India, Indonesia, China, the U.S., and Thailand.

Another important and valuable group of Crustacea is the crab. Caught usually by traps, they form a base for the canning industry, particularily in the U.S., the U.S.S.R., and Japan. Crabs are also sold fresh and frozen. Of all crabs, Pacific snow crabs *Chionoecetes* spp. and king crabs *Paralithodes* spp. are the most important species.

Lobsters are considered a delicacy all over the world and are thus highly priced. Due to their edible quality, lobsters are sold unprocessed, commonly alive, but as a majority fresh or frozen. There are many different species of lobsters of which spine lobsters *Panulirus* spp., rock lobsters *Jasus* spp., American lobster *Homarus americanus,* and European lobsters *H. gammarus* are the most important ones. Coldwater lobsters of *Homarus* spp. differ significantly in shape from the first ones inhabiting warm waters. The *Homarus* spp. have strong claws and can reach the size of a few kilograms.

There are also vast quantities of small pelagic crustacea *Euphausidacea* of which antarctic krill *Euphausia superba* form the largest concentrations, thus enabling efficient catches.[4] Commercial exploitation of this species began in mid-1970s, but so far catches did not exceed 0.5 million tons. The main obstacles in utilization of krill is its small size, about 7 cm and several grams of weight, and thus the necessity to develop new processing machines. Significant progress in this area has been reached in the U.S.S.R., Japan, and Poland. In mid-1980s, peeled krill, frozen or canned, appeared on the market in these countries.

Due to large and still unexploited resources, krill is considered as future object for fisheries not only for food but also as a feed. Important natural polymers, chitin and chitosan, can be extracted on a commercial scale from krill shell. These polymers may be applied in the food industry, waste water treatment, pharmacy, medicine, and the cosmetic industry.

D. FISH
1. General Biological Characteristics

Different species of commercially exploited fish vary in regard to abundance, availability for catch, distribution, size, and biological characteristics.

Most of the species have a streamlined shape. Good swimmers such as salmon, herring, cod, mackerel, shark, or tuna are torpedo or spindle shaped. A laterally or dorsoventrally flattened body is characteristic of bottom dwellers. There are also fish of rod-like shape, e.g., the eel. Many species of fish, less valuable as food sources, have most peculiar forms of the body.

The body of most fish species is covered with scales that are deep-seated in the skin. The scales are covered with epidermis containing many mucous cells which excrete a slime forming a protective layer on the fish body. The color of the fish skin is caused by silvery crystals of guanine, located in the outer layer of the scales. Furthermore, there are skin chromatophores containing yellow and red carotenoid lipochromes, brown or black melanophores containing melanines, and yellow flavine pigments.

The skeleton of bony fish consists of the backbone, the head skeleton, and the bones supporting the fins. Some fish also have a large number of thin intramuscular bones which are a nuisance for the processor and consumer. In the cartilaginous fishes, i.e., sharks, dogfishes, skates, and rays, the skeleton consists of cartilage.

Most fish species have paired pectoral and pelvic fins, a large vertical tail fin, and unpaired fins under the tail and along the back (Figure 5). The fins are of different shape and the unpaired fins differ in number in various species.

The bulk of the trunk musculature in fish consists of two large lateral muscles running on both sides of the body from head to tail. Each muscle is divided by a horizontal septum of connective tissue into the dorsal and ventral part. Details on the structure of the muscles are given in Chapter 3.

The digestive system of the fish varies somewhat from species to species, depending on the specific mode of feeding. Some predatory fish can open their jaws very wide to catch the prey of a size nearly equalling their own. The teeth in predatory species are located not only in the jaw, but also in the throat. They are used for biting the prey and smashing the hard shells of crustaceans. The plankton-eating fish filter off their fine food from water. Fish usually swallow their food without masticating it. The alimentary tract of predatory fish is short and has a distinct stomach, capable of extensive stretching. The stomach is

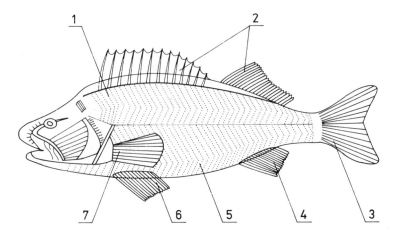

FIGURE 5. The main fins and muscles of fish. (1) Large lateral muscle, dorsal part; (2) dorsal fins; (3) caudal fins; (4) anal fin; (5) large lateral muscle, ventral part; (6) ventral fin; and (7) pectoral fin.

supplied by very active digestive juices. In the bony fish, digestive enzymes are also produced in the pyloric appendices, branching from the tract near the bottom of the stomach. In plankton-feeding fish, the digestive tract is longer and has no stomach.

The liver, pancreas, kidneys, and reproductive organs in fish play a similar role as in mammals. The liver in some fish, apart from its other metabolic functions, also serves as a large store of fat. The kidneys lay in the form of reddish-brown ribbons of soft tissue along the backbone. The ovaries and testes change their shape and size according to the stage of sexual maturity of the fish and are classified as juvenile, mature, and spent. In the mature state, the individual eggs and the fluid semen containing the sperm can be easily pressed out from the roe and the milt, respectively. Most bony fish produce several million eggs during spawning, while in cartilaginous fishes usually a few dozen large eggs are formed.

Many species of bony fish are provided with a swim bladder which plays the role of a buoyancy organ.

Fish breathe with gills and through the skin surface. The gills are thin, strongly vascularized membrane lobules, located under the gill covers at the base of the head. The total surface of the gills is about equal to that of the whole fish. In some species, there is additionally a strongly vascularized upper segment of the intestine that allows oxygen to be absorbed from the air swallowed above the water surface. In these tissues, oxygen is taken up by the blood. Fish have generally less blood than mammals — about 2% of the body weight against about 7%. Breathing is inhibited in most fish species when the oxygen concentration in water is below 2 cm^3/dm^3. However, some species are more demanding in this respect.

The heat produced in the fish organism as the result of metabolism is easily dissipated into the environment, so that the bodies of most fish, while resting, have a temperature of the surrounding water. On swimming, the body temperature generally increases only very little, up to about 1°C. Tuna, on the other hand, belongs to species that keep a constant temperature of about 9°C above that of the water. These species have also very particular requirements as to the temperature of the environment.

The sensory organs of fish are well adapted to living in water. Fish have a superbly developed sense of smell and taste, located in the mouth cavity, on the lips, the head, in the skin especially along the lateral line, and on the fins. They also have a well-functioning sense of touch and can detect small changes in currents which are generated by underwater obstacles or swimming objects.

2. Fish Families of Commercial Importance[5]

a. *Clupeidae and Engraulidae*

These pelagic, shoaling, plankton-eating fish occur in a range of species, adapted to living in cold as well as warm waters. Most Clupeidae are small sized, e.g., sprat, pilchard, and anchovy are 11 to 20 cm long, and the herring may reach 40 cm in length and about 400 g. They have whitish-gray or dark flesh and are suitable for salting, smoking, marinating, and canning. Many species of Clupeidae, especially the menhaden and the pilchard, as well as of *Engraulidae*, mainly the Peruvian anchovy, the anchovy fished off the U.S. west coast, and the Cape anchovy, are extensively used for the manufacture of fish oil and fish meal.

b. *Gadidae*

These predominantly bottom and predatory fish live mainly in cold waters. They range in size from about 30 to about 150 cm. The commercially most important species are cod, 30 to 150 cm long; haddock, 30 to 110 cm; pollock, 40 to 120 cm, fished in large quantities in the North Atlantic; many species of hake abundant both in the Atlantic and Pacific; and the Alaska pollack of the Pacific. The Gadidae have lean white meat, suitable especially to be sold as fresh or frozen fillets. For the manufacture of fish sticks or fish fingers, they are frozen in form of blocks of fillets or mince. They are also used for drying, smoking, and canning.

c. *Serranidae*

These are fish of tropical and warm shelf waters, ranging in size from about 30 to 220 cm. They feed mainly on smaller bottom-dwelling fish and benthonic crustaceans. The commercially most important species are the grey grouper, 30 to 90 cm long, the red grouper, 45 to 55 cm, and the marbled rockfish, 70 to 90 cm. Many *Serranidae* are highly valued fish because of their lean, white, tasty meat.

d. *Carangidae*

This family consists of over 200 species of fish, from medium sized to large, that live in temperate and warm pelagic waters. Some of them form shoals. They feed mainly on small fish but also on pelagic plankton crustaceans. The most important for fishery are several species of *Trachurus,* mainly the horse mackerel, 25 to 50 cm long, and jack mackerel, 25 to 70 cm. The medium fatty meat of many species of *Carangidae* is whitish to grayish-pink with appealing flavor. It is used as fresh fish and is suitable for smoking and canning.

e. *Lutianidae*

These are small to medium-sized predatory fish, living in tropical shelf waters. They are important for commercial fisheries and some species are also valued objects of game fishing. Here belong several species of snapper, such as the grey snapper, 30 to 90 cm, and John's snapper, 30 to 70 cm. The snappers are highly priced, sold mainly as fresh round fish, but are also used for salting, smoking, and drying.

f. *Sparidae*

This family consists of a range of species important for the fisheries in the Central Atlantic shelf waters. They feed on small fish and benthonic crustaceans and mollusks. The species fished in largest quantities are the white stumpnose, 20 to 55 cm; common sea bream, 30 to 70 cm; and red bream, 30 to 60 cm. Many Sparidae have white, lean, and very tasty meat, suitable for every kind of preparation and preservation.

g. *Scienidae*

These are also fish of warm coastal waters, ranging in length from about 30 to 180 cm.

They feed on small fish such as herring and menhaden but also on benthonic crustaceans and mollusks. Species important for fisheries are the Japanese meagre, 70 to 180 cm long, gray weakfish, 60 to 100 cm, croaker, about 30 cm, and the drum, 27 to 40 cm, fished along the coast of Brazil, Uruguay, and Argentina. The Scienidae have lean gray meat, rather tasty, which is used fresh, smoked, salted, or dried.

h. Nototheniidae

This family of demersal fish, living in cold subantarctic waters, feeding mainly on krill, gained importance for international fisheries during the past decade. They are medium sized and have white, fatty, and very tasty meat. Here belong the marbled notothenia, 30 to 90 cm, and the blue notothenia, 25 to 80 cm.

i. Scombridae

These are medium sized and very large, mainly predatory, pelagic fish of warm and tropical waters. To this family belong many highly valuable species of great importance for the world fisheries such as mackerel, 30 to 50 cm long; striped Spanish mackerel, 70 to 180 cm; painted mackerel, 50 to 180 cm; Atlantic and Pacific bonito, 30 to 70 cm; frigate mackerel, 30 to 60 cm; bluefin tuna that can grow to a maximum size of 3.5 m and 800 kg; southern bluefin tuna, 60 to 150 cm; albacore, 60 to 150 cm; bigeye tuna, 80 to 200 cm; and skipjack, 40 to 100 cm. Many Scombridae are prized as the object of game fishing. Their main outlet, however, is the manufacture of canned products and fish sausages. They are also used as fresh fish and for smoking. Their flesh contains distinct layers of very fatty dark red muscles and the rest of the meat is lighter in color, grayish pink or whitish.

k. Scorpenidae

To this family belong medium-sized predatory fish, living in temperate and warm waters on continental shelves and slopes, some to about 900 m deep. Here belong the ocean perch, 30 to 90 cm long; rosefish, 30 to 70 cm; and Pacific rosefish, 25 to 50 cm. Their meat is white, lean, and very tasty. Scorpenidae are sold mainly in the form of skinned fresh or frozen fillets.

l. Bothidae, Pleuronectidae, and Soleidae

These are fish flattened laterally, living in cold, temperate, and warm zones, in shallow and deep waters. They are bottom-dwelling predatory animals, feeding mainly on benthonic fauna. The average length of most of the commercial flatfish is about 40 cm, while the largest species, i.e., the halibut, grows up to 4.5 m and 400 kg, although the extremely large specimens are already depleted. Important for the fisheries are the nothern fluke, 40 to 90 cm; turbot, 40 to 100 cm; several species of halibuts; the sand dab, 20 to 50 cm; plaice, 30 to 90 cm, and the sole, 30 to 60 cm. The meat of most of the flatfish is white and rather on the lean side. It is highly priced because of its exquisite flavor and texture and is generally sold as fresh or frozen whole fish or skinned fillets.

m. Salmonidae

These are predatory migratory fish, spawning in fresh waters. The most important are the Atlantic salmon, 60 to 150 cm, and several species from the Pacific, mainly the pink salmon, 45 to 80 cm; silver salmon, 50 to 100 cm; red salmon, 50 to 65 cm; and the king salmon, 50 to 150 cm. The Salmonidae are highly valued as game fish. They are also sold as fresh, as cold-smoked sides, or canned. The eggs of salmonid fish are salted as red caviar.

n. Selachii

There are about 300 species of sharks living in all oceans, but mainly in warm pelagic waters. Most of them are predators, although the largest species are plankton-feeding fish.

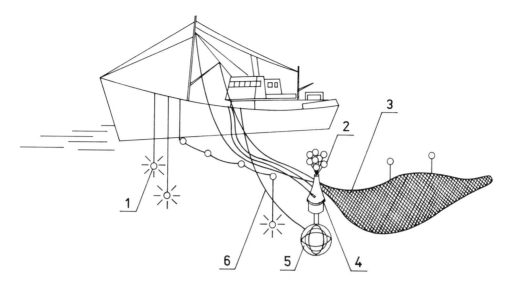

FIGURE 6. Electric fishing unit. (1) underwater lamp, (2) floats, (3) bag, (4) fishpump, (5) electrode, and (6) electric cable.

Sharks range in size from the small *Squalidus,* 15 cm long, to the largest *Rhincodon typus* or whale shark that grows up to 15 m. The commercially most important species fished for human food are the mako or bonito shark, the spiny dogfish, the thresher shark, the soupfin shark, and the mackerel shark. The flesh of sharks is lean, may be dark or light depending on the species, and is generally coarser and more strongly flavored than that of the majority of telost fish. Because of a large content of trimethylamine oxide and urea, it tends to develop off-odors and off-flavors early after catch. Shark meat is utilized mainly as steaks, fillets, and smoked fish and is also used for fish and chips as well as for manufacturing fish sausages. In many developing countries, shark meat is also salted and dried.

III. FISHING GEAR AND BOATS

A. FISHING GEAR
1. Development

Over the centuries, many types of gear have been developed to assist the fishermen in catching fish. As the application of various fishing techniques and gear depends on the general standard of technology in the given society, the fisherman of a developing country may still use the most primitive techniques in his in-shore fishery, while the highly organized commercial fleets of big industrial vessels have sophisticated equipment for precise underwater monitoring of moving shoals of fish and most efficient mechanized catching gear. Many research projects are under way aiming at developing new efficient methods of fishing, e.g., by applying electric current or light for concentrating the fish and by pumping the catch on board without using nets (Figure 6). Satellites are also used recently to locate fish shoals.

2. Wounding Gear and Fishing Lines

The simplest technique is manual picking of shellfish and mollusks left on the shore during the ebb tide, or diving to catch fish or pick abalone by hand. While hunting for a large fish, the fisherman may make use of a harpoon. Tuna is caught by using large fishing rods with or without bait from the deck of vessels, known as tuna clippers. Very popular are different types of hooks on lines, used by individual fishermen and also on big commercial vessels. They are used for catching large nonshoaling fish and also on rocky grounds, inaccessible for drag nets. The lines with hooks may be anchored or may drift at any depth between the surface and the bottom of the sea. Pelagic drifting tackles with dead bait, e.g., frozen sauries, in sets of total length of 80 to 110 km, are used for fishing tuna and other large fish.

3. Fish Traps

This type of gear is used for coastal fishing for many valuable species. The fish or crustaceans can easily enter the traps but cannot find the escaping route (Figure 7). In some countries, this type of gear is applied in coastal fishing of tuna. Traps are especially popular and efficient for catching crustaceans. They can be used individually or after being connected by long lines.

4. Nets

There are several types of nets differing in mode of action and in efficiency. Gill nets are set either as walls or screens, anchored at various distances from the sea bottom, or are operated as sets of floating drift nets, forming a barrier. The barrier causes the migrating fish of proper size to get entangled in the mesh. Drifting gill nets, about 5 km long, were used extensively in the great days of the herring and mackerel fishery in the North Sea.

Other types of nets are used for surrounding or encircling the fish found in a given area. Seine nets are employed in inshore fisheries. One end of the net is fixed on shore, while the other is being taken out in a boat. After encircling the planned area close to the sea bed or in the pelagial, the seine is brought back to the shore. The fish surrounded by the screen get concentrated in a pocket of the net and are taken out on the shore. The purse seine is used mainly in deep-sea fisheries to encircle shoals of fish (Figure 8). For efficient fishing, the shoal must be precisely located and the direction and speed of its movement should be monitored. A very large purse seine is 500 to 1000 m long. It can bring as much as 500 tons of fish in a single successful haul. The catch is taken out of the closed corral by using dip nets or by pumping.

Among dragged nets, trawls, which can be employed for bottom fishing as well as for midwater or pelagic work, are very popular. Large trawls (Figure 9) used on industrialized factory and freezer trawlers, can catch as much as 100 tons of fish in a single haul in 1 to 2 h.

B. FISHING BOATS
1. Introduction

A very large variety of fishing craft is being operated by world fisheries. The vessels differ in size, shape, and construction of the hull, type of propulsion, the range of operation and speed of traveling, the gear employed for fishing, the equipment and facilities on board available for processing and preservation of the catch, the navigation and fish location aids, the efficiency and versatility of operation, the size and standard of the accommodation for the crew, and the provisions securing the personal safety of the fishermen.

In in-shore fisheries, small and very versatile multipurpose boats are mainly employed, while in industrialized deep-sea operations the fleets consist of rather highly specialized large vessels.

2. Coastal Fishing Boats

Small boats under about 14 m in length comprise the majority of the world fishing fleet, not only in developing countries. They are used for catching the most valuable species of fish and crustaceans. These are open wooden vessels that may be built by local carpenters, but can also be steel launches or have hulls molded of glass-reinforced polyesters. The size of the craft depends on the type of fishing, the cost of construction bearable by the fishermen,

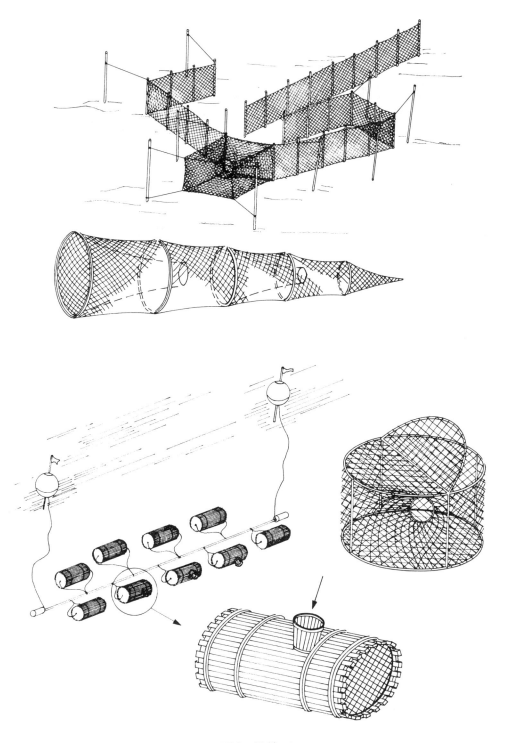

FIGURE 7. Fishing traps.

and the traditions prevailing in the specific region. These small craft can operate from harbors or else if fishing is carried out from open beaches, they can be beached and launched by manpower or by winches. A large proportion of these vessels are rowboats and sailing boats. Among the motorboats, a great many are powered by outboard engines. These small craft are used for diving operations in search of abalone, for trapfishing, especially for crustaceans,

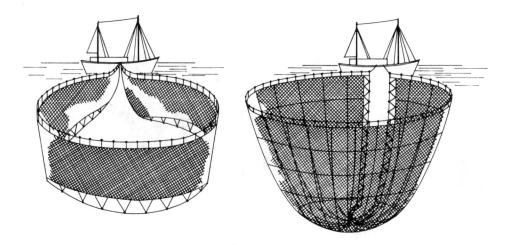

FIGURE 8. The purse seine.

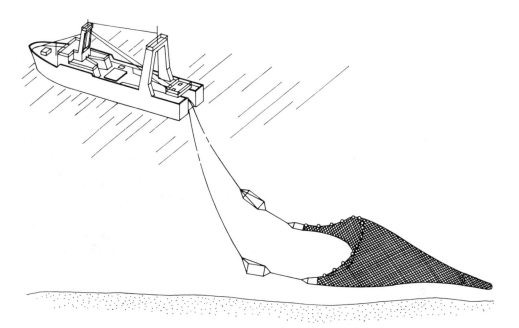

FIGURE 9. Trawling.

for gill netting, for coastal trolling for tuna, and for exercising many other fishing techniques. The catch is kept in wells, ice boxes, or chilled sea water. Because of their small size and very limited living accommodations for the crew on most of the smallest boats, these vessels generally make only daily trips out of their ports or beaches.

3. Tuna Clippers and Long Liners

Modern high seas clippers are about 30 to 55 m long yacht-like wooden or steel vessels, able to make 10,000 to 12,000 mi-long trips. In addition to the necessarily large supplies of oil and provisions, they must also carry live bait in tanks. The tuna, in dense pelagic shoals attracted by the bait thrown overboard, are fished with the help of short lines with hooks, attached to poles. The caught tuna is preserved ungutted by brine freezing.

For catching tuna feeding in midwater, long liners are usually employed. The smaller vessels, about 45 m long, are used for autonomic fishing. Larger ships, up to 60 m in length, are equipped with two to four small catchers. The catch is preserved on board by freezing, as the vessels stay in the fishing ground for several months.

4. Trawlers

The craft used for trawling can be classified into several categories according to their size, range of operation, and the techniques used for preserving the catch. While on the old-type side trawlers the net had to be laboriously hauled and shot over the side, on modern stern ramp vessels only the cod end is raised to be emptied.

The near water trawlers are small vessels, 25 to 35 m long, equipped with fish rooms for storing iced fish in boxes or bins. Their trips last up to several days. Very small trawlers, up to about 25 m in length, are called cutters in some countries. They are mainly employed in in-shore fisheries, making 2- to 3-d trips, but can participate also in long distance expeditions in cooperation with a factory ship. Middle water trawlers are 35 to 40 m long and have a travel range of at least 25 d. They are often equipped with facilities for freezing round fish on board, or else have chilled fishrooms. Deep-sea trawlers are large vessels up to about 130 m long and 4500 DWT, staying in the distant fishing grounds for several months. They are built to withstand the rough weather prevailing in the North Atlantic, Pacific, or Antarctic waters and also to offer suitable working conditions regardless the climatic zones. They may have installations for rapid chilling of large catches in retention tanks prior to processing, for gutting and filleting of the fish, for freezing and storage at $-30°C$ or lower, for canning, and also for processing the offal and trash fish to fish meal and oil. They are categorized as freezing trawlers.

5. Other Vessels Employed in Fisheries

Besides the above-described types of boats, there are many other specialized vessels, serving in various parts of the world, e.g., the salmon-herring seiners, the halibut long liners, and the purse seiners.

Typical one-purpose specialized vessels may be regarded as wasteful, as they can be employed only in specific fishing seasons and grounds. In order to minimize the losses, resulting from the vessels being kept idle in off-seasons, several types of combination fishing vessels have been used, e.g., the near water drifter trawlers that served extensively in the herring and mackerel fishing in the North Sea. There are also the Pacific combination boats used to purse seine for pelagic fish, trawl for bottom fish, long line for halibut, and pole fish or troll for tuna. Also known are the Japanese pole and line fishing boats.

The largest fishing enterprises, operating their fleets in waters very distant from their home ports, employ mother ships that process and store the catch from their own fleet of small catchers. They also have base ships that supply all necessary provisions, materials, and services to autonomic trawlers and take care of their catch, as well as refrigerated cargo vessels, designed for cooperation with flotillas of catchers and factory trawlers.

During the FAO International Fishing Boat Congress in Paris in 1953, Mogens Jul reflected on the fishing boat of the future:[6] "Some have said that the factory ship is the fishing boat of the future. People have also said that the aeroplane is the means of transport of the future. Both may be true, but only in this sense: for a long time to come the world will probably have cargo liners, river barges, bicycles and mules as well as aeroplanes. In the same way it will have factory ships along with trawlers, purse seiners, longliners, catamarans and other fishing craft." Now 35 years later, this opinion is still valid and there are signs indicating that, after a period of huge investments in very large fishing trawlers and factory ships, the trend is rather towards increasing the efficiency and safety of operations of small and medium-sized versatile craft.

IV. ACCESSIBILITY AND LIMITATIONS OF RESOURCES

A. BIOLOGICAL FACTORS

Many environmental factors influence the migrations of fish and fluctuations of the stock. The knowledge of fish migrations is helpful in selecting the most suitable fishing methods and gear, as well as in observing efficient rules of conservation of the stock.

Fish migrate to the spawning ground, where they find proper conditions of salinity, temperature, and depth necessary for the development of the fertilized eggs. Spawning concentrations of shoaling fish are suitable to be fished with large efficient gear. Fish migrate also in pursuit of their living food resources. Many species move to the deeper layers of water during the day and upward during the night, following the movements of plankton organisms. Therefore, such a pelagic species as the herring can be caught, depending on the time of day, either by drifting pelagic gill nets or by bottom trawls.

There are many biological and environmental factors that can influence the strength of the fish populations on different grounds. Unfavorable weather conditions during the spawning and hatching period, lower than usual turbulence of the shelf waters impairing the growth of plankton, epidemic diseases of fish or lower organisms in the food chain, or even long-term climatic changes can decrease the stock size in the particular area. Furthermore, considerable damage can also be done by overfishing, or by the use of too heavy gear that can destroy the natural habitat of the fish. In order to make the best use of the living sea resources, an equilibrium between the biological production of the particular stock and the yearly catch must be sustained. The optimum catch depends mainly on the biology of the species and the influence of the environmental conditions. In the case of short-living and rapidly growing fish, like pilchard, laying a large number of eggs, slight overfishing does not significantly jeopardize the productivity of the stock. However, in species such as halibut or sturgeon that attain sexual maturity very late or lay a small number of eggs, such as salmon or the sharks, overfishing can permanently damage the equilibrium.

The 1986 world catch of fish, mollusks, and crustaceans is about 92 million tons (Table 1). According to opinions of specialists, the total catch of traditional species could be increased to about 100 million tons without damaging the biological power of the stock. Furthermore, by using new methods and gear, additionally about 50 million tons of less popular species of fish and mollusks could be taken, as well as more than that of Antarctic krill.

B. TECHNICAL FACTORS

In order to achieve an increase in total world catch, many fisheries should be better supplied with technical equipment for

- Efficient detecting and monitoring of fish shoals on the oceanic waters
- Concentrating of dispersed fish and squid of the open oceanic waters
- Directing the concentrated shoals into nets or pumping facilities
- Catching of unconventional resources known to exist in large concentrations on the continental slope, 1000 to 1500 m deep
- More efficient exploitation of underutilized demersal resources on inaccessible grounds

Furthermore, to make good use of the increased catch, consisting in a large part of unconventional species, and to avoid losses due to spoilage, rational preservation and processing methods must be applied both on board and on shore.

TABLE 1
World Landings of Fish, Crustaceans, Mollusks, and Other Aquatic Animals

Species	Year (Tons · 10^3 live weight)	
	1980	1986
World total	72,128	91,457
Catches in marine fishing areas	64,460	80,345
Herrings, sardines, anchovies	15,501	23,943
Cods, hakes, haddocks	10,757	13,493
Jacks, mullets, sauries	7,322	7,188
Redfishes, basses, congers	5,362	5,966
Mackerels, snoeks, cutlass-fishes	4,631	4,033
Tunas, bonitos, billfishes	2,638	3,418
Flounders, halibuts, soles	1,084	1,308
Salmons, trouts, smelts	828	1,011
Shrimps, prawns	1,670	1,954
Clams, cockles, arkshells	1,232	1,843
Squids, cuttlefishes, octopuses	1,542	1,667
Oysters	972	1,011
Seaspiders, crabs	795	987
Mussels	672	829

Data from *FAO Yearbook Fishery Statistics. Catches and Landings,* Vol. 62, Food and Agriculture Organization, Rome, 1988, 91, 96, and 97.

REFERENCES

1. **Demel, K.,** *The Life of the Seas,* 4th ed., Wydawnictwo Morskie, Gdańsk, 1974, (in Polish).
2. *FAO Yearbook Fishery Statistics. Catches and Landings,* Vol. 62, Food and Agriculture Organization, Rome, 1988, 91, 96, and 97.
3. **Kreuzer, R.,** *Cephalopods: Handling, Processing and Products,* FAO Fish. Tech. Paper (254), Food and Agriculture Organization, Rome, 108.
4. **Budziński, E., Bykowski, P., and Dutkiewicz, D.,** *Possibilities of Processing and Marketing of Products Made of Antarctic Krill,* FAO Fish. Tech. Paper (268), Food and Agriculture Organization, Rome, 46.
5. **Rutkowicz, S.,** *Encyclopedia of Marine Fish,* Wydawnictwo Morskie, Gdańsk, 1982, (in Polish).
6. **Jul, M.,** Aspects of factory ship operations, in *Fishing Boats of the World,* Traung, J. O., Ed., Fishing News, London, 1955, 551.

Chapter 3

THE NUTRITIVE COMPOSITION OF THE MAJOR GROUPS OF MARINE FOOD ORGANISMS

Zdzisław E. Sikorski, Anna Kołakowska, and Bonnie Sun Pan

TABLE OF CONTENTS

I.	The Muscles of Marine Fish and Invertebrates	30
II.	The Gross Chemical Composition	31
III.	Water	33
IV.	Proteins	34
	A. Total Contents and Composition	34
	1. The Crude Protein and Protein Fractions	34
	2. The Amino Acid Composition	34
	B. The Sarcoplasmic Proteins	35
	1. General Description and Contents	35
	2. The Enzymes	37
	C. The Myofibrillar Proteins	37
	1. General Characteristics	37
	2. Myosin and Paramyosin	38
	3. Actin	38
	4. Other Myofibrillar Proteins	38
	D. The Proteins of the Stroma	39
	1. Composition	39
	2. Collagen	39
	3. Proteins of the Ligaments	40
V.	Lipids	41
	A. Composition of Marine Lipids	41
	B. Fatty Acid Composition of Marine Lipids	41
	C. The Effect of Polyunsaturated Fatty Acids on Human Health	42
	D. The Distribution of Lipids in Seafoods	44
VI.	Flavor Compounds of Seafoods	44
	A. Nitrogenous Compounds	44
	1. Amino Acids	44
	2. Dipeptides	45
	3. Nucleotides	45
	4. Guanidine Compounds	45
	5. Quaternary Ammonium Bases	45
	B. Volatile Compounds of Seafoods	46
	1. Sulfur-Containing Compounds	46
	2. Aldehydes, Ketones, and Alcohols	46
VII.	Vitamins	47
	A. The Fat-Soluble Vitamins	47

	B.	The Water-Soluble Vitamins	47
VIII.	Mineral Components		49
	A.	General Considerations	49
	B.	Macroelements	49
	C.	Microelements	49
		1. The Contents in Marine Foods	49
		2. Mercury	49
		3. Cadmium	51
		4. Lead and Arsenic	51
		5. Fluoride	52
References			52

I. THE MUSCLES OF MARINE FISH AND INVERTEBRATES

The main edible portion of a marine animal is composed of the largest muscles of the body. However, many other parts are also used as food, especially the skin, liver, milt, roe, the fins of shark, and the alimentary tract of squid.

The muscles that form a fish fillet are known as the large lateral muscles, which run on both sides of the body. They are covered by thinner layers of muscles, stretching beneath the skin. The large lateral muscles are generally off-white or whitish. They are called the white or ordinary muscles. The subcutaneous muscle contains much myoglobin and is called the red or dark muscle. The amount and distribution of the dark meat in the body of fish is characteristic for different species.

The fish muscles are divided by thin connective tissue membranes, known as myocommata, into segments called myotomes. The thickness of the myocommata depends on the species, the age or length, and the nutritional state of the fish. The number of the myotomes corresponds to that of the vertebrae in the backbone. Each myotome is composed of numerous cells, called muscle fibers, which run approximately parallel to the long axis of the fish. The muscle fibers are generally less than 20 mm long and 0.02 to 1.0 mm in diameter. Each fiber is surrounded by a membrane, called sarcolemma, which contains thin collagenous fibrils. These fine fibrils merge with the myocommata at the myotome-myocommata junction.[1]

A muscle fiber contains all components typical for a cell of an eukariotic organism. Most of the cell volume, however, is taken up by a bundle of myofibrils, each up to 5 μm in diameter, running parallel to the long axis of the fiber (Figure 1). The myofibrils are segmented into sarcomeres, which are composed of thin and thick myofilaments and are bordered by z-lines. The interactions of the myofilaments form the basis for muscle contraction and post-mortem stiffening of the body.

The ultrastructure of the adductor muscle of scallop was described in detail by Morrison and Odense.[3] The muscle consists of uninucleate cells, containing a single striated fibril. The fibril is formed of thick and thin myofilaments, arranged in sarcomeres. Each thick filament is surrounded by eight thin ones. The muscle fiber contains also a sarcotubular system. No large amounts of connective tissue were visible between the cells and this led Morrison and Odense to the conclusion that the fibers were loosely connected.

The structure of the muscle of squid mantle, as revealed by Otwell and Giddings,[4] is

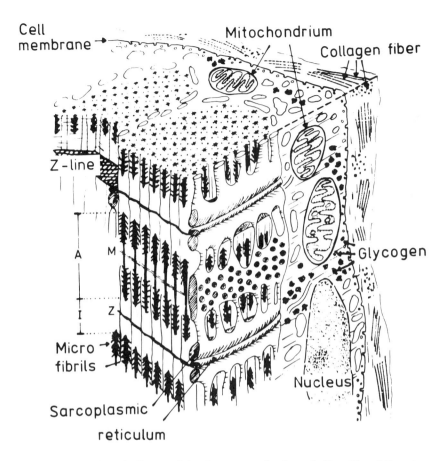

FIGURE 1. A schematic diagram of the ultrastructure of cod muscle fiber. (From Liljemark, A., *Livsmedelsteknik*, 10, 3, 1968. With permission.)

quite different. The muscle fiber layer, which makes up 98% of the mantle thickness, consists of sheets of circumferential bands, 0.1 to 0.2 mm thick, sandwiched between thin, 0.010- to 0.015-mm radial bands (Figure 2). Each fiber contains on the peripheries a number of myofibrils. The center is taken by the sarcoplasm with mitochondria and nuclei. The average diameter of the muscle fiber is 3.5 μm. The muscle fiber layer is placed between the outer and inner tunic of connective tissue, the fibers of the radial band being connected with the tunics. The outer tunic, consisting of layers of collagenous fibers, is adjacent to an outer lining, composed also of connective tissue fibers, which lies just below the skin. The inner tunic, which has loosely bound and interwoven fibrous aggregates, is covered by a nonfibrous visceral lining.

II. THE GROSS CHEMICAL COMPOSITION

The nutritive and commercial value of various fish and marine invertebrates depends on the structure of the flesh and other edible parts, on the proportions of these parts in the total mass of the specimen, on the chemical composition of the meat, gonads, liver, etc., and on factors related to fishing and handling procedures.

The main chemical components of fish meat are water, crude protein, and lipids. Together they make up about 98% of the total mass of the flesh. These components have the largest impact on the nutritive value, the functional properties, the sensory quality, and the storage stability of the meat. The other constituents, i.e., carbohydrates, vitamins, and minerals,

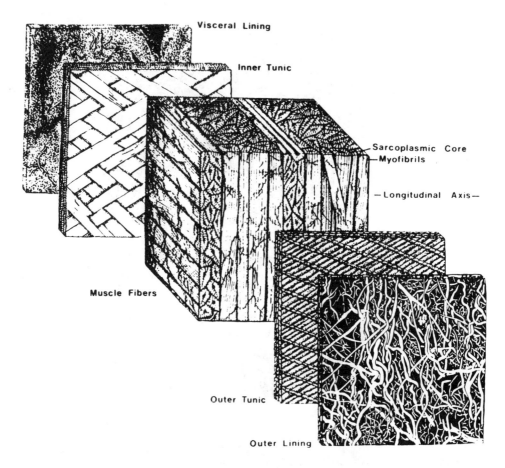

FIGURE 2. Artist's rendition of the tissue composition in the mantle of squid (*Loligo pealei*). The view of an expanded cube cut from the entire thickness of the mantle. Skin has been removed from the outer lining, and the profuse sarcoplasmic tubular network typically surrounding the surface of the muscle fibers has been omitted to reveal muscle fiber structure. The longitudinal axis refers to the head to tail axis of the squid mantle. (From Otwell, W. S. and Giddings, G. G., *Mar. Fish. Rev.*, 42(7-8), 67, 1980. With permission.)

although minor in quantity, also play a significant part in the biochemical processes taking place in the tissues post-mortem. They are coresponsible for the sensory properties, nutritive value, and wholesomeness of the product.

The contents of the main components in the fish body depend primarily on the species, the stage of maturity, and the nutritional condition of the animal. Thus, they change very much with the annual feeding and reproduction cycle. The most dramatic changes regard the contents of water and fat in the fatty species (Table 1). The concentration of other components depends also on the pollution of the habitat, e.g., the contents of heavy metals, and on the post-mortem conditions, effecting the contents of carbohydrates, nucleotides, and volatile odoriferous compounds. There are also significant differences in composition between various muscles and organs. The red muscles are especially rich in chromoproteins and contain about two to five times more lipids than the white muscles. The composition of the internal organs differs very much from that of the muscles in the contents of all main components, the most characteristic being the large content of lipids in the liver of some species of fish and of various enzymes in the liver, kidneys, and spleen.

The commercially exploited species can be classified according to the contents of fat and protein in the flesh of fish in good condition (Table 2). In respect to crude protein, which does not change seasonally so much as the contents of fat, four groups of fish have

TABLE 1
The Main Components of the Flesh of Fish and Edible Marine Invertebrates (Mean Values and Range)

Species	% Wet weight		
	Protein	Fat	Moisture
Herring, Atlantic	18.2	15.7	60.1
Clupea harengus	15.2—21.9	2.4—29.1	52.6—78.0
Cod	17.9	0.3	81.1
Gadus morhua	16.5—20.7	0.1—0.8	78.2—82.6
Tuna, bluefin	24.7	3.9	70.4
Thunnus thynnus	23.3—27.5	1.2—8.0	67.7—72.6
Halibut, Pacific	21.1	1.1	77.9
Hipoglossus stenolepis	20.3—22.0	0.6—3.6	77.3—78.7
Salmon, pink	19.4	5.3	74.0
Oncorhynchus gorbuscha	17.2—20.6	2.0—9.4	69.0—78.3
Lobsters	19.6	1.3	76.0
Panulirus spp.	16.2—21.6	0.6—1.9	71.5—81.2
Crab, blue	16.1	1.0	81.2
Callinectes sapidus	11.9—19.2	0.4—1.5	77.4—86.7
Oysters	7.8	1.5	84.8
Ostreidae spp.	5.5—14.3	0.7—2.6	76.0—93.0
Clams	11.7	1.4	83.0
Mixed spp.	7.6—19.0	0.3—4.8	73.7—87.9
Scallops	17.2	0.7	79.2
Pectinidae spp.	15.2—20.1	0.3—1.6	74.6—85.6
Abalone	14.9	0.5	76.9
Haliotis kamtschatkana	10.4—18.2	0.3—0.7	72.6—82.4

Data from Sidwell, V. D., Foncannon, P. R., Moore, N. S., and Bonnet, J. C., *Mar. Fish. Rev.*, 36(3), 21, 1974.

TABLE 2
Categories of Fish and Marine Invertebrates According to Oil and Crude Protein Contents

Type	Contents in flesh (% wet weight)		Typical species
	Oil	Protein	
Low oil-high protein	< 5	15—20	Cod, croaker, flounder, mullet, crab, lobster, scallop
Medium oil-high protein	5—15	15—20	Anchovy, mackerel, sablefish, sockey salmon
High oil-low protein	> 5	< 15	Siscowet lake trout
Low oil-very high protein	< 5	> 20	Albacore, halibut, skipjack tuna
Low oil-low protein	< 5	< 15	Clam, oyster

Data from Stansby, M. E. and Hall, A. S., *Fish. Ind. Res.*, 3(4), 29, 1967.

been proposed, containing below 10%, 10 to 15%, 15 to 20%, and above 20% crude protein, i.e., N·6.25, in the flesh. The sum of water + lipids in the fish meat is roughly constant. For 153 species, the following relationship was established[7] between the contents, in percent, of water (W), crude protein (P), and lipids (L): W + L = 98.8 − 1.01 P.

III. WATER

The muscles of marine fish and edible invertebrates contain from about 50 to about 85%

water, depending on the species and the nutritional status of the animal. Starvation, which is common in many fish species during spawning, depletes the energy reserves of the tissues and consequently increases the water content of the flesh.

In muscles and other tissues, water plays the important part of a solvent for a host of organic and inorganic solutes, provides the environment for biochemical events in the cells, is an active partner in many reactions, and has a large impact on the conformation and reactivity of proteins. The hydration of proteins is responsible for the rheological properties and juiciness of muscle foods.

The state of water in the fish flesh depends upon various interactions of water structures with different solutes and especially with proteins. The hydrophilic amino acid residues participate in H-bonding with water molecules and structures, while the hydrophobic groups in proteins and lipids act as structure makers, i.e., they induce around themselves layers of highly ordered water structures. Thus, in fish meat, only a part of the aqueous medium can be regarded as bulk water. The rest of it is in a different extent involved in water-protein-lipid-solute interactions.

The bulk phase of free water does not exude freely from the tissues, even after comminution, as it is entrapped in the structure of the material. It has the largest translational freedom within the meat, behaves like a dilute salt solution during freezing, and is the first to evaporate from the tissues at low air humidity. The portion of water, which is held in capillary spaces and is bound by small structure-forming solutes, is called the interfacial water. It is not uniform in its characteristics, as it interacts with various active groups of the solutes with different binding energies. Thus, due to changes in the structure of the tissues, effected by processing, a part of the interfacial water may turn into bulk water and hence increase its translational freedom. The most restricted in mobility is the constitutional water forming the monolayer on hydrophilic groups in proteins.

Changes in the immobilization and contents of water in the flesh, induced by processing, effect the rheological properties, nutritive value, and sensory quality of the fish meat. These changes also have a large impact on the shelf life of different products.

IV. PROTEINS

A. TOTAL CONTENTS AND COMPOSITION
1. The Crude Protein and Protein Fractions

In tables of food composition, the content of proteins refers usually to the crude protein. This represents proteins and other nitrogenous compounds, such as nucleic acids, nucleotides, trimethylamine (TMA) and its oxide (TMAO), free amino acids, urea, etc. The flesh of fish and marine invertebrates contains usually from about 11 to 24% crude protein, depending on the species of the animal, the nutritional condition, and the type of muscle. Cod flesh contains from about 2.1 to about 3.0% of protein nitrogen.

The muscles are composed of several groups of proteins: the components of the sarcoplasmic fraction which perform the biochemical tasks in the cells, the myofibrillar proteins of the contractive system, and the proteins of the connective tissues, responsible mainly for the integrity of the muscles. The relative amounts of these groups of proteins depend upon the sexual development and depletion of the fish and may fluctuate in the annual cycle within a few percent. The yield of these fractions is affected by the conditions of extraction, mainly the procedure of grinding, mixing, and centrifuging, pH, salt concentration, and dilution, as well as on the degree of denaturation and loss in solubility of the proteins due to storage and processing of the fish.

2. The Amino Acid Composition

The total muscle proteins, i.e., of the whole skinned fillet, of various fish species, do not differ much in the amino acid composition (Table 3). The histidine content, however,

TABLE 3
Amino Acid Composition of Fish Muscle Proteins

Amino acid	Mean[a] (% N·6.25)	Range (% N·6.25)
Alanine	7.91	7.7—8.8
Arginine	5.95	5.7—6.3
Aspartic acid	10.34	9.9—10.9
Cystine	1.04	0.9—1.1
Glutamic acid	14.91	14.3—15.4
Glycine	4.60	4.2—5.4
Histidine	2.01	1.8—2.2
Isoleucine	6.03	5.5—6.3
Leucine	8.41	7.8—9.1
Lysine	8.81	7.9—9.5
Methionine	2.97	2.8—3.2
Phenylalanine	3.92	3.7—4.1
Proline	3.52	3.3—3.7
Serine	5.14	4.6—6.0
Threonine	4.62	4.4—5.0
Tryptophan	0.96	0.9—1.0
Tyrosine	3.27	3.1—3.4
Valine	5.95	5.6—6.2

[a] Mean values for ten species of fish: cod, coalfish, haddock, redfish, catfish, plaice, halibut, ling, torsk, and mackerel. The mean for histidine does not include the value for mackerel.

Data from Braekkan, O.R. and Boge, G., *Reports on Technological Research Concerning Norwegian Fish Industry,* Vol. 4, Fiskeridirectorates Skrifter, Bergen, Norway, 1962.

is exceptionally large in the proteins of mackerel, being 4.37 to 4.60 g/100 g N·6.25.[8] The nutritive value of fish proteins is very high because of the favorable essential amino acid pattern (Table 4). The *in vivo* digestibility of the proteins of raw fish meat is in the range 90 to 98% and that of shellfish about 85%.[9] High nutritive value of the protein of raw fish and marine invertebrates has been confirmed in biological experiments (Table 5).

The amino acid composition of different proteins of the muscle and skin is not identical, as these proteins, having to perform different tasks, must differ in their properties.

B. THE SARCOPLASMIC PROTEINS
1. General Description and Contents

The term sarcoplasmic proteins usually refers to the proteins of the sarcoplasm, the components of the extracellular fluid, and the proteins contained in the small particles of the sarcoplasm. The truly intracellular soluble fraction makes up 90 to 95% of the total proteins of the extract obtained by homogenizing the muscle tissue with water or solutions of neutral salts of ionic strength below 0.15.[10] The sarcoplasmic proteins are also soluble in more concentrated salt solutions.

Generally the sarcoplasmic fraction makes up about 30% of the total amount of proteins in fish muscles. The contents of sarcoplasmic proteins is higher in pelagic than in demersal fish muscles.

The group of fish albumins is composed of over 100 various proteins with a wide range of molecular weights and isoelectric points. Most of these proteins have enzymatic activity.

TABLE 4
Predicted Protein Quality Values for Raw Flesh of Various Classifications of Seafoods

Seafood group	Amino acid score	Chemical score	EAA index	DC-PER	Computed digestibility
Clupeiformes: Clupeoidei					
Include pilchard, anchovy, herring	100	72	90	2.74	90.2
Clupeiformes: Salmonoidei					
Include trout, salmon, whitefish, smelt	99	62	79	2.85	98.5
Gadiformes					
Include cod, hake, haddock, ling, torsk	100	75	90	2.76	92.6
Galiformes					
Include shark	100	65	88	2.82	92.5
Perciformes: Scombroidei					
Include tuna, mackerel, swordfish, skipjack, albacore	96	61	80	2.88	98.9
Perciformes, other orders					
Include goby, mullet, meagre, dorado, perch	100	70	84	2.77	98.1
Pleuronectiformes					
Include sole, flounder, turbot	94	57	86	3.18	93.3
Crustaceans	96	70	83	3.19	89.8
Mollusks	100	75	87	2.73	93.9
Average	98	67	85	2.88	94.2

Note: These values were calculated from the essential amino acid concentrations given by Food and Agriculture Organization, in FAO Nutritional Studies No. 24, Rome, 1970, using an assigned concentration of 1.40 g NH_3 per 100 g protein in the DC-PER method.

After Acton, J. C. and Rudd, C. L., *Seafood Quality Determination,* Kramer, D. E. and Liston, J., Eds., Elsevier, Amsterdam, 1987, 453. With permission.

TABLE 5
Protein Efficiency Ratios of Raw Flesh of Fish and Shellfish

Sample	Relative PER
Mackerel, *Scomber scombrus*	149
Croaker, *Micropogon undulatus*	120
Cod, *Gadus morhua*	113
Rockfish, *Sebastodes,* five species	103
Surf clam, *Spissula solidissima*	102
Squid, *Loligo pealei*	99

Data from Acton, J. C. and Rudd, C. L., *Seafood Quality Determination,* Kramer, D. E. and Liston, J., Eds., Elsevier, Amsterdam, 1987, 453.

Here also belong the proteins bonded to nucleic acids, the components of lipoproteins, as well as the chromoproteins of muscle and blood.

Dark muscles, both superficial and deep-seated, contain more hemoglobin, myoglobin, and cytochrome *c* than the white muscles (Table 6).

Some Antarctic and Artic fish have in their blood serums characteristic proteins, known

TABLE 6
Chromoproteins in Dark and Ordinary Muscles of Fish

	(mg/100 g wet weight)					
	Hemoglobin and myoglobin		Myoglobin		Cytochrome c	
Species	Dark	Ordinary	Dark	Ordinary	Dark	Ordinary
Black marlin *Makaira mazara*	1020	14	510	0	12.3	0.1
Chub mackerel *Scomber japonicus*	980	10	390	—	13.0	0.1
Saury *Cololabis saira*	510	36	27	1	42	2.0
Yellowtail *Seriola quinqueradiata*	400	12	150	2	17.2	0.9
Japanese tuna *Thunnus orientalis*	810 5090[a]	240	320 1910[a]	70	0.9 14.0[a]	0.3

[a] Deep-seated red muscle.

Data from Matsuura, F. and Hashimoto, K., *Bull. Jpn. Soc. Sci. Fish.*, 20, 4, 1954.

as antifreeze glycoproteins, containing galactosyl-*N*-acetylgalactosamine units, linked glycosidically to threonine residues.[12] In the colorless blood of the Antarctic hemoglobin-free fish, the protein concentration is five to ten times lower than in the blood of red-blooded fish.[13]

2. The Enzymes

Among the sarcoplasmic enzymes influencing the quality of fish as food are mainly the enzymes of the glycolytic pathway and the hydrolytic enzymes of the lysosomes.

Various proteinases were isolated from the muscles of fish of different species and of marine invertebrates. The maximum activity of these enzymes toward endogenous and other substrates falls within the acidic, neutral, or alkaline range of pH, the activity of the acid proteinases being generally the highest. The activity of Antarctic krill neutral and alkaline proteinases is about ten times higher in the cephalothorax than in the tail meat.

In the sarcoplasmic fraction there are also enzymes catalyzing further degradation of nitrogenous compounds, e.g. oligopeptidases, tri- and dipeptidases, transaminases, amidases, glutamate dehydrogenase, carnosinase, arginase, nicotinamide adenine dinucleotidase, adenosine triphosphatase (ATPase), adenosine deaminase, trimethylamine demethylase, and thiaminase. In the sarcoplasmic fraction of several crustaceans, high activity of catechol oxidase was found. Extracts of Antarctic krill are rich in various polysaccharide degrading enzymes and in lipases. Lysozyme activity was found in the mucus, mantle muscle, and internal organs of mollusks.[14]

The activity of the sarcoplasmic enzymes depends upon the species of the fish, the condition of the animal, and the kind of muscle.

C. THE MYOFIBRILLAR PROTEINS
1. General Characteristics

These proteins can be extracted from the comminuted fish meat with neutral salt solutions of ionic strength above 0.15, usually ranging from 0.30 to 1.0. The fraction of the myofibrillar proteins, which can be precipitated by tenfold dilution of the centrifuged supernatant with distilled water, makes up from 40 to 60% of the total amount of N·6.25 in the fish meat.

The composition of the myofibrillar fraction and the structures and properties of these proteins have been investigated since the early 1940s. Most of these proteins are described in details in biochemistry and food chemistry textbooks. The myofibrillar proteins participate in the post-mortem stiffening of the tissues (rigor mortis). Changes in these proteins lead later to resolution of the stiffness while during long-term frozen storage they may cause toughening of the meat. The myofibrillar proteins are also mainly responsible for the water-holding capacity of fish, for the characteristic texture of fish products, as well as for the functional properties of fish minces and homogenates, especially the gel-forming ability.

2. Myosin and Paramyosin

Myosin makes up 50 to 58% of the myofibrillar fraction. It can be extracted from the minced muscle in 1 to 3 min, while other components, especially actin, need much longer extraction times. The extraction and purification of squid mantle myosin is difficult because of high activity of squid cathepsins, low resistivity of the squid myosin to proteolytic attack, and contamination with paramyosin. There is published information on the amino acid composition of fish and marine invertebrate myosin. According to Buttkus,[15] myosin isolated from the muscles of rabbit and trout under conditions preventing oxidation contains 42 mol of SH groups per $5 \cdot 10^5$ g protein. According to other publications, the contents of SH groups in myosin from various species of fish, range from 29 to 40 mol/$5 \cdot 10^5$ g protein.[16] The fish myosin ATPase in KCl solution is in many respects similar to that of rabbit myosin ATPase. However, its activity is generally lower than that of rabbit myosin, known exceptions being the ATPase of tuna and skipjack.[16] The ATPase of squid myosin is activated not only by Ca^{2+} but slightly also by Mg^{2+} and has two pH maxima of activity.[17] At 30°C, the heat inactivation of squid Ca-ATPase is about 50 times more rapid than that of rabbit myosin.[18]

Paramyosin occurs in the striated and smooth muscles of invertebrates and has been extracted from various species of marine mollusks. The salt-soluble protein fraction of the foot muscle of abalone *Notohaliotis discus* contains about 65% paramyosin.[19] In squid muscle, paramyosin makes up 14% of the myofibrils. Paramyosins isolated from the muscles of various mollusks are similar in amino acid composition and in molecular weight.[20]

3. Actin

Actin makes about 15 to about 20% of the total quantity of N·6.25 in the muscles of cod. The water-extractable actin which can be obtained from the acetone-dried powder of the purified myofibrillar fraction is in the monomeric form called G-actin. It polymerizes in the presence of neutral salts to the filamentous F-actin. When minced fish meat is treated with neutral salt solutions, actin is extracted together with myosin in form of actomyosin. This complex exhibits the Ca^{2+} activated ATPase characteristics, just like myosin, but is also activated by Mg^{2+}.

Incubation of fish and squid actomyosins at temperatures as low as 25°C brings about after 60 min a significant decrease in ATPase activity. The thermal stability of krill ATPase is about 100 times lower than that of Alaska pollack actomyosin.[21]

4. Other Myofibrillar Proteins

A number of other proteins, involved in the structure of the myofibrils and in the interactions of the contractile proteins, together make a little over 10% of the myofibrillar fraction, the main constituents being tropomyosin and the troponins. Many literature data are available on the amino acid composition and structure of these proteins isolated from the muscles of various fish and marine invertebrates.

Biochemical investigations continue to detect minor components of the myofibrillar fraction.

Maruyama et al.[22] isolated and characterized an elastic protein called connectin, present in the myofibrils, known also as titin. In carp, the connectin contents are from 0.4% in the dark muscle to 0.8% in the white muscle.[23] In the amino acid composition, connectin is similar to actin. Traces of hydroxyproline residues found in this protein preparations were probably the result of residual contamination with collagen. Kimura et al.[24] separated by sodium dodecylsulfate-polyacrylamide gel electrophoresis bands of connectin, much larger in molecular weight than the heavy chain of myosin, from the muscles of several fish, including mackerel, yellowtail, and Pacific marlin. These bands were not found in extracts from striated and smooth myofibrils of scallop adductor nor in the striated muscles of lobster tail and the mantle of cuttlefish.

D. THE PROTEINS OF THE STROMA
1. Composition

The residue after extraction of the sarcoplasmic and myofibrillar proteins, called the stroma, is composed of the main connective tissue proteins — collagen and elastin, of reticulin, and of denatured aggregated myofibrillar and possibly sarcoplasmic proteins, which lost their characteristic solubility. The stroma, insoluble in dilute solutions of hydrochloric acid or sodium hydroxide, constitutes about 3% of the total muscle proteins of teleosts and up to 10% of elasmobranchs.[25]

2. Collagen

The contents of collagen in the muscles depends upon the species as well as on the state of maturation and feeding of the fish. In starving fish, the sarcoplasmic and myofibrillar proteins undergo gradual degradation, while the connective tissues are not utilized, or extra collagen is even deposited in the myocommata and in the skin.[26] Generally, however, the contents of collagen in fish muscles range from about 1 to 12% of the crude protein, i.e., 0.2 to 2.2% of the wet weight of the meat, and 1.7 to 4.6% of collagen nitrogen in the fish skin.[27,28] Raw fish meat rich in collagen is tougher than that containing less collagen. The muscle tissues of some edible marine invertebrates contain somewhat larger amounts of collagen.[27] In the skinned mantle and skinned arms of squid *Illex argentinus,* collagen has been found by Sadowska[29] to constitute 2 to 11% and 2 to 16% of true proteins, respectively.

Fish muscle and skin collagens differ from bovine meat and hide collagens in having significantly higher contents of seven essential amino acids and a considerably lower concentration of hydroxyproline residues (Table 7). A characteristic property of shrimp collagen is a high content of tryptophan residue. Thompson and Thompson[34] suggested that in shrimp collagen this amino acid partly replaced the residues of imino acids, as the total contents of hydroxyproline, proline, and tryptophan is similar to that in collagen from other sources. The collagens of edible marine invertebrates are characteristic for a high content of carbohydrates.[35] Some fish and invertebrate collagens also contain, besides the sugars listed in Table 8, small amounts of arabinose, xylose, and ribose residues. The carbohydrates are mainly linked O-glycosidically to hydroxylysine residues as glucosylgalactosylhydroxylysine units. These hydroxylysine-linked carbohydrates may have an impact on the structure of the fibrils in the invertebrate collagens.

The connective tissues have a large effect on the properties of muscles as food. Collagen, the main component of these tissues, is responsible for their considerably low nutritional value. At the same time, however, it mostly contributes to the tensile strength of the muscles and has a significant influence on the functional and rheological properties of the meat. Collagen is important for the meat technologist, as it controls the background toughness of beef. For the fish processor, however, toughness of a cooked fresh fillet from a valuable fish species is never a problem. On the other hand, the mantle of some species of squid may get tough and rubbery after cooking. Thermal changes in collagen are also important factors in hot smoking of fish, in high-temperature, short-time sterilization of canned fish containing bony parts, and in utilization of fish wastes.[27] A significant deterioration in the

TABLE 7
Amino Acid Composition of Muscle Collagens of Marine Fish and Invertebrates

Amino acid	Residues per 1000 residues			
	Cod[30]	Squid[31]	Spiny lobster[32]	Bovine L. dorsi[33]
Alanine	106.0	88.8	43	107
Arginine	59.1	59.0	54	45
Aspartic acid	42.3	57.7	47	34
Cystine	—	1.8	0	—
Glutamic acid	82.2	86.4	102	83
Glycine	313.6	308	324	336
Histidine	16.3	7.4	7	5
Hydroxyproline	40.7	89.3	90	109
Hydroxylysine	8.2	16.1	24	8
Isoleucine	18.6	20.9	20	12
Leucine	32.3	33.9	46	25
Lysine	36.9	15.3	15	23
Methionine	20.4	7.7	12	5
Phenylalanine	14.5	11.5	8	14
Proline	87.6	96.0	108	113
Serine	62.9	46.9	49	36
Threonine	25.8	26.2	27	17
Tyrosine	6.0	4.5	4	3
Valine	26.1	21.1	20	25

TABLE 8
Main Neutral Sugars in Collagens of Marine Fish and Invertebrates

Collagen source	Total sugars (%)	Glucose (%)	Galactose (%)	Mannose (%)	Fucose (%)
Bigeye tuna, skin	0.40	0.17	0.19	0.01	0.02
Carp, skin	0.43	0.18	0.20	0.01	0.02
Octopus, body wall	2.89	1.50	1.00	0.05	0.18
Squid, body wall	3.96	2.16	1.44	0.10	0.26
Abalone, foot part	4.18	2.19	1.32	0.13	0.48
Spiny lobster, subcuticular tissue	10.19	5.76	3.84	0.17	0.22
Blue crab, subcuticular tissue	12.45	6.90	4.82	0.52	0.21

Data from Kimura, S., *Bull. Jpn. Soc. Sci. Fish,* 38, 1153, 1972.

quality of fresh and frozen fish can result from post-mortem changes in collagen, which lead to disintegration of the fillet during handling and processing.

3. Proteins of the Ligaments

These are proteins capable of forming rubber-like elastic fibers. A typical representative is elastin. It constitutes most of the material of the ligaments in mammals, is present in large amounts (up to 60% of total protein) in the walls of blood vessels, and has been found in small concentration in the skin. A protein called abductin, similar to the elastic properties to elastin, is in the triangular hinge ligament of pecten.[36] It differs from elastin in the amino acid composition, which is unusually high in glycine and phenylalanine — 630 and 93 residues per 1000 residues, respectively. It is insoluble in standard protein solvents, including 6 M urea, but may be solubilized in 0.1 M NaOH solution at 98°C.

V. LIPIDS

A. COMPOSITION OF MARINE LIPIDS

Lipids belong to the basic components of marine organisms. Although present in all tissues, they are concentrated mostly in the subcutaneous fatty layer of marine mammals and fatty fish, in the liver of lean fish, in the muscle tissue, and in mature gonads. Marine lipids are composed of phospholipids, sterols, triacylglycerols, wax esters, minor quantities of metabolic products of these, as well as small amounts of unusual lipids, such as glyceryl esters, glycolipids, sulfolipids, and hydrocarbons.

Phospholipids and sterols occur in small but relatively constant amounts of 0.2 to 0.3% wet weight of the tissues. They play an important structural role in biomembranes and participate in basic cellular functions. The remaining lipids are essentially energy stores and are important for buoyancy. Their amounts are therefore different and variable. An average fish phospholipid fraction contains about 60% phosphatidylcholine, 20% phosphatidylethanolamine, and several percent phosphatidylserine and sphingomyeline, while the rest is made up by other phospholipids. Invertebrate phospholipids contain less phosphatidylcholine. The lowest content of phosphatidylcholine is found in marine plants.

Crustaceans, e.g., shrimp, contain much sphingomyeline, the compound being abundant also in the liver of most marine animals. Under special conditions, phospholipids may also be used as a source of energy, which is the case with Antarctic krill, whose phospholipid contents make up as much as 5% wet weight of the tissues.

The marine sterols, free and esterified, consist almost exclusively of cholesterol. Most fish contain about 20 to 40 mg cholesterol per 100 g meat, 250 to 650 mg/100 g roe, and even more in the liver.[37] Crustacean and molluskan meat contains two to three times more steroids. The lipids of marine algae are particularly rich in various sterols.[38]

In many marine organisms, wax esters serve to increase buoyancy. They are accumulated in the organisms which have to endure a long-lasting starvation period, e.g., during the polar winter, and those living in deep waters. Wax esters are present in numerous food fish such as orange roughy, codfish (*Moridae*), mullets, sharks, and in some crustaceans and mollusks. In castor oil fish (*Ruvettus presiosus*) and coelacanths (*Latimeria chalumnae*), wax esters make up more than 70% of total lipids.[39]

Marine animals also contain small amounts of alkyl glycerol ethers, sulfolipids, and glycolipids. Some shark oils are very rich in hydrocarbons, particularly in squalene.

B. FATTY ACID COMPOSITION OF MARINE LIPIDS

The fatty acid composition of marine lipids is much more complex than that of lipids of terrestrial plants and animals. The carbon chain length is generally from C_{14} to C_{24}, although C_{12} and C_{26} are found as well. The marine fatty acids are particularly highly unsaturated. Even the C_{14} and C_{16} acids have unsaturated bonds, while the C_{20} and C_{22}; acids contain four, five, and six double bonds (Table 9). Most of the polyunsaturated fatty acids (PUFAs) of fish lipids occur as the n-3 type. The n-6 acids make up only a few percent of the total. Fish lipids contain also some fatty acids with odd carbon numbers in the chain, C_{15}, C_{17}, and C_{19}. The usual content of these fatty acids is 1 to 3%, but at least in one species, the mullet, it may be even above 10% or more.[40]

The lipids of some fish, e.g., yellowfin tuna, and of marine mammals also contain branched chain fatty acids, such as the iso-16:0 and iso-18:0 acids.

The distribution of fatty acids in lipids is far from uniform. The polyenoic acids occur mainly in phospholipids, while the monounsaturated acids in triacylglycerols. Thus, at least 50% of the fatty acids in phospholipids are polyenoic, basically the $C_{20:5}$ and $C_{22:6}$, n-3, the first occurring preferably in phosphatidylcholine, the latter in phosphatidylethanolamine. The triacylglycerols compose 50% of the monoenoic fatty acids, the rest being more or less equally divided between saturated and polyenoic acids.

TABLE 9
Fatty Acids in Seafood Lipids

Saturated	Monoenoic	Polyenoic
\multicolumn{3}{c}{Percent of Total Fatty Acids}		
25	35	40
	30—60	10—60
\multicolumn{3}{c}{Main Components}		
C_{16}	C_{18}	$C_{20:5}$
C_{14}	C_{16}	$C_{22:6}$
C_{18}	C_{20}	
	C_{22}	

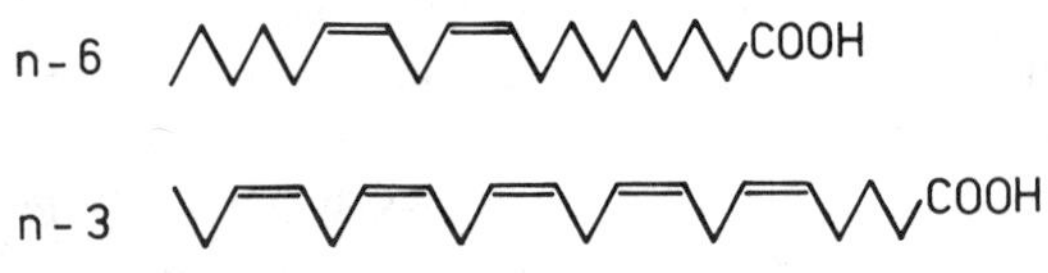

FIGURE 3. The structure of essential fatty acids.

The contents of different fatty acids in fish lipids depend on numerous factors, such as the diet, geographic location, environmental temperature, season of the year, body length, lipid content, etc. The lipid composition of freshwater fish is intermediate between that of terrestial mammals and marine fish. The polyenoic to saturated acids ratio in marine and freshwater fish is 1:3 and 1:0, respectively. Freshwater fish contain more n-6 PUFAs, about 15% of total fatty acids, and less n-3 acids than marine fish. Therefore, the n-3 to n-6 ratio allows to differentiate between freshwater and marine fish, the respective ranges being 0.5 to 4 and 5 to 15. The lipids of cultured fish and shellfish contain more n-6 and less n-3 PUFAs than the lipids of wild fish. Seals and dolphins contain similar amounts of the two types of acids. Tropical fish are richer in n-6 acids than the northern hemisphere fish. Generally, a decrease in ambient temperature is accompanied by an increase in the degree of unsaturation of fatty acids and by an increase in the contents of the lipids.

The two most important n-3 PUFAs are the $C_{20:5}$ and $C_{22:6}$. The first is typical of marine algae and the other originates from zooplankton. The proportion of the two acids in lipids depends on the feeding habits of marine organisms. Most fish feed on zooplankton or are predators; thus, their lipids contain more $C_{22:6}$ than $C_{20:5}$ acid. The case is similar with squids. On the other hand, most shellfish show either a prevalence of the $C_{20:5}$ acid or the contents of the two acids are similar. The Antarctic fish living under the sea ice and feeding on algae contain more $C_{20:5}$ than $C_{22:6}$.

C. THE EFFECT OF POLYUNSATURATED FATTY ACIDS ON HUMAN HEALTH

Polyenoic acids are recognized as important dietary components. The fatty acids presented in Figure 3 are essential, since the double bonds at the third and sixth carbon atoms from the methyl group cannot be synthetized in the animal body and have to be derived from food. On the other hand, the chain may be elongated and desaturated. The n-6 acids are essential for man, as they serve to generate the eicosanoids (Figure 4) — modulators of important metabolic functions. Arachidonic acid is present in cellular membrane phospholipids of every human cell.

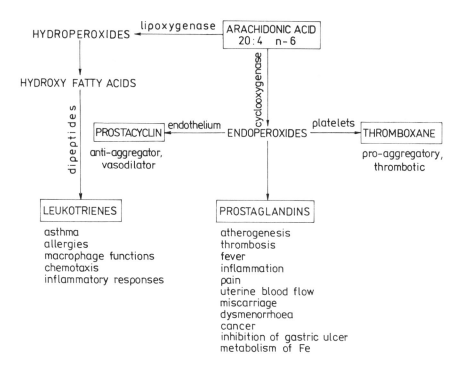

FIGURE 4. The conversion of n-6 fatty acids to metabolic regulators.

Arachidonic acid $C_{20:4}$, n-6, from phospholipid reserves in the organism, from the diet, or obtained by elongation and desaturation of the $C_{18:2}$, n-6 acid which is more frequent in foods, is oxidized, in the presence of lipoxygenase or cyclooxygenase, to linear or cyclic peroxides (endoperoxides). The hydroperoxides participate in the formation of hydroxy fatty acids which form leukotrienes with dipeptides. A cyclic peroxide is transformed in blood platelets to thromboxane TXA_2 and in the endothelium of blood vessels to prostacyclin PGI_2 and various prostaglandins.

A healthy organism produces extremely low quantities of eicosanoids. Large amounts are synthetized by pathological tissues and in pathologic conditions, e.g., inflammation, arthritis, bleeding, vascular injury, tumorigenesis, and cancer. This concerns prostaglandins, leukotrienes, thromboxane, and free radicals from peroxides. Particularly important are the antagonistic effects of thromboxane, enhancing platelet aggregation, and the prostacyclin which not only inhibits aggregation, but also disperses the aggregates. The development of sclerosis is related to prostacyclin deficits.

PUFAs provided with the diet reduce the level of blood cholesterol and the low-density lipoproteins, but at the same time the presence of large quantities of n-6 PUFAs may result in overproduction of eicosanoids and peroxides. Higher contents of the latter inhibit prostacyclin synthesis.

The n-3 PUFAs $C_{20:5}$ and $C_{22:6}$ are easily incorporated into phospholipids instead of arachidonic acid and pass through the whole cycle to produce appropriate eicosanoids or docosanoids.

The n-3 PUFAs, compared to arachidonic acid, are poor hydroperoxide generators. They are false substrates for cyclooxygenase, inhibiting thus the synthesis of further eicosanoids. While the $C_{20:5}$ acid inhibits both the thromboxane and prostacyclin synthesis, the $C_{22:6}$ acid preferentially inhibits the thromboxane synthesis. This may mean that this acid is a better antithrombotic factor. Furthermore, TXA_3 formed from n-3 PUFAs is a much weaker proaggregatory factor than the thromboxane TXA_2 produced from arachidonic acid.

The discussion above is an attempt to explain the particularly beneficial effects of fish-rich diets in terms of inhibiting ischemic heart diseases and thrombosis as well as tumorigenesis and cancer. Such diets involve a favorable high-density/low-density lipoprotein ratio, low triacylglycerol and cholesterol contents, and a low content of very low-density lipoproteins in the blood serum. It is recommended to substitute a part of dietary n-6 PUFAs with n-3. Thus, out of the advised 30% of energy provided by fat, 8% should be supplied by saturated lipids, 12% by monounsaturated, and 10% by the n-6 and n-3 PUFA. It is also simply recommended to eat 5 g of fish oil daily.[41]

D. THE DISTRIBUTION OF LIPIDS IN SEAFOODS

The average lipid content in green algae is below 0.1% and in marine invertebrates from below 1% to about 2% wet weight. The lipid content in the meat of marine mammals, excluding the subcutaneous adipose tissue, is generally similar to that in medium-fat marine fish. The dark muscles of fish contain more lipids than the white muscles due to higher contents of triacylglycerols necessary as energy reserves for swimming. Generally, pelagic fish have more dark muscles and are fattier, while less mobile demersal fish are usually lean, with white meat.

The lean fish meat contains less than 1% lipids; these are actually the structural lipids only, 8% of them being the n-3 PUFA-rich phospholipids. The reserve lipids are stored in the liver which is rather large and rich in triacylglycerols.

The liver of medium-fat and fat fish is small and relatively nonoily. The lipids in such fish are stored in the muscles and during feeding periods are also located in the subcutaneous fat layer. Salmon produces an adipose hump for the purpose of the spawning migration; during the migration, lipids in the hump are successively substituted by water.

The fish reserve lipids are utilized in various parts of the body when needed during, for example, starvation, overwintering, fast movements, reproduction, and growth. During gonad maturation, lipids are transported from the liver and muscles to the gonads. During the spawning period, a rapid decrease in lipid content is observed. After spawning, the fish assumes intensive feeding and the lipid content increases in the meat and liver and decreases in the gonads. The range of variations depends on the fat metabolism, maturity stage, environmental temperature, food availability, stress, and other factors. The range may be very large in fatty fish, from 1% to more than 25% wet weight. Consequently, the lipid content of a fish belonging to the "fat" group may be, over certain periods, equal to that of a lean fish. The lipid content and composition in lean fish vary only slightly, more pronounced variations being observed in the liver.

As the amount of phospholipids does not usually exceed 1% tissue wet weight, all that is above that value may be regarded as triacylglycerols or else wax esters. Variations, seasonal and other, in lipid content involve the reserve lipids. The phospholipid fraction remains relatively stable, its amount and composition being independent of diet and other variables. Consequently, the composition of total lipids and their nutritive value depend on the dilution of the phospholipids by triacylglycerols and/or other reserve lipids.

The fish lipids, being highly unsaturated, are very sensitive to oxidation. Although the oxidation process is chemical, the endogenous skin lipoxygenase and microsomal peroxidation system may constitute a significant source of initiating radicals.[42,43]

VI. FLAVOR COMPOUNDS OF SEAFOODS

A. NITROGENOUS COMPOUNDS
1. Amino Acids

Amino acids, peptides, nucleotides, guanidine compounds, and quaternary ammonium compounds are the major contributors to the taste of seafoods.

Glycine, alanine, serine, and threonine taste sweet, while arginine, leucine, valine, methionine, phenylalanine, histidine, and isoleucine give bitter taste. The sweetness of fresh prawn and crab is contributed to by the abundance of free glycine in their muscle. The high content of free arginine in crustaceans enriches the sweet taste with complexity and fullness and yields a seafood-like flavor. Taurine, proline, and alanine are among the major free amino acids in crustaceans. Free methionine, isoleucine, leucine, tyrosine, and phenylalanine were not found in the instantly killed grass prawn (*Penaeus monodon*) but occur and increase in content during chilled storage.

Histidine and taurine are the most abundant free amino acids in some species of fish. Migratory fish such as tuna and mackerel are high in free histidine. Taurine in fish muscle is probably derived from cysteine. Different genera of the same species may not contain the same amount of taurine. Higher taurine content leads to more active Maillard reaction during fish drying.

The amino acids in 66 fish and shellfish were compiled by Konosu and Yamaguchi.[44]

2. Dipeptides

Only three dipeptides have been identified in the muscle of fish and shellfish. Carnosine was found in the hepatopancreas and the first leg meat of male Alaska king crab, but was not found in snow crab, blue crab, or horsehair crab. The muscle of chum salmon contains 4 to 8 mg carnosine per 100 g. Also eel and skipjack accumulate carnosine in the muscle. Anserine is abundant in tuna, skipjack, salmon, trout, and some species of sharks. The content ranges between 300 and 600 mg/100 g. Balenine was found high in whales.

3. Nucleotides

The palatable meaty taste, being called shean by the Chinese and umami by the Japanese, is mainly produced by the nucleotides in the muscle.

ATP is the predominant nucleotide present in the muscle of live animals. Post-mortem, ATP is degraded by endogenous enzymes. Mollusks have considerably higher content of ATP and other nucleotides than fish.

4. Guanidine Compounds

Creatine is present in the muscle of fish in the range of 300 to 700 mg/100 g. Creatinine is present in a much lower concentration, 10 to 50 mg/100 g. Shrimp also has much higher content of creatine than of creatinine.

Arginine predominates in the muscle of invertebrates. A decrease in arginine content concurs with an increase in octopine in squid, octopus, and scallop.

5. Quaternary Ammonium Bases

TMAO is one of the most abundant nonprotein nitrogenous constituents in fish. It ranges from 156 mg/100 g in puffer fish, about 400 mg/100 g in flathead flounder, to around 1000 mg/100 g in Alaska pollack and cod, and 750 to 1480 mg/100 g in the muscle of sharks and rays. A thorough review on the occurrence and content of TMAO in fish and shellfish was compiled by Hebard et al.[45]

The muscle of elasmobranchs contains much more TMAO than of marine teleosts. The level of TMAO fluctuates with size of fish, the season, and the environmental conditions. Freshwater teleosts contain only a negligible amount of TMAO.

Marine invertebrates also have high TMAO content. Squid contains 728 to 884 mg/100 g, crabs 564 to 863 mg/100 g, and marine prawn 820 to 846 mg/100 g. Since TMAO is responsible for osmoregulation of muscle, decreases in the salinity of the culture water or the natural environment result in lower TMAO concentration in the animal muscle. TMAO contributes a sweet taste to fresh shrimp.

Homarine was found in the tissue of marine invertebrates with seasonal changes. The content of homarine in the liver is higher than in the muscle of squid, top-shell, and female crab. However, in abalone, pearl oyster, and sea cucumber, the content in the adductor muscle is higher than that in the viscera or in the liver.

B. VOLATILE COMPOUNDS OF SEAFOODS
1. Sulfur-Containing Compounds

The volatile sulfur-containing compounds in seafoods fall mainly into four groups: linear sulfides, cyclic sulfides, methyl-thioesters, and nitrogen-containing sulfur compounds.

Linear sulfides are predominant sulfur compounds of fish oils. Dimethyl disulfide, the single sulfur compound quantitatively dominant, possibly results from oxidation of methanethiol formed by bacterial degradation of methionine in raw fish. Dimethyl trisulfide is also present in the volatiles of contaminated fish, and in the off-flavor prawn. The trisulfides possess a remarkably low odor threshold, 0.01 ppb in water; therefore, they are readily noticeable.

Convincing evidence shows that the formation of H_2S and methanethiol in spoiling fish are the results of bacterial decomposition of cysteine and methionine, respectively.

The occurrence of trithiolane and thialdine derivatives in raw and fermented shrimp indicates that these compounds are formed from the reaction of free amino acids, ammonia H_2S, lipids, and other precursors of aldehydes. The cyclic and/or nitrogen-containing sulfur compounds usually contribute to a distinctive note of the flavor of seafoods. The 3,5-dimethyl-1,2,4-trithiolane has an onion-like odor. Replacing the methyl groups with one or two ethyl groups modifies the odor to garlic-like. Dimethyltrithiolanes in dilute concentration has a meaty aroma. When it is concentrated, it gives a sulfide odor.

Trimethylarsine also contributes to the off-flavor of some species of prawn. bis-Methylthio-methane was found in relation to the offensive odor of prawns and sand lobster. Propyl thioacetate is an off-flavor component in Antarctic krill.

2. Aldehydes, Ketones, and Alcohols

Hexanal was found in the volatiles of all raw fishes, while 2-hexenal, 2-octenal, 2-nonenal, and 2,6-nonadienal were only present in freshwater fish. These unsaturated aldehydes, together with some unsaturated 8-carbon alcohols, contribute to the sweet melon-like aroma in fresh white fish.

Saturated ketones including 2-alkanones containing 5, 7, 8, 9, 10, 11, and 15 carbons and 3-alkanones of 7 and 8 carbons have been reported to occur in the volatiles of fresh fish. 2,3-Octanedione was found in freshwater fish.

Unsaturated ketones such as 1-penten-3-one were found in Pacific oyster, and 1-octen-3-one and 1,5-octadien-3-one in freshwater fish but not in saltwater fish.

Alkyl-substituted and cyclic alkenones have also been reported as volatile components of seafood flavor.

Alcohols contained in the fish of different species possess a characteristic flavor of that species. The flavor is highly susceptible to change upon exposure of the oil to even low levels of oxygen at very low temperature for a relatively short period of time.

The naturally occurring key-note flavor of menhaden oil is similar to that of *cis*-3-hexen-1-ol.

Unsaturated alcohols such as 1-octene-3-ol, 1,5-octadien-3-ol, and 2,5-octadiene-1-ol were found in both Pacific oyster (*Crassostrea gigas*) and Atlantic oyster (*C. virginica*). The individual unsaturated alcohol content was more than twice higher in the former than in the latter. In addition, 3,6-nonadien-1-ol was found in the volatile fraction of Pacific oyster but not in that of the Atlantic oyster. The high concentration of these unsaturated alcohols contributed to the melon-like aroma of the Pacific oyster, while the Atlantic oyster

TABLE 10
Vitamin A and D in Fish Liver Oils

Species	Oil (%)	Vitamin A (IU 10^3/g)[a]	Vitamin D (IU 10^3/g)[b]
Soupfin shark	25—72	42—200	0.005—0.025
Dogfish	30—80	Trace-210	0.005—0.025
Haddock	40—85	0.2—3	0.05—0.075
Halibut	8—30	5—250	0.55—20
Pink salmon	3—6	10—40	0.1—0.6
Yellowfin tuna	3—5	35—90	10—45
Albacore	7—20	10—60	25—250

[a] IU of vitamin A equal to 0.3 µg of retinol.
[b] IU of vitamin D equal to 25 mg of vitamin D_3.

Data from Higashi, H., *Fish as Food,* Vol. 1, Borgstrom, G., Ed., Academic Press, New York, 1961, 411.

lacked this aroma. Other unsaturated alcohols, i.e., 1-pentene-3-ol, and cyclic alcohol, i.e., cyclopentanol, were abundant in the two varieties of oyster.

VII. VITAMINS

A. THE FAT-SOLUBLE VITAMINS

Fish flesh, oils, and offals are very rich in vitamins. The fat-soluble vitamins are present in especially high concentrations in the liver oils of some species, whereas the body oils, obtained from whole fish or fish viscera and other filleting offals, contain lower amounts of vitamin A, D, and E. The concentration of vitamin A in fish liver oils depends upon the species (Table 10) and on several other biological factors. In many fish species, the concentration of vitamin A in the liver oil increases with the size of the fish and with depletion of oil in the liver. There are also seasonal variations related to the spawning cycle of the fish, climatic conditions, and availability of feed. The tocopherol content in fish liver oils is in the range 20 to 60 mg/100 g.

The amount of fat-soluble vitamins in the flesh of marine animals is effected by the concentration of fat. It varies therefore both between and within the species. Thus, the flesh of the lean white fish, such as cod, haddock, and pollock, contains from 25 to 50 IU of vitamin A per 100 g, while in the fatty species such as herring there is from 100 to about 4500 IU of this vitamin in 100 g of meat. The content of vitamin D in sardines and pilchards and in tuna is in the range 530 to 5400, and 700 to 2000 IU per 100 g, respectively. According to a few available literature data, the contents of vitamin E in the edible parts of fish and marine invertebrata range from about 0.2 to 270 mg/100 g wet weight.[47]

B. THE WATER-SOLUBLE VITAMINS

The amount of water-soluble vitamins in marine foods is less dependent upon the species. The average content of thiamine in 155 species, as compiled by Sidwell et al.,[47] was in the range from 4 mg/100 g in needlefish to 388 mg/100 g in turbot. Generally a serving of seafoods may significantly contribute to satisfying the human daily needs for B vitamins (Tables 11 and 12).

The contents of both groups of vitamins in the final products depend also on the losses which occur due to oxidation and leakage as the result of industrial processing and culinary preparation.

TABLE 11
The Water-Soluble Vitamins in the Edible Portion of Raw Fish

	Mean values and range			
Vitamin	Codfishes Gadidae	Halibuts Pleuronectidae	Herrings Clupeidae	Tunas Scombridae
Thiamin	71	83	46	120
(μg/100 g)	18—150	40—180	6—170	10—434
Riboflavin	121	80	261	164
(μg/100 g)	11—325	44—185	50—1000	13—660
Niacin	2.5	7.5	3.8	9.7
(mg/100 g)	0.2—6.7	2.8—14.2	0.6—9.6	0—23.4
Pyridoxine	221	400	310	647
(μg/100 g)	170—288	347—430	160—450	190—920
Panthothenic	163	303	2427	917
acid (μg/100 g)	96—400	111—595	970—9500	186—3280
Biotin	1.2	8.5	—	1.5
(μg/100 g)	0.2—2.6	6.6—9.5		
Folic acid	5.0	2.6	10.3	2.1
(μg/100 g)	1.8—6.7	2.0—2.9	1.7—14	0.6—3.2
Cobalamines	0.6	0.8	11.4	6.2
(μg/100 g)	0.1—2.0	0.7—1.0	1.4—34	0.2—47
Ascorbic acid	—	0.0	9.0	2.6
(mg/100 g)			0.0—27.7	0.0—10.7

Data from Sidwell, V. D., Loomis, A. L., Foncannon, P. R., and Buzzell, D. H., *Mar. Fish. Rev.*, 40(12), 1, 1978.

TABLE 12
The Water-Soluble Vitamins in the Raw Edible Portion of Marine Invertebrates

	Mean values and range			
Vitamin	Clams (mixed species)	Oysters Ostreidae	Lobsters and crayfishes (mixed species)	Shrimps and prawns (mixed species)
Thiamin	49	153	99	41
(μg/100 g)	2—139	9—300	7—165	10—143
Riboflavin	238	188	64	76
(μg/100 g)	12—780	16—340	10—130	13—190
Niacin	1.3	1.8	2.3	2.7
(mg/100 g)	0.2—2.3	0.7—7.1	1.2—4.3	0.7—4.9
Pyridoxine	75	166	210	66
(μg/100 g)	0—350	30—320		16—125
Pantothenic acid	531	365	410	278
(μg/100 g)	440—620	184—530	410—410	165—372
Biotin	2.3	41	5.0	1.0
(μg/100 g)		10—72	4.8—5.2	
Folic acid	25.1	84.4	0.6	5.2
(μg/100 g)	2.7—58	3.7—240	0.6—0.6	3.0—7.4
Cobalamines	9.8	17.2	1.6	3.8
(μg/100 g)	0.2—62.3	11.5—33	0.5—2.7	0.9—8.1
Ascorbic acid	11.2	10.7	3.0	1.5
(mg/100 g)	2.0-30	0—38.1	0—5.0	0—3.0

Data from Sidwell, V. D., Loomis, A. L., Foncannon, P. R., and Buzzell, D. H., *Mar. Fish. Rev.*, 40(12), 1, 1978.

VIII. MINERAL COMPONENTS

A. GENERAL CONSIDERATIONS

Marine foods are very rich sources of mineral components. The total content of minerals in the raw flesh of marine fish and invertebrates is in the range 0.6 to 1.5% wet weight. The final concentration of these components in the ready dishes depends upon the addition of salt for preservation or sensory purposes, on the losses due to leakage, on the weight loss during culinary preparation, and on whether the final product is eaten together with the bony parts, e.g., canned sardines or sprats.

The mineral components are contained in food as macro- and microelements. The macroelements are present in quantities of several to hundreds of milligrams per 100 g wet weight. The microelements are contained in the flesh in quantities not larger than that of iron, i.e., from below 0.1 to a few tens of micrograms per 1 g. The components of both groups are important in human nutrition. Some of them are highly desirable in large quantities, while others are required in small amounts but may be toxic in higher concentrations. The human nutritional requirements depend upon the biological state of the organism and on the efficiency of utilization of the elements of the diet. The availability of the elements is effected by the form in which they are present in the food, as well as by other food constituents, which can promote or impede the absorption. The concentration and speciation, i.e., the determination of the forms of existence of the minerals in seafoods, as well as the bioavailability of F, Fe, Se, and Zn contained in marine products have been recently discussed by Gordon.[48]

B. MACROELEMENTS

The range of contents of the macroelements in the flesh of fish and marine invertebrates, in milligrams per 100 g wet weight, is according to available published data: sodium, 25 to 620; potassium, 25 to 710; magnesium, 10 to 230; calcium, 5 to 750; iron, 0.01 to 50; phosphorus, 9 to 1100; sulfur, 100 to 300; and chlorine 20 to 500.

The content of sodium is of special interest because of the current efforts of nutritionists to lower the dietary intake of this element. The average amount of sodium in the flesh of 122 species of fish and marine invertebrates, calculated from the data compiled by Sidwell et al.,[49] is 120 mg/100 g, the average for clams, cockles, mussels, oysters, scallops, snails, squid, octopuses, crabs, crayfish, shrimps, and prawns being 188 mg/100 g.

C. MICROELEMENTS

1. The Contents in Marine Foods

An average serving of fish or marine invertebrates can satisfy the total daily human requirements for essential microelements (Table 13). However, the presence of some microelements in considerably high concentrations in various marine foods evokes public concern because of the possible toxic effects. This especially regards mercury, cadmium, arsenic, and fluorine.

2. Mercury

Although some fish and marine invertebrates belong to foods richest in mercury, the content of this element in the flesh of many popular food fishes is very low, usually in the range 0.02 to 0.2 µg/g wet weight. The mean values found in over 1500 samples of herring, 500 samples of mackerel, and 1430 samples of bluefin tuna were, respectively, 0.07, 0.15, and 0.7 µg/g wet tissue.[51] The mean concentration of mercury in the edible parts of 87 species of crustaceans, fish, and mollusks, calculated from the data compiled by Sidwell et al.[50] is 0.5 µg/g wet weight, but the mean does not exceed 0.4 µg/g in 69% of the species. Higher means than the current U.S. Food and Drug Administration action level of 1 ppm

TABLE 13
Microelements in the Edible Portion of Marine Fish and Invertebrates

	Wet weight, mean values, and range (µg/g)			
Element	Codfishes Gadidae	Flounders Pleuronectidae	Crayfishes (mixed species)	Oysters (mixed species)
Vanadium	0.6	0.1	2.9	0.1
	0.0—1.6	0.0—0.5	0.0—8.5	
Chromium	0.1	0.1	0.1	0.1
	0.1—0.3	0.0—0.2		0.1—0.1
Molybdenum	3.0	0.2	0.2	—
		0.0—0.4		
Manganese	0.2	0.4	1.5	3.3
	0.0—0.6	0.0—1.8	0.1—4.2	0.1—6.5
Cobalt	0.3	0.8	1.5	0.2
	0.0—1.2	0.5—1.2	0.1—2.8	
Nickel	0.0	1.0	0.1	0.5
		0.0—3.3	0.0—0.1	
Copper	2.6	1.7	20.4	79.3
	1.1—19.4	0.1—7.0	0.1—167	0.3—606
Silver	0.0	0.0	0.3	—
Zinc	17	4.6	27.0	844
	2.8—52.5	0.8—14.2	1.5—66	71—2000
Cadmium	0.1	0.0	0.1	—
	0.0—0.5		0.0—0.2	
Mercury	0.2	0.2	0.2	0.1
	0.0—0.8	0.0—0.8	0.0—0.5	0.0—0.2
Aluminum	4.1	11.0	45.9	13.4
	0.1—21.8	10.0—32.3	1.4—90.3	
Tin	1.4	0.9	1.2	0.1
	0.0—3.7	0.0—3.2	0.9—1.5	
Lead	0.5	0.4	1.6	24.9
	0.2—1.6	0.2—0.5	0.3—11.6	0.2—100
Arsenic	2.3	2.5	12.8	9.1
	0.3—9.8	0.1—4.5	0.4—44.5	0.5—42.7
Selenium	0.7	0.7	0.7	0.7
	0.4—1.2	0.3—1.4		
Fluorine	3.8	0.4	—	1.1
	0.7—7.0			0.7—1.6
Iodine	1.5	0.4	1.0	0.6
	0.1—6.0	0.1—1.0	0.3—1.4	0.1—1.3

Data from Sidwell, V. D., Loomis, A. L., Loomis, K. J., Foncannon, P. R., and Buzzell, D. H., *Mar. Fish Rev.*, 40(9), 1, 1978.

were found only in 12.5% of the investigated species. Generally, the concentration of mercury in the flesh of fish from unpolluted ocean waters is highest in large, long-lived, and predator species, especially Pacific halibut, sharks, swordfish, and some tunas. In most fish species, 80 to 95% of the total mercury in the tissues is present as methyl mercury, which is more toxic than inorganic mercury. In human populations, consuming habitually large amounts of fish with high natural contents of mercury, slightly above 1 µg/g, no toxic effects have been found. The human organism is capable of converting methyl mercury to mercury, and the effectiveness of this process increases with the amount of introduced methyl mercury.[52] Furthermore, there may be some involvement of selenium contained in the fish flesh. Selenium is known to diminish the toxicity of mercury.[53] In fish from heavily polluted estuarian waters, the concentration of mercury in the edible parts may be as high as 25 µg/g wet weight. Such highly contaminated fish were the cause of fatal mercury poisonings in Japan.

TABLE 14
Cadmium in the Flesh of Fish and in Marine Invertebrates

Species	Cadmium (μg/g wet weight)	Number of samples	Locality	Ref.
Cod, *Gadus morhua*	0.005	201	Baltic Sea	54
Herring, *Clupea harengus*	0.009	181	Baltic Sea	55
Flounder, *Platichthys flessus*	0.013	103	Baltic Sea	56
Sprat, *Sprattus sprattus*	0.031	208	Baltic Sea	57
Sea mullet, *Mugil cephalus*	0.05	57	Cockburn Sound	58
Yellow finned whiting, *Silago schomburgkii*	0.06	29	Cockburn Sound	58
Scallop *Pecten alba*		60	Port Philip Bay	59
Adductor muscle	1.04			
Gonad	0.94			
Inedible viscera	7.73			
Scallop, *Placopecten magellanicus*		33	Browns Bank	60
Adductor muscle	1.69		Georges Bank	
Mantle	1.09		Navy Island	
Gill	1.19			
Viscera/rest of soft tissue	46.40			

3. Cadmium

Data from several sources indicate that the flesh of marine fish contains usually below 0.1 μg cadmium per 1 g wet weight (Table 14). This value is of the same order as in most other foods like grain, potatoes, fruit, eggs, cheese, and meat. Significantly higher, however, is the concentration of cadmium in marine invertebrates, although still lower than in beef kidney (619 ± 663 μg/g) and liver (123 ± 136 μg/g).[61] The content of Cd in mussels and oysters is proportional to the concentration of the metal in the sea water. In the Derwent estuary at 7.4 μg Cd per cubic decimeter water, the oysters *Crassostrea gigas* contained 30 μg Cd per gram wet weight.[62] Cd is not uniformly distributed in the body of animals, but is selectively accumulated in the liver, kidney, and viscera.

4. Lead and Arsenic

The average content of lead in the flesh of 40 species of marine crustaceans, fish, and mollusks, calculated from the data compiled 10 years ago by Sidwell et al.,[50] is 0.9 μg/g wet weight. This considerably high average does not include the mean for oysters, which was 24.9 μg/g, with a total range of 0.2 to 100.0 μg/g in 12 samples. Newer data, obtained by using atomic absorption spectrometry, indicate that many valuable food fish contain significantly lower amounts of lead. In the flesh of 201 samples of Baltic cod, 208 sprats, and 187 herrings, the contents of lead, in micrograms per gram wet weight, was 0.086 (range not detectable to 0.45), 0.10 (0.029 to 0.31), and 0.079 (0.06 to 0.50), respectively.[54,55,57] This indicates that marine fish are not likely to contribute much to the tolerable human intake of lead, for which the FAO/WHO provisional weekly value has been set at 3 mg per person.

The edible parts of marine invertebrates have been known for a long time as a rich source of arsenic. However, not very many analytical data regarding the concentration of inorganic and organic arsenic in marine foods are available. In the flesh of food fishes, the total content of arsenic is usually below 0.5 μg/g. Flanjak found in 45 samples of the edible portion of the eastern common crayfish 0.12 to 0.41 μg and 11.9 to 54.1 μg of inorganic and organic arsenic, respectively, per 1 g wet weight.[63] The organic arsenic compounds ingested with the food are excreted in the urine of mammals.

5. Fluoride

Fluoride is present in the muscles of fish, crab, shrimp, and prawns from the North Sea in amounts from about 1 to 4 µg/g wet weight. About five times higher concentrations were found in the muscles of krill-feeding fish from the Antarctic waters. The average fluoride content in the Antarctic fish *Notothenia gibberifrons* and *N. rossii marmorata* was in the fillet, skin, and backbone, respectively, 13.5, 92.5, and 1606 µg/g wet weight.[64] The Antarctic krill contains exceptionally large amounts of fluoride: about 1000 µg/g dry weight in the whole animal, 70 µg/g dry weight of muscle, and 1958 µg/g dry weight of the exoskeleton.[65] After catch, a rapid migration of fluoride from the exoskeleton into the muscle takes place.

REFERENCES

1. **Love, R. M., Yamaguchi, K., Creach, J., and Lavety, J.,** The connective tissues and collagens of cod during starvation, *Comp. Biochem. Physiol. B,* 55, 487, 1976.
2. **Liljemark, A.,** Electron microscopy of fish musculature, *Livsmedelsteknik,* 10, 3, 1968.
3. **Morrison, C. M. and Odense, P. H.,** Ultrastructure of the striated muscle of the scallop *(Placopecten magellanicus), J. Fish. Res. Board Can.,* 25, 1339, 1968.
4. **Otwell, W. S. and Giddings, G. G.,** Scanning electron microscopy of squid, raw, cooked and frozen mantle, *Mar. Fish. Rev.,* 42(7-8), 67, 1980.
5. **Sidwell, V. D., Foncannon, P. R., Moore, N. S., and Bonnet, J. C.,** Composition of the edible portion of raw (fresh or frozen) crustaceans, finfish, and mollusks. I. Protein, fat, moisture, ash, carbohydrate, energy value, and cholesterol, *Mar. Fish. Rev.,* 36(3), 21, 1974.
6. **Stansby, M. E. and Hall, A. S.,** Chemical composition of commercially important fish of the United States, *Fish. Ind. Res.,* 3(4), 29, 1967.
7. **Levanidov, I. P.,** Interrelation of the main components of the chemical composition of fish flesh, *Rybn. Khoz.,* 8, 62, 1980, (in Russian).
8. **Braekkan, O. R. and Boge, G.,** A comparative study of amino acids in the muscle of different species of fish, *Reports on Technological Research Concerning Norwegian Fish Industry,* Vol. 4, Fiskeridirectorates Skrifter, Bergen, Norway, 1962.
9. **Acton, J. C. and Rudd, C. L.,** Protein quality methods for seafoods, in *Seafood Quality Determination,* Kramer, D. E. and Liston, J., Eds., Elsevier, Amsterdam, 1987, 453.
10. **Scopes, R. K.,** Characterization and study of sarcoplasmic proteins, in *The Physiology and Biochemistry of Muscle as a Food,* Vol. 2, Briskey, E. J., Cassens, R. G., and Marsh, B. B., Eds., University of Wisconsin Press, Madison, 1970, 471.
11. **Matsuura, F. and Hashimoto, K.,** Chemical studies on the red muscle of fishes. II. Determination of the content of hemoglobin, myoglobin, and cytochrome C in the muscles of fishes, *Bull. Jpn. Soc. Sci. Fish.,* 20, 4, 1954.
12. **Feeney, R. E., Osuga, D. T., Ahmed, A. J., and Yeh, Y.,** Antifreeze proteins from fish bloods. Relationship of the function to structure, solvent, and freezing conditions, *Lebensm. Wiss. Technol.,* 14, 171, 1981.
13. **Suzuki, M.,** Blood proteins of the Antarctic hemoglobin-free fish *Neopagetopsis ionah, Bull. Jpn. Soc. Sci. Fish.,* 46, 1027, 1980.
14. **Mochizuki, A. and Matsuchiya, M.,** Lysozyme activity in shellfishes, *Bull. Jpn. Soc. Sci. Fish.,* 49, 131, 1983.
15. **Buttkus, H.,** The sulfhydryl content of rabbit and trout myosins in relation to protein stability, *Can. J. Biochem.,* 49, 97, 1971.
16. **Suzuki, T.,** *Fish and Krill Protein: Processing Technology,* Applied Science, London, 1981, chap. 1.
17. **Tsuchiya, T., Yamada, N., and Matsumoto, J. J.,** Extraction and purification of squid myosin, *Bull. Jpn. Soc. Sci. Fish.,* 44, 175, 1978.
18. **Kimura, I., Yoshitomi, B., Konno, K., and Arai, K.,** Preparation of highly purified myosin from mantle muscle of squid *Ommastrephes sloani pacificus, Bull. Jpn. Soc. Sci. Fish.,* 46, 885, 1980.
19. **Pyeun, J. H., Hashimoto, K., and Matsuura, F.,** Isolation and characterization of abalone paramyosin, *Bull. Jpn. Soc. Sci. Fish.,* 39, 395, 1973.
20. **Horie, N., Tsuchiya, T., and Matsumoto, J. J.,** Studies on ATP-ase activity of actomyosin of squid mantle muscle, *Bull. Jpn. Soc. Sci. Fish.,* 41, 1039, 1975.

21. **Nishita, K., Takeda, Y., and Arai, K.,** Biochemical characteristics of actomyosin from Antarctic krill, *Bull. Jpn. Soc. Sci. Fish.,* 47, 1237, 1981.
22. **Maruyama, K., Matsubara, S., Natori, R., Nonomura, Y., Kimura, S., Ohashi, K., Murakami, F., Handa, S., and Eguchi, G.,** Connectin, an elastic protein of muscle. Characterization and function, *J. Biochem.,* 82, 317, 1977.
23. **Kimura, S., Akashi, Y., and Kubota, M.,** Carp connectin — its contents in white and dark muscles, *Bull. Jpn. Soc. Sci. Fish.,* 45, 237, 1979.
24. **Kimura, S., Miyaki, T., Takema, Y., and Kubota, M.,** Electrophoretic analysis of connectin from the muscles of aquatic animals, *Bull. Jpn. Soc. Sci. Fish.,* 47, 787, 1981.
25. **Dyer, W. and Dingle, J. R.,** Fish proteins with special reference to freezing, in *Fish as Food,* Vol. 1, Borgstrom, G., Ed., Academic Press, New York, 1961, 275.
26. **Love, R. M.,** *The Chemical Biology of Fishes,* Academic Press, London, 1970, 323.
27. **Sikorski, Z. E., Scott, D. N., and Buisson, D. H.,** The role of collagen in the quality and processing of fish, *Crit. Rev. Food Sci. Nutr.,* 20, 301, 1984.
28. **Sato, K., Yoshinaka, R., Sato, M., and Shimizu, Y.,** Collagen content in the muscle of fishes in association with their swimming movement and meat texture, *Bull. Jpn. Soc. Sci. Fish.,* 52, 1595, 1986.
29. **Sadowska, M.,** unpublished data, 1989.
30. **Yamaguchi, K., Lavety, J., and Love, R. M.,** The connective tissues of fish. VIII. Comparative studies on hake, cod and catfish collagens, *J. Food Technol.,* 11, 389, 1976.
31. **Kimura, S., Nagaoka, Y., and Kubota, M.,** Studies on marine invertebrata collagens. I. Some collagens from crustaceans and molluscs, *Bull. Jpn. Soc. Sci. Fish.,* 35, 743, 1969.
32. **Kimura, S. and Tanaka, H.,** Partial characterization of muscle collagens from prawns and lobster, *J. Food Sci.,* 51, 330, 1986.
33. **McClain, P. E., Wiley, E. R., and McCague, K. E.,** Species variation in the cross-linking characteristics of collagen from the intramuscular connective tissues of striated muscles *(Bos taurus, Ovis aries, Sus scrofa), Int. J. Biochem.,* 2, 167, 1971.
34. **Thompson, H. C. and Thompson, M. H.,** Isolation and amino acid composition of the collagen of the white shrimp *Penaeus setiferus, Comp. Biochem. Physiol.,* 27, 127, 1968.
35. **Kimura, S.,** Studies on marine invertebrate collagens. V. The neutral sugar composition and glucosylated hydroxylysine contents of several collagens, *Bull. Jpn. Soc. Sci. Fish.,* 38, 1153, 1972.
36. **Kelly, R. E. and Rice, R. V.,** Abductin: a rubber-like protein from the internal triangular hinge ligament of pecten, *Science,* 155, 208, 1967.
37. **Iwasaki, M. and Harada, R.,** Cholesterol content of fish gonads and livers, *Bull. Jpn. Soc. Sci. Fish.,* 50, 1623, 1984.
38. **Okano, M., Mizu, F., Funaki, Y., and Avatani, T.,** Seasonal variation of sterol, hydrocarbon, fatty acid and phytol fractions in *Enteromorpha prolifera* (Muller) J. Agardh, *Bull. Jpn. Soc. Sci. Fish.,* 49, 621, 1983.
39. **Benson, A. A., Lee, R. F., and Nevenzel, J. C.,** Wax esters: major marine metabolic energy source, *Biochem. Soc. Symp.,* 35, 175, 1972.
40. **Stansby, M. E.,** Properties of fish oils and their application to handling of fish and to nutritional and industry use, in *Chemistry and Biochemistry of Marine Food Products,* Martin, R. E., Flick, G. J., Hebard, C. E., and Ward, D. R., Eds., AVI Publishing, Westport, CT, 1982, 75.
41. **Lands, W. E. M.,** *Fish in Human Health,* Academic Press, Orlando, FL, 1986.
42. **German, J. B. and Kinsella, J. E.,** Lipid oxidation in fish tissue. Enzymatic initiation via lipoxygenase, *J. Agric. Food Chem.,* 33, 680, 1985.
43. **Slabyj, B. M. and Hultin, H. O.,** Lipid peroxidation by microsomal fractions isolated from light and dark muscles of herring *(Clupea harengus), J. Food Sci.,* 47, 1395, 1982.
44. **Konosu, S. and Yamaguchi, K.,** The flavor components in fish and shellfish, in *Chemistry and Biochemistry of Marine Food Products,* Martin, R. E., Flick, G. J., Hebard, C. E., and Ward, D. R., Eds., AVI Publishing, Westport, CT, 1982, 367.
45. **Hebard, C. E., Flick, G. J., and Martin, R. E.,** Occurrence and significance of trimethylamine oxide and its derivatives in fish and shellfish, in *Chemistry and Biochemistry of Marine Food Products,* Martin, R. E., Flick, G. J., Hebard, C. E., and Ward, D. R., Eds., AVI Publishing, Westport, CT, 1982, 149.
46. **Higashi, H.,** Vitamins in fish, in *Fish as Food,* Vol. 1, Borgstrom, G., Ed., Academic Press, New York, 1961, 411.
47. **Sidwell, V. D., Loomis, A. L., Foncannon, P. R., and Buzzell, D. H.,** Composition of the edible portion of raw fresh or frozen crustaeceans, finfish, and mollusks. IV. Vitamins, *Mar. Fish. Rev.,* 40(12), 1, 1978.
48. **Gordon, T.,** Minerals in seafoods: availability and interactions, in *Seafood Quality Determination,* Kramer, D. E. and Liston, J., Eds., Elsevier, Amsterdam, 1986, 517.
49. **Sidwell, V. D., Buzzell, D. H., Foncannon, P. R., and Smith, A. L.,** Composition of the edible portion of raw (fresh or frozen) crustaceans, finfish, and mollusks. II. Macroelements: sodium, potassium, chlorine, calcium, phosphorus, and magnesium, *Mar. Fish. Rev.,* 39(1), 1, 1977.

50. **Sidwell, V. D., Loomis, A. L., Loomis, K. J., Foncannon, P. R., and Buzzell, D. H.,** Composition of the edible portion of raw (fresh or frozen) crustaceans, finfish, and mollusks. III. Microelements, *Mar. Fish. Rev.*, 40(9), 1, 1978.
51. **Schreiber, E.,** Mercury content of fishery products: data from last decade, *Sci. Total Environ.*, 31, 283, 1983.
52. **Margolin, S.,** Mercury in marine seafood: the scientific medical margin of safety as a guide to the potential risk to public health, *World Rev. Nutr. Diet.*, 34, 182, 1980.
53. **Burk, R. F.,** Selenium in nutrition, *World Rev. Nutr. Diet.*, 30, 88, 1978.
54. **Falandysz, J.,** Trace metals in cod from the southern Baltic, 1983, *Z. Lebensm. Unters. Forsch.*, 182, 228, 1986.
55. **Falandysz, J.,** Trace metals in herring from the southern Baltic, 1983, *Z. Lebensm. Unters. Forsch.*, 182, 36, 1986.
56. **Falandysz, J.,** Trace metals in flatfish from the southern Baltic, 1983, *Z. Lebensm. Unters. Forsch.*, 181, 117, 1985.
57. **Falandysz, J.,** Trace metals in sprats from the southern Baltic, 1983, *Z. Lebensm. Unters. Forsch.*, 182, 40, 1986.
58. **Plaskett, D. and Potter, I. C.,** Heavy metal concentration in the muscle tissue of 12 species of teleost from Cockburn Sound, Western Australia, *Aust. J. Mar. Freshwater Res.*, 30, 607, 1979.
59. **Walker, T. I., Glover, J. W., and Powell, D. G.,** Effects of length, locality and tissue type on mercury and cadmium content of the commercial scallop *(Pecten alba* Tate) from Port Philip Bay, Victoria, *Aust. J. Mar. Freshwater Res.*, 33, 547, 1982.
60. **Ray, S., Woodside, M., Jerome, V. E., and Akagi, H.,** Copper, zinc, cadmium, and lead in scallops *(Placopecten Magellanicus)* from Georges and Browns Banks, *Chemosphere*, 13, 1247, 1984.
61. **Diehl, J. F. and Boppel, B.,** Dietary intake of cadmium: a re-evaluation, *Trace Elements Med.*, 2(4), 167, 1985.
62. **Cooper, R. J., Langlois, D., and Olley, J.,** Heavy metals in Tasmanian shellfish. I. Monitoring heavy metal contamination in the Dervent estuary: use of oyster and mussels, *J. Appl. Toxicol.*, 2, 99, 1982.
63. **Flanjak, J.,** Inorganic and organic arsenic in some commercial East Australian crustacea, *J. Sci. Food Agric.*, 33, 579, 1982.
64. **Manthey, M.,** Fluoride-content in the Antarctic fish, *Information für die Fischwirtschaft*, 27(6), 261, 1980, (in German).
65. **Boone, R. J. and Manthey, A.,** The anatomical distribution of fluoride within various body segments and organs of Antarctic krill *(Euphausia superba Dana)*, *Arch. Fischwiss.*, 34, 81, 1983.

Chapter 4

POSTHARVEST BIOCHEMICAL AND MICROBIAL CHANGES

Zdzisław E. Sikorski, Anna Kołakowska, and James R. Burt

TABLE OF CONTENTS

I. The General Course of Events 56

II. Degradation of Organic Phosphates and Carbohydrates 56
    A. The Effect of Catching 56
    B. Degradation of Organic Phosphates 56
    C. Changes in Carbohydrates 59
    D. Change in pH of the Flesh 59

III. Rigor Mortis 60
    A. Stiffening 60
    B. The Biophysical Mechanism 61
    C. The General Course of Rigor in Fish Flesh 61
    D. The Effect of Rigor on Fish Quality 62

IV. Changes in Nitrogenous Compounds 63
    A. Causes and Effects 63
    B. Degradation of Nonprotein Compounds 63
    C. Changes in Proteins 64

V. Degradation of Lipids 64
    A. Lipolysis 64
    B. Oxidation of Lipids 65

VI. Microbial Contamination and Spoilage 65
    A. The Microflora of Fresh Seafoods 65
        1. The Total Count 65
        2. The Spoilage Microflora 66
        3. Pathogenic Organisms 66
    B. The Growth of Bacteria on Seafoods 66
    C. Bacterial Activity and Spoilage 67

VII. The Functional Properties of Fish Meat 67
    A. Interactions with Food Components 67
    B. The Hydration of Proteins 68
    C. The Interactions with Lipids 68

VIII. Changes in Sensory Properties 68
    A. Color 68
    B. Texture 69
    C. Odor and Flavor 69

IX. The Assessment of Freshness of Seafoods 69
    A. Sensory Assessment of Freshness 69

B. Objective Freshness Tests 70
     1. Indicators of Freshness and Spoilage 70
     2. Hypoxanthine 70
     3. The K-Value 70
     4. Trimethylamine 71
     5. Total Volatile Bases 71
     6. Diamines and Histamine 71
     7. Volatile Sulfur Compounds and Reducing Substances 72
     8. Rancidity 72
     9. Physical Methods 72

References 72

I. THE GENERAL COURSE OF EVENTS

The postharvest biochemical and microbial changes in fish tissues depend very sigificantly upon the factors which effect the concentration of substrates and metabolites in the tissues of the live fish, the activity of the endogenous enzymes, the microbial contamination, and the conditions after catching. Of great importance for the quality of fish as food are the circumstances of capture. They can either induce anaerobic metabolism and acidity in the muscles of the struggling fish, if the exercise is very strenuous, or else allow for excretion of the metabolic acid at longer capture times at low levels of activity. They also have a significant effect on the initial bacterial contamination of the catch and on the conditions controlling the rate of growth of the microflora. The biochemical post-mortem changes, involving the main chemical constituents of the tissues, bring about various structural alterations in the tissues, including rigor mortis, and different degrees of disintegration of the muscle ultrastructure. In well-rested, rapidly killed, and refrigerated fish, all stages of changes presented in Table 1 can be distinguished, while in an exhausted specimen from warm waters on deck the rigor mortis phenomenon may not be marked and bacterial spoilage may take over within hours. The degradation of the different constituents of the skin and muscles leads to gradual development of staleness and spoilage of fish and shellfish. The temperature of holding is of supreme importance.

II. DEGRADATION OF ORGANIC PHOSPHATES AND CARBOHYDRATES

A. THE EFFECT OF CATCHING

The contents of organic phosphates and carbohydrates in the flesh of freshly caught fish are affected mainly by the conditions prevailing before and during capture of the animal. Fatigue of the fish due to vigorous struggling manifests itself, on the molecular level, by exhaustion of the resources of high energy phosphates, i.e., ATP and creatine phosphate, as well as of glycogen (Figure 1). Thus, a fish in poor condition, tired on the hook or in the fishing net, contains less organic phosphates and glycogen than the muscles of well-fed fish killed instantaneously. In anoxic conditions in the flesh, the organic phosphates and carbohydrates continue to be metabolized under the action of the tissue enzymes and, subsequently, degraded by bacteria.

B. DEGRADATION OF ORGANIC PHOSPHATES

The main route of ATP degradation in fish muscles post-mortem involve gradual and stepwise dephosphorylation to AMP and deamination to inosine monophosphate (IMP),

TABLE 1
Sequence of Changes in the Main Components of the Muscles of Caught Fish

Stage after catch	Changes in main components		
Struggle in the fishing gear and on board	Ante-mortem exhaustion of reserves		
Asphyxia	Gradual formation of anoxial condition in the muscles		
	Organic phosphates and glycogen	**Nitrogenous compounds**	**Lipids**
Early enzymatic processes	Dephosphorylation formation of glucose, sugar phosphates, and lactic acid; decrease in pH	Changes in blood proteins; decomposition of urea	Hydrolysis and initiation of oxidation
Rigor mortis		Interaction of the contractile system, release of hydrolases, decrease in hydration	
Loss of freshness	Further enzymatic breakdown; utilization of the degradation products by microflora	Early stages of autolysis; decomposition of TMAO; formation of volatile bases; increase in pH	Hydrolysis and oxidation; effect of microbes
Rapid bacterial growth	Utilization by microflora	Bacterial decomposition; increase in hydration; formation of volatile compounds	Inhibition of oxidation by some metabolites
Bacterial spoilage	Accumulation of volatile odorous products, formation of discolored slime, increase in plasticity of the muscles		

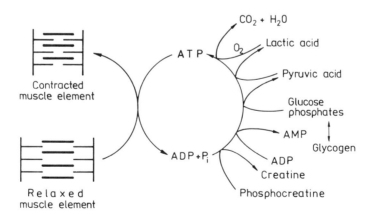

FIGURE 1. Organic phosphates and glycogen as energy sources for muscle contraction.

although deamination of ATP and adenosine (Ado) has also been established.[1] The AMP-Ado route is common in shellfishes.[2]

The first steps of the degradation of ATP in the meat of fish and marine invertebrata (Figure 2) are catalyzed by endogenous tissue enzymes and proceed rapidly. In refrigerated fish, the hydrolysis of ATP to IMP is nearly complete in the first 2 d after catch (Figure

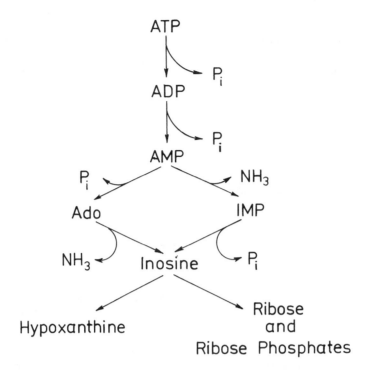

FIGURE 2. A simplified summary of nucleotide degradation.

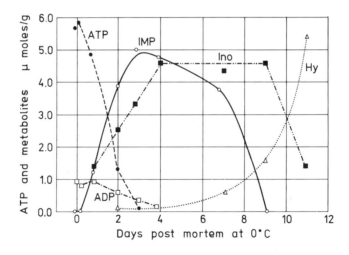

FIGURE 3. Nucleotide degradation in the flesh of well-rested cod. (From Fraser, D. J., Dingle, J. R., Hines, J. A., Nowlan, S. C., and Dyer, W. J., *J. Fish. Res. Board Can.*, 24, 1837, 1967. With permission.)

3). Further stages are less rapid, although in the breakdown of inosine (Ino) besides tissue enzymes bacteria are also involved. The gradual disappearance of IMP is to a large extent responsible for the loss of the typical, desirable flavor of fresh fish. The rate and pattern of post-mortem metabolism of the adenine nucleotides in marine fish and invertebrata differ between the species and muscles.

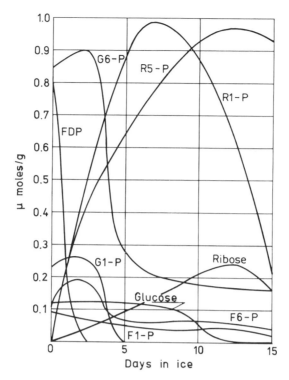

FIGURE 4. Sugars and sugar phosphates in the muscles of cod during ice storage. Glucose × 10^{-1}, ribose and ribose phosphates × 10^3. (From Jones, N. R., *Proc. 2nd Int. Congr. Food Science and Technology*, Tilgner, D. J. and Borys, A., Eds., Wydawnictwo Przemyslu Lekkiego i Spozywczego, Warsaw, 1967, 109. With permission.)

C. CHANGES IN CARBOHYDRATES

The post-mortem degradation of glycogen in fish muscles proceeds by the Embden-Meyerhof-Parnas pathway and by the amylolytic route, catalyzed by endogenous enzymes.[3-6]

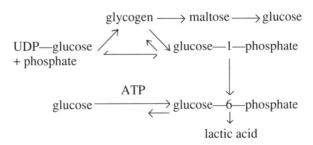

The changes in the concentration of sugars and sugar phosphates in the muscles (Figure 4) contribute to the gradual loss of the sweet, meaty character of the flavor of very fresh fish.

D. CHANGE IN pH OF THE FLESH

Lactic acid generated in anoxic conditions from glycogen is the principal factor in lowering the post-mortem pH in the fish muscles. The change in acidity depends also on the liberation of inorganic phosphate and ammonia due to the enzymatic degradation of ATP, and on the inherent buffering capacity of the muscles. A decrease in pH by 1 unit

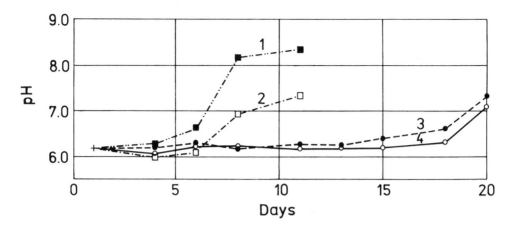

FIGURE 5. The pH of dogfish muscle stored in ice at different temperatures. 1, not gutted, 10°C; 2, not gutted, 5°C; 3, not gutted, iced; and 4, gutted, iced. (From Biliński, E., Jonas, R. E. E., and Peters, M. D., *J. Food Sci.*, 48, 808, 1983. With permission.)

can be caused by the accumulation of about 60 and 120 μg lactic acid per 1 g of fish and rock lobster muscle, respectively.[7] Generally, the ultimate pH in commercially caught cold-water fish is not lower than 6.2; as in most cases, the glycogen reserves are not high enough to cause extensive accumulation of lactic acid. In cod, although for most of the year the average ultimate post-mortem pH is above about 6.7, a short seasonal drop to about 6.3 during the heavy feeding period immediately after starvation was observed by Love.[8] Very low levels of pH, reaching 5.4, were found in tuna and halibut. In large tuna, caught by methods allowing for hauling the fish on board within minutes after hooking, the strenuous struggling in conditions impairing oxygen supply may induce acidosis in the muscles. As it is difficult to chill such large fish very rapidly, symptoms of burned tuna may develop. In anaerobic conditions, at low pH and temperatures above 26°C, the myoglobin may be oxidized to metmyoglobin, and protein denaturation may occur. The burned tuna meat appears pale muddy brown or turbid. It is soft and has a sour taste and a stringent aftertaste. These undesirable changes make such tuna unsuitable for being eaten raw as sashimi.[9]

During the later stages of post-mortem changes, the decomposition of nitrogenous compounds leads to an increase in pH in the fish flesh. The rate of pH change depends on temperature (Figure 5). In the muscles of scampi *Nephrops norvegicus* stored in ice, the pH increased from the initial value of 6.3 just after killing to 7.9 after 13 d.[11]

III. RIGOR MORTIS

A. STIFFENING

The catabolic processes taking place in a dead animal body lead to stiffening of the muscles known as rigor mortis. The flesh, which just after death is pliable, limp, and elastic under light stress, turns stiff, hard, and inextensible, causing the body of the fish in rigor often to have a bent form. The stiffness of a fish in rigor is a sure sign of freshness. However, it may have an adverse effect on the suitability of the fish for mechanical or even hand filleting. After several hours, the rigid fish gradually softens and becomes pliable again, although the extension of the muscles under stress is not reversible and the muscle has no ability to respond to electrical stimuli. The biochemical state of the postrigor muscles is different from that of the prerigor flesh. The postrigor fish does not display the signs of prime freshness.

B. THE BIOPHYSICAL MECHANISM

Rigor mortis as a biophysical phenomenon has been studied for many decades. As it has a significant impact on the quality of red meats, many contributions to the knowledge of its nature and consequences have been made by meat researchers. The actual view of the biomechanical events taking place in rigor mortis is based on the sliding theory of muscle contraction of Huxley and Hanson.[12] Accordingly, the sarcomeres contract as a result of axial displacement of the myosin microfibrils relative to the actin filaments, leading to formation of cross-bridges between the filaments. Although, in an alternative proposal by Obendorf,[13] the displacement is due to a screw motion of the myosin filament, the biochemical reactions, nevertheless, led also to the formation of cross-bridges. When rigor develops, a number of the muscle fibers contract, while in the rest of the fibers the formation of cross-bridges between the filaments is not accompanied by contraction.

According to the present understanding rigor mortis is caused by bonding of the myosin heads, extending radially from the thick microfibrils, to the active centers in actin units of the thin filaments. This leads to the formation of a rather rigid structure of interconnected myofilaments. This reaction between these major muscle proteins is made possible by changes in the regulatory proteins. These changes are in turn induced by an increase in the concentration of Ca^{2+} in the sarcoplasm. In a resting muscle, the concentration of free Ca^{2+} in the sarcoplasm is lower than $10^{-7} M$ because the action of various calcium pumps, located in the cell membrane and in the sarcoplasmic reticulum, drives the Ca^{2+} out of the sarcoplasm, against the concentration gradient. The calcium pumps work at the expense of energy from ATP hydrolysis. After the death of the animal, a gradual depletion of ATP in the muscles takes place, due to exhaustion of the creatine phosphate and glycogen reserves. This impairs the action of the calcium pumps and increases the concentration of Ca^{2+} in the sarcoplasm. At ATP concentrations below $10^{-4} M$ and that of Ca^{2+} above $10^{-6} M$, rigor mortis sets in. As the individual muscle fibers contain different quantities of ATP, they do not enter rigor at the same time post-mortem. Thus, stiffness in a muscle sets in gradually. In some fibers, which still have sufficient reserves of ATP, several cycles of cross-bridging, contraction, and detachment are possible before, at low ATP concentration, persistent bonds between the myosin heads and actin are formed.

Resolution of rigor mortis commences after a certain time due to the action of different endogenous proteinases, attacking various structural muscle proteins. The intensity of these degradative changes increases with the time of aging of the muscle.

C. THE GENERAL COURSE OF RIGOR IN FISH FLESH

Generally stiffness in fish begins in the head region and spreads gradually towards the caudal muscles. However, a reverse sequence has also been observed. In fish of some species, the whole body stiffens gradually at the same time.

The intensity of rigor mortis, changing in time, can be assayed by measuring the hardness of the muscles, the development of tension and shortening, and the extension of the muscles under load, using various rigorometers. The extent of shortening of the muscle depends on the state of the tissues and the environmental conditions. In mackerel, scad, and hake, shrinkage in length of the fillets, excised just after hauling on board, is 6 to 17%, depending on the duration of the trawling and the load of the fish in the net.[14] In some deep-water species, about 40% shortening of the fillets was observed.[15] However, in rock lobster or prawn, physical examination is often ineffective in following rigor, as no apparent stiffening of the body is detectable. Experiments with isolated sections of rock lobster muscles have shown that a slight shortening during rigor has usually been immediately followed by lengthening.[16]

The time after which the onset of rigor is noticeable, the degree of change in the rheological properties of the fish body, and the duration of the stiff condition depend upon

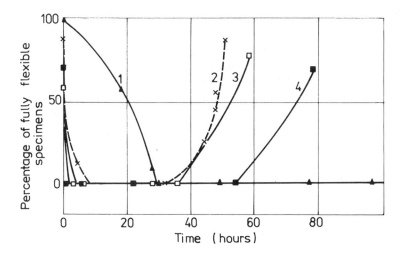

FIGURE 6. The evolution of rigor in fish of different species. Fish obtained by bottom trawling, 30 min, boxed in ice, and stored around 0°C. 1, grenadier; 2, hake; 3, sea bream; and 4, anchovy. (From Trucco, R. E., Lupin, H. M., Giannini, D. H., Crupkin, M., Boeri, R. L., and Barassi, C. A., *Lebensm. Wiss. Technol.*, 15, 77, 1987. With permission.)

factors influencing the biochemical state of the muscles at the time of death and on the rate of post-mortem processes. In cold-water species, all factors decreasing the rate of depletion of the energy reserves in the fish muscles extend the time between death and the onset of rigor and increase the duration of the stiff condition. Thus, in well-nourished, not exhausted, large, refrigerated fish, rigor develops later, is more intensive, and lasts longer than in small fish of poor physical condition kept at ambient temperature. Destruction of the brain of fish, which have not been subject to prolonged struggle, delays significantly the onset of rigor. In rapidly caught kahawai *Arripis trutta* immediately chilled in ice-seawater, spiking in the brain delayed rigor by about one third.[17] Slaughtering of large fish soon after catch favors an intensive and long lasting rigor state. There is a distinct influence of species and temperature on the time course of rigor (Figure 6). On a vessel fishing in warm regions, a part of the catch after some 4 h of trawling may already be in rigor, while a slightly stiff condition, even in rapidly chilled fish, may last not longer than at best a few hours.[19] In some tropical fish, a rigor mortis-like stiffening can occur within minutes when the fish are iced. The experiments of Curran et al.[20] have shown that at 0°C, tilapia, a tropical freshwater fish, stiffened in a few minutes and were fully rigid within 8 h, although the rate of ATP degradation was similar to that at 22°C. This cold-shock stiffening was not accompanied by muscle contraction.

D. THE EFFECT OF RIGOR ON FISH QUALITY

The quality of fish, regardless of the species characteristics, is effected both by the freshness and the appearance of the fillet. As long as the fish is in the prerigor or rigor state, its freshness is impeccable. The biochemical and biophysical processes involved in rigor may, however, influence the appearance of the fillet and the amount of fluid lost due to freezing/thawing and cooking.

Under the contraction associated with rigor mortis, some myosepta, connecting the myotomes of the muscles, break, yielding to the tension, and the flakes come apart. The gaping is severe if the tension is strong and the connective tissue is weakened, especially when rigor mortis sets in at high ambient temperature.[21] For cod, the critical temperature above which gaping increases sharply is 17°C.[22] The extent of gaping is higher in well-nourished and not exhausted fish than in spent specimens. Rough handling of fish in rigor increases the incidence of gaping. Fillets cut from well-nourished fish just after catch shrink at high ambient temperature due to rigor mortis by as much as 30 to 40% of the initial length. Their cut surface is rough and corrugated.

Fish entering rigor at high ambient temperatures loose much drip on thawing and may be tough and stringy after cooking.[23]

IV. CHANGES IN NITROGENOUS COMPOUNDS

A. CAUSES AND EFFECTS

The post-mortem metabolism of nitrogenous compounds in fish flesh is mainly responsible for the gradual loss of the fresh appearance of the catch and for the development of the signs of putrefaction. This is due to decomposition of some nonprotein components which contribute to the desirable flavor of seafoods, formation of volatile odorous compounds, and partial degradation and changes of proteins causing undesirable rheological properties and color of the muscles. During the first days of storage in ice, endogenous enzymes are mainly involved and the process is called autolysis. Later, bacterial metabolism predominates and leads to final spoilage. Many of the decomposition reactions can be catalyzed both by the endogenous and bacterial enzymes. Thus, it is not possible to distinguish precisely between autolytic and bacterial changes.

B. DEGRADATION OF NONPROTEIN COMPOUNDS

Among the changes leading to the formation of volatile odorous compounds, the bacterial reduction of TMAO to TMA:

$$NADH + H^+ + (CH_3)_3NO \rightarrow NAD^+ + (CH_3)_3N + H_2O$$

and the endogenous enzymatic breakdown of TMAO to DMA and formaldehyde:

$$(CH_3)_3NO \rightarrow (CH_3)_2NH + HCHO$$

have been most extensively investigated. Both reactions contribute to the gradual increase in total volatile bases in fish muscles post-mortem, although the production of DMA and formaldehyde in iced fish takes place mainly in anaerobic conditions.[24]

In the muscles of sharks and rays, even in fresh fish, ammonia may accumulate due to the activity of endogenous urease:

$$(NH_2)_2CO + H_2O \rightarrow 2NH_3 + CO_2$$

Large amounts of ammonia are also generated in fish muscles upon deamination of AMP.

Many odorous compounds are formed by degradation of the components of the free amino acid pool and from amino acids liberated by enzymatic and bacterial proteolysis or other reactions. In the abdominal muscles of rock lobster, about 27% of the total free amino acids, on a molecular basis, is made up of arginine, which is also rapidly generated by enzymatic dephosphorylation of phosphoarginine.[7,16] This amino acid is then broken down by bacteria into ornithine and ammonia. The products of amino acid metabolism, i.e., amines, aldehydes, sulfides, mercaptans, and short-chain fatty acids, have distinct, undesirable, putrid odors. Some decarboxylation products, formed mainly due to the action of bacteria, may induce health risks, such as the nonvolatile biogenic amines:

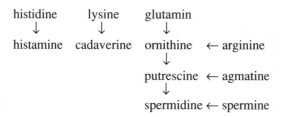

In fishery products, the most important of these amines is histamine. The histidine decarboxylase of fish flesh exhibits a relatively low activity. Under aseptic conditions, only negligible amounts of histamine are formed in the muscles of white fish, while in mackerel, bonito, and sardine 10 to 15 mg histamine in 100 g accumulate even under optimum conditions of temperature and pH. On the other hand, many strains of bacteria are known histamine producers.

Tyrosine liberated during proteolysis in shrimp and lobster muscle undergoes oxidation to dihydroxyphenyl alanine and leads further to the formation of melanin pigments.

C. CHANGES IN PROTEINS

Post-mortem protein degradation in fish muscles, catalyzed by tissue proteinases described in Chapter 3, as well by bacterial proteinases, leads to slow changes in the rheological properties of refrigerated fish. This is due to partial fragmentation of the molecules and loosening of the structure. Changes in the muscle structure and proteins occurring post-mortem have been investigated particularly in beef with respect to aging of meat. So far it has been found that aging increases the quantity of actinin soluble in salt solutions, brings about some disintegration of the myofibrillar structure within the Z-linc and loss of lateral adhesion between adjacent myofibrils, and promotes mechanical fragmentation of the myofibrils.

The susceptibility of the myofibrils to fragmentation caused by standard homogenization is a characteristic of various fish species. It is higher in fish which rapidly loose their freshness than in species known for their long shelf life.[25] With the time of storage in ice, the resistance of the myofibrils to fragmentation decreases, the species specificity being retained.

The autolytic changes in small uneviscerated fish are caused not only by the endogenous muscle enzymes but also by kidney and liver cathepsins, as well as by the digestive enzymes of the alimentary tract. The effect depends on the activity of the enzymes, pH in the muscles, properties of the connective tissues, and the presence of proteinase inhibitors.[26] Advanced proteolytic breakdown mainly caused by enzymes released from the digestive tract may lead to belly burst in small, heavily feeding fish such as herring, sprat, and capelin. The role of proteolytic bacteria in the degradation of the muscle proteins early after catch is negligible, as they constitute in fresh cod only about 10% of the total aerobic bacterial population on the skin, while the flesh is sterile, except for injured places.[27]

Post-mortem protein changes in tuna involve also oxidation of the desirable red myoglobin and oxymyoglobin of the red muscles to brown metmyoglobin. The rate of oxidation depends on the species of the fish and on the storage temperature.[28]

V. DEGRADATION OF LIPIDS

A. LIPOLYSIS

Post-mortem lipid degradation proceeds mainly due to enzymatic hydrolysis. Under the conditions of chill storage, the oxidation of lipids is of minor importance. About 20% of lipids is hydrolyzed during the shelf life of iced fish. The amount of free fatty acids is more or less doubled during that period. Phospholipids are hydrolyzed most readily, followed by triacylglycerols, cholesterol esters, and wax esters. Phosphatidylcholine is most rapidly degraded, more than half of its amount in cold-stored cod and krill being hydrolyzed after about 20 d and 72 h, respectively.[29,30] Changes in fatty acids, including n-3 polyunsaturated fatty acids (PUFAs) during refrigerated storage of fish and krill, are insignificant, the maximum losses amounting to about 10%. The hydrolytic changes in lipids in iced fish are accelerated after a few days. No release of lipase from lysosomes occurs during 7 d in rainbow trout held in ice.[31] On the other hand, phospholipase A_2 release may be triggered by enzymatic and nonenzymatic peroxidation.[32] During the later stages of storage, significant activity of bacterial lipases as well as of digestive enzymes can be expected.

B. OXIDATION OF LIPIDS

Lipid oxidation in wet fish concerns basically fatty species. These fish contain more free lipids and more dark muscles in which oxidation proceeds several times faster than in white muscles.[33] Particularly susceptible to oxidation, because of a closer contact with lipoxygenase present in the skin and with atmospheric air, are the lipids of the subcutaneous layer and of the skin.

It is thought that lipid oxidation does not occur if bacerial spoilage takes place. Autoxidation may also be retarded by the products of phospholipid hydrolysis and by a number of nonprotein nitrogenous compounds.

Furthermore, in the presence of bacterial spoilage, rancidity is imperceptible. To give but one example: a sensory panel is not able to detect any rancid taste or odor in iced Baltic herring, even when the oxidation level is as high as that which disqualifies frozen herring because of rancidity.

The oxidation of the tissue lipids has a very large effect on the quality of frozen stored fish (see Chapter 7).

VI. MICROBIAL CONTAMINATION AND SPOILAGE

A. THE MICROFLORA OF FRESH SEAFOODS
1. The Total Count

In fish from clean waters, just after catch, the microbial contamination is generally comparable in magnitude to that in dressed carcasses of beef, pigs, and poultry. It depends mainly on the pollution and temperature of the environment, on the method of catching, and on the conditions of handling on board vessel. The water in the open sea contains very small numbers of bacteria, i.e., a few colony-forming units (cfu) per 1 cm^3, while the coastal regions and the sediments there may be heavily polluted, up to about 10^6 cfu per cubic centimeter. For a recent review, see Reference 34.

Fish captured individually in clean, cold, surface waters contain on the skin from one to ten bacteria per 1 $cm.^2$ On the other hand, the total surface count on fish from commercial bottom catches may reach numbers as high as $10^5/cm^2$. The number of bacteria present on the surface of crustaceans is similar to that on fish. The bacterial load of the gills is usually one or two orders higher and that of the intestines is 10 to 10^9, depending on the feeding status of the fish.

Zaleski and Lojkiewicz[35] reported the stomach and middle-intestine of the Baltic cod, caught during the spawning season, to be free of bacteria, while the total plate count of the contents of the back intestine and esophagus of the same fish was 10^3 to $10^4/g$. Whole Antarctic krill frozen immediately after catch may contain from 10 to 10^4 cfu per gram, while the contents of the krill alimentary tract range from 10^2 to 10^7 cfu per gram.[36] The microbial population of bivalve mollusks decreases during depuration i.e., holding in tanks with clean, flowing sea water. The muscle tissue of fresh healthy fish is sterile.[37]

2. The Spoilage Microflora

The skin microflora of fresh fish taken from cold waters is composed predominantly of Gram-negative bacteria, mainly *Psychrobacter, Acinetobacter, Alteromonas, Psudomonas, Flavobacterium,* and *Vibrio*.[34] In freshly frozen krill, the bacterial population comprises *Alcaligenes, Micrococcus, Flavobacterium, Arthrobacter,* and *Moraxella*-like species.[36] The microflora of fish from warm waters is dominated by Gram-positive forms, especially micrococci, coryneforms, and bacilli. The surface bacteria of cold-water fish are mainly psychrotrophic, while warm-water fish carry on their skin and gills more mesophilic species. According to Kochanowski and Maciejowska,[38] among the organisms isolated from fish taken in subtropical and tropical African waters, only 15% were able to grow at 0°C and 17% of the species were inactivated. Among the surface microflora of fish and shellfish, several genera of yeasts may also be present, mainly *Rhodotorula, Torulopsis,* and *Candida*. Molds are rarely associated with fresh healthy marine animals.

The fish alimentary tract contains generally *Vibrio,* organisms identified formerly as *Achromobacter, Pseudomonas, Xanthomonas,* and Gram-positive microflora, mainly *Clostridium* and other spore-forming bacteria.[34,37,39]

3. Pathogenic Organisms

Much attention has been paid to the occurrence of microorganisms of public health significance on marine foods. Although marine fish and crustaceans from unpolluted areas are generally free of salmonellae and staphylococci just after catching, they may become contaminated with pathogenic bacteria during subsequent handling and processing.

The catch from coastal waters may carry pathogens of marine origin, among them several species of *Vibrio,* mainly *V. parahaemolyticus* and to a minor extent 01 *V. cholerae,* non-01 *V. cholerae, V. vulnificus,* and *V. mimicus*. Some of these organisms are widely distributed in bays and estuaries.[40] Their occurrence is known to undergo seasonal fluctuations. Although many strains of *V. parahaemolyticus* have been isolated from warm coastal waters worldwide, only less than 1% of these strains have been found to be virulent. *Aeromonas hydrophila* has been frequently found in many estuaries, as well as in fish and shellfish. Its potential role as a causative agent in seafood-associated gastroenteritis must be considered, especially as *Aeromonas* are facultative anaerobes and psychrotrophic organisms.[41] *C. botulinum* type E is widespread, albeit in low numbers, in marine sediments in temperate zones. It is not normally present in large numbers in freshly caught fish and shellfish, though its incidence can occasionally be high. Growth of this organism, and toxin production in fish is almost always due to faulty handling and processing.[34]

Food poisoning caused by pathogenic bacteria of marine origin is usually associated with eating raw oysters, uncooked, smoked, fermented, and salted fishery products, or recontaminated cooked seafoods.[42] Raw and undercooked shellfish have also been implicated in virus-associated cases of gastroenteritis.[43]

B. THE GROWTH OF BACTERIA ON SEAFOODS

Handling and storage of the catch on ice brings about a change in the number, distribution, and composition of the microflora of seafoods. The growth of bacteria on fish can be generally represented by a typical pattern. The initial lag period lasts usually until the resolution of rigor mortis, although no increase in the total surface bacteria has been reported on snapper *Chrosophrys auratus* during 10 d of chilling on ice or in air, regardless of a noticeable decrease in the freshness of the fish.[44] During the early days on ice, the population is concentrated on the surface. Slow penetration into the muscle tissue occurs mainly in places where skin cuts and abrasions facilitate the migration. The rate of penetration into the muscles depends also on the barrier properties of the skin. These may differ as much as, for example, in sprat and redfish. In whole, uneviscerated fish, the muscles are also invaded, in the stage of autolysis, by bacteria of the alimentary canal. The exposed muscle layers of fillets are especially vulnerable to bacterial penetration.

The increase in the size of the population results to a large extent from a very rapid growth of *Alteromonas* and *Pseudomonas*, as they are well adapted to refrigeration conditions and effectively utilize the extractives of fish flesh.[37] As a consequence, during the later period of storage on ice, about 90% of the population may be made up to *Alteromonas* and *Pseudomonas*. The other principle groups are *Moraxella, Psychrobacter, Acinetobacter,* and *Flavobacterium*.

C. BACTERIAL ACTIVITY AND SPOILAGE

The metabolic processes of the microflora contribute partly to the gradual loss of taste substances from the iced fish and lead ultimately to spoilage due to partial proteolysis and accumulation of unpleasant metabolites.

The involvement of bacteria in the degradation of many components of fish flesh has been indicated in earlier sections of this chapter. Many bacteria are capable of producing trimethylamine (TMA), responsible mainly for the fishy odor, as they have the ability of using trimethylamine oxide (TMAO) as a terminal electron acceptor. The TMAO-reducing capacity was found in most species of Enterobacteriacae, in *V. parahaemolyticus,* and in certain species of *Pseudomonas, Shewanella, Alteromonas,* and *Campylobacter*. The N-oxide reductase of *Escherichia coli* can be inhibited by tetrasodium ethylenediaminetetra-acetate, benzoic acid, and methylparaben. Sorbic acid, which has been proposed as an antimicrobial agent for iced fish, decreases the production of TMA by suppressing the growth of bacteria.[45]

The objectionable putrid odors developing in spoiling cod and haddock held under refrigeration are generated by *P. fragi, P. putida,* and possibly *Shewanella putrefaciens*. According to investigators from Torry Research Station, only about 10 to 20% of the total fish microflora is responsible for these spoilage phenomena.[46] In shrimp, *Pandalus jordani,* held at different temperatures, the accumulation of large amounts of idole was associated with high numbers of *Proteus* in the bacterial population.[47]

A very important bacterial metabolite in some fish, mainly scombroid and mahimahi, is histamine. About 1% of the total microbial population typical for fresh fish has the ability to decarboxylate histidine. These are especially *P. morgani* and *Enterobacter aerogenes,* but at least 13 other species of histamine-producing bacteria have been isolated from marine fish.[48] The optimum temperature for histamine accumulation in fishery products depends upon the histamine-forming bacterial species and the properties of the fish, but is generally in the range 20 to 45°C. At refrigeration temperatures, the formation of histamine is usually negligible, as long as the sensory quality of the fish is acceptable. However, Okuzumi et al.[49] found a halophilic Gram-negative strain of coccobacilli capable of producing, at 5°C, large quantities of histamine, up to 4 mg/cm^3 of the medium.

Bacterial spoilage is mainly a surface phenomenon. In the early days of storage, not the bacteria but the products of their metabolism penetrate into the deeper layers of the flesh. During advanced stages of spoilage, the proportion of proteolytic bacteria to the total aerobic count in the muscles of cod may be about 30%; thus, bacteria may play a significant part in protein hydrolysis in evidently spoiling fish.[27]

VII. THE FUNCTIONAL PROPERTIES OF FISH MEAT

A. INTERACTIONS WITH FOOD COMPONENTS

The total quality of fish as food depends on the nutritive value of the meat, its sensory attributes, and the technological value or functional properties, i.e., on the ability to contribute to the desirable sensory characteristics of food products by interactions with water and other food components. In fish flesh, the technological value depends mainly on the proteins. The functional properties attributed to proteins of the fish flesh comprise hydration, which is reflected in solubility, dispersibility, water retention, swelling, and gel-forming ability, as well as interaction with lipids, i.e., emulsifying capacity and emulsion stability. These properties depend on the composition and conformation of proteins. They change during storage and processing of the fish.

B. THE HYDRATION OF PROTEINS

The solubility and dispersibility of the proteins contained in fresh fish flesh is characteristic for different proteinaceous components of the muscles and has been described in Chapter 3.

Changes in pH as well as denaturation and aggregation due to freezing storage and processing may cause an undesirable decrease in solubility and thus deterioration of other functional properties of the proteins.

The water-retaining properties of fish flesh can be measured in different ways, mainly as the loss of juice from a sample due to, for example, pressing or centrifugation, or as the water-binding capacity, i.e., the amount of water, bound by comminuted meat with added water, in the pellet after centrifugation.[50] These properties in muscle foods depend upon many factors, especially the characteristics of the proteins, the pH level, the concentration of post-mortem metabolites and added salts, as well as the changes in the proteins due to storage and processing. All aspects of the water-holding capacity of meat have been investigated and discussed by Hamm,[51,52] while water retention in fish flesh has been presented by Regenstein and Regenstein.[50]

The gel-forming ability of proteins is responsible for the characteristic texture of cooked fish and of the different jellied fish products. For many food proteins, it has been found to depend mainly on the surface hydrophobicity and the concentration of SH groups and disulfide bridges.[53] The gel-forming ability can be determined as the least concentration endpoint, at which the hydrated protein or meat slurry, after heating, forms in standardized conditions a gel firm enough not to flow out of a test tube, or by measuring the rheological properties, e.g., the yield limit of the gels.

C. THE INTERACTIONS WITH LIPIDS

The interaction of fish proteins with lipids is especially important in fish sausages, as high emulsifying capacity and emulsion stability is required in the sausage batters. These attributes as well as other functional properties have a special impact on the quality of fish protein concentrates and preparations which are intended to be used as structure forming components of different food products.[54,55] The emulsifying properties have optimum values at a specific balance between the hydrophilic and lipophilic response and are significantly related to the surface hydrophobicity and solubility of the proteins.[53]

VIII. CHANGES IN SENSORY PROPERTIES

A. COLOR

Changes in the surface coloration of fish and shellfish, as well as the altered color of the flesh, result mainly from enzymatic and nonenzymatic oxidation. The yellow, orange, and red color, or colorlessness, of fish and shellfish is caused by oxidation of carotenoids present in large amounts in the skin, shells, or exoskeletons. The dark-brown to black pigmentation of fish skin, induced by melanines, fades away, the skin becoming lusterless, and loses its iridescent appearance. Crustaceans become darker on storage, particularly the cephalothorax near the legs. Traumatism or molting may effect this deficiency more than the storage conditions.[56] The "black spots" in shrimps, lobster tails, and crabs, the bluing in crabs, darkening of krill, and quinone-tanning of muscles are caused by melanines of a similar nature. These compounds are formed from phenols, mainly from tyrosine, by oxidation, as well as by enzymatically initiated and metal-catalyzed polymerization.

The color of the white fish flesh changes from light creamy to gray. Due to chemical enzymatic oxidation of heme pigments, the dark red muscles become brown. On the other hand, the colorless meat of scampi turns pink. The flesh of fresh fish is translucent, but in stale fish it tends to be opaque. The slime on the skin, initially watery and clear, becomes cloudy, clotted, and discolored as a result of increased bacterial growth.

B. TEXTURE

The changes in texture of the fish involve loss of springiness and increase in softness, causing the spoiled fish to become smeary. Such a paste-like texture can be sometimes encountred in fresh fish, e.g., in muscles strongly infected with protozoans or in salmon undergoing spawning migration, due to increased activity of proteinases.[57]

In the initial stage of storage, the increase in softness results from the structural disintegration brought about by weakening of the connective tissue and fragmentation of myofibrils rather than by proteolytic changes in myofibrilar proteins.[58] These proteins are significantly effected by endogenous and bacterial proteinases only in the stage of advanced spoilage.

C. ODOR AND FLAVOR

Fresh fish exude a fresh seaweedy or shellfishy odor which, on storage, becomes less intense, neutral, and flat-sweet until off-odors appear, indicating intensive malodorous spoilage.

The smell of fresh fish is caused by carbonyl compounds and alcohols with six, eight, and nine carbon atoms: hexanal, 1-octan-3-ol, 1.5-octadien-3-ol, and 2.5-octadien-1-ol. The carbonyl compounds dominate, their thresholds being 10,000 times lower than those of the corresponding alcohols. The fresh odor gets weaker and changes from the sweetish melon-like aroma of 3.6-nonadien-1-ol to sweet and insipid. This is caused by the increase in alcohol fractions and the presence of short-chain esters.[59] In fat fish the carbonyl compounds dominate all the time. Later other odors appear, mainly musty, milky, bready, malty, beery, sour, acetic, and strong fishy, the last as a result of accumulations of volatile fatty acids from bacterial deamination of amino acids and accumulation of volatile amines.

The most unequivocal smell-related signs of spoilage are provided by offensive odors associated with the presence of $(CH_3)_2S$, CH_3SH, and H_2S formed from cysteine and methionine. These smells are perceived as musty, mouse-like, stale cabbage-like, and turnipy. Ultimately a clear hydrogen sulfide smell can be perceived. Putrid smells are caused by the presence of indol, putrescine, cadaverine, and other diamines from bacterial degradation of amino acids. Fat fish may exude greasy, oily, and rancid odors associated with the presence of carbonyl compounds from autoxidized PUFAs.

The sweetish flavor, typical of fresh fish and shellfish, weakens on storage, until the seafoods become insipid, flavorless, and finally bitter and rancid, beyond the limit of acceptability.

IX. THE ASSESSMENT OF FRESHNESS OF SEAFOODS

A. SENSORY ASSESSMENT OF FRESHNESS

Sensory freshness assessment involves determining the advancement of post-mortem changes in fish and shellfish by using the senses of smell, sight, and touch, with reference to a code containing minimum requirements and frequently also the criteria of quality grades. The most frequently used quality grades are the following: fresh, marketable, unfit; or extra, A, B, C. The grade limits do not fully coincide with freshness stages. The first grade usually covers very fresh fish and those with reduced freshness but without any signs of spoilage.

In the class of marketable fish are seafoods showing the first signs of spoilage. The rejection limit is not well defined, either. This results from the difficulties in assessment, particularly with regard to sensory discrimination between fresh and somewhat less fresh fish. To render the assessment more definite, most often five- or ten-point scales are used. They all stem from that of Shewan et al.[60] prepared for the assessment of gadoids. That scale allows one to evaluate some of the most important characters only, such as raw odor or flavor or by adding the partial assessment scores, to arrive at the final grade. It should take into consideration the relative importance of various characters. Shewan's scale allows for the maximum score of 10 for odor and flavor, 5 being the maximum for the remaining characters. In uniform scales, the total score is calculated by applying weighting coefficients. Another type of grading involves assessing defects and their intensity. Each quality class corresponds to a certain score or allowed amount of defects. However, a proper sensory analysis is as troublesome as are other laboratory assays. It calls for a team of several persons trained for many weeks.[61] On the other hand, a simple consumer assessment does not allow one to distinguish, after cooking or frying, between fish stored for 2 and 7 to 8 d. Thus, everyday quality control is carried out by one to three professionally experienced inspectors. Attempts are made to combine sensory assessment with objective microbiological, chemical, or physical tests.

B. OBJECTIVE FRESHNESS TESTS
1. Indicators of Freshness and Spoilage

It is required of a freshness test that it be fast, reliable, consistent with sensory assessment, and preferably applicable to all seafoods. This is very difficult to achieve in view of the variety of species and biochemical changes.

Microbiological freshness assays based on the determination of the total number of bacteria are of little use. Generally the composition of microflora is determined, e.g., the number of psychrotropic Gram-negative organisms, hydrogen sulfide producers, and indicator bacteria.

Chemical indices, indirectly related to bacterial activity, are often employed in assessing freshness. Out of numerous proposed indicators such as ammonia, TMA, total volatile bases (TVB), volatile acids, volatile reducing substances (VRSs), pH, buffering capacity, sulfides, nucleotide breakdown products, and others,[62] only a few proved useful. No single indicator, however, is sufficient to qualify a seafood as fresh. Most often at least two tests are used, one to determine the loss of freshness, if any, and the other to detect bacterial spoilage.

Hypoxanthine (Hx) and K-value are the most useful indicators of loss of freshness, in spite of the fact that their increase is due to enzymatic degradation as well as to bacterial activity. To evaluate bacterial spoilage, better tests are known. Statistical relationships between certain sensory and nonsensory freshness tests have been examined for cod and grading schemes based on freshness tests have been constructed.[63-67]

2. Hypoxanthine

The content of Hx increases linearly with the time of storage to about $5 \mu m/g$ wet weight and subsequently declines or remains at that level. A significant increase of Hx in squids and prawns occurs after bacterial spoilage has begun. The contents of Hx correlates well with sensory assessment, the flavor in particular. The following values are proposed as a limit of acceptability of fish and shellfish: 2 to 3 $\mu m/g$ for cod, 2 to 2.5 $\mu m/g$ for herring, 1 to 1.2 $\mu m/g$ for mackerel,[68] 2 $\mu m/g$ for shrimps,[69] and 2 to 4 $\mu m/g$ for squids.[70]

3. The K-Value

Many fish, e.g., two thirds of 98 species examined by Ehira and Uchiyama,[71] accumulate inosine instead of hypoxanthine. Thus, the K-value, i.e., percent ratio of inosine and Hx to the sum of ATP and all the products of ATP degradation, is a more useful indicator for them:

$$K\% = \frac{Hx + Ino}{ATP + ADP + AMP + IMP + Ino + Hx} \cdot 100$$

The initial value of K, immediately after capture, does not exceed 10% and at first increases gradually due to enzymatic degradation. Later, usually after an inflection point, it shows another rapid increase, caused by bacterial action.

The K-value of 20% is regarded as a freshness limit, 60% being the rejection point.[72] The following quality criteria are proposed for tuna:

- Class I — very good quality; up to 3.5%
- Class II — good quality; up to 18.7%
- Class III — rather good, restaurant quality; up to 52%

The rate of increase in K values allows one to identify the fish which have a longer shelf life. The differences in time of ice storage of different fish until the K-value reaches 20% may be as high as 10 d. This difference is presumably related to the species-dependent pH maximum of IMP-degrading enzymatic activities and depends on handling during capture.[73] The K-value increases more rapidly in cold-water fish and in squid than in fish. The increase is five times faster in dark than in white muscles.[74]

4. Trimethylamine

Changes in TMA content in fish with time of storage are correlated with the bacterial count and the sensory score, particularly with raw odor. The rejection limit is usually 5 to 10 mg TMA N per 100 g. Connell[62] has proposed 10 to 15 mg TMA N per 100 g as rejection limit for fish and Hebard et al.[75] proposed 5 mg TMA N per 100 g for shrimp. TMA is regarded as a good indicator for gadoids, although the results are variable even for these fish. On the other hand, in numerous fatty fish and shellfish the concentration of TMA N never reaches the limit of 5 mg/100 g, whereas in some other shellfish the value of 5 mg TMA N per 100 g may be exceeded long before spoilage.

5. Total Volatile Bases

The TVB include ammonia, TMA as well as small amounts of DMA, and methylamine. Ammonia is produced by bacterial as well as tissue enzymes. In shellfish, the increase in ammonia and TVB begins sooner than in fish. A significant increase of TVB both in fish and shellfish coincides with bacterial spoilage.

Most often, the TVB content of 30 mg N per 100 g is regarded as the fish acceptability limit. A slightly lower value of about 20 mg N per 100 g is proposed for fatty fish such as herring and mackerel,[68,76] 17 mg N per 100 g for oysters,[77] and as much as 45 mg N per 100 g for squids.[78]

6. Diamines and Histamine

The presence of significant quantities of diamines, mainly of putrescine and cadaverine, and of histamine, is sound proof of spoilage of fish and shellfish. Properly refrigerated fresh fish contain only trace amounts of these compounds. Their content increases with bacterial spoilage and after about 1 week at 5°C may reach 40 to 60 mg N per 100 g. Practically, however, such stale fish can be easily rejected by sensory assessment. On the other hand, due to the hazard of scombroid poisoning, the requirement of histamine determination in scombroids has been introduced in many countries, although histamine is present during the period of acceptability only in trace amounts. Generally the recommended limit for histamine in pelagic fish is less than 5 mg/100 g wet weight. Different countries accept various limits within a range 1 to 5 mg/100 g,[79] while Sweden will permit levels up to 20 mg/100 g in fish products.[80] The U.S. has established a hazard action level of 50 mg/100 g for histamine in tuna.[81] This is based on the experience acquired from the investigation of a number of poisoning episodes, but scombroid poisoning is believed to be a result of the synergistic action of histamine and other substances, possibly including diamines.

Indol is a useful spoilage indicator in shrimps. Its content should not exceed 25 µg/100 g. Refrigerated shrimp may get spoiled before this limit is exceeded.[82]

7. Volatile Sulfur Compounds and Reducing Substances

Volatile sulfur compounds, although important in sensory assessment, are seldom determined as freshness indices. Instead, particularly in the tropics, the bacteria capable of producing these compound are identified and determined.

The VRSs indicate bacterial spoilage. Their content is well correlated with sensory score, especially odor. The assay involves reducing $KMnO_4$ by the volatile compounds, usually stripped from a sample by air. The indicator, once popular, has been replaced by more modern techniques of determining the amount and composition of aromatic substances.

8. Rancidity

Hydroperoxide determination in refrigerated fish is of little use. Most often a test with 2-thiobarbituric acid is used. This test correlates well with sensory score, most probably because, as a highly nonspecific rancidity indicator, it combines lipid oxidation measurement and evaluation of bacterial spoilage of other tissue components.

9. Physical Methods

Among physical methods of freshness assessment, texture measurement is applied most often. Texture features can be determined simply by one parameter, e.g., the puncture force, or by measuring the rheological changes brought about by the applied force. The problems associated with instrumental measurements in freshness assessment are mainly related to the difficulty of finding the sensory equivalent to the measured physical parameters.

For rapid estimation of fish freshness, especially on board vessel and in the fish market, different electronic devices are available, e.g., the Torry fish freshness meter or the Intellectron fish tester. These gadgets are simple to operate and some of them can be applied even to fish in the box. Their readings can be given in freshness units or directly in days of remaining shelf life in ice.[83,84]

REFERENCES

1. **Tugai, V. A., Sakhnenko, I. V., Akulin, V. I., and Epstein, L. M.,** AMP-aminohydrolase activity and adenine nucleotide content in fish muscles, *Prikl. Biokhim. Mikrobiol.,* 19(4), 541, 1983 (in Russian).
2. **Jones, N. R.,** Observtions on the relations of flavour and texture to mononucleotide breakdown and glycolysis in fish muscle, in *Proc. 2nd Int. Congr. Food Science and Technology,* Tilgner, D. J. and Borys, A., Eds., Wydawnictwo Przemyslu Lekkiego i Spozywczego, Warsaw, 1967, 109.
3. **Fraser, D. J., Dingle, J. R., Hines, J. A., Nowlan, S. C., and Dyer, W. J.,** Nucleotide degradation, monitored by thin-layer chromatography, and associated post-mortem changes in relaxed cod muscle, *J. Fish. Res. Board Can.,* 24, 1837, 1967.
4. **Burt, J. R.,** Glycogenolytic enzymes of cod (*Gadus callarias*) muscle, *J. Fish. Res. Board Can.,* 23, 527, 1966.
5. **Burt, J. R. and Stroud, G. D.,** The metabolism of sugar phosphates in cod muscle, *Bull. Jpn. Soc. Sci. Fish.,* 32, 204, 1966.

6. **Tarr, H. L. A.**, Post-mortem changes in glycogen, nucleotides, sugar phosphates, and sugars in fish muscles — a review, *J. Food Sci.*, 31, 846, 1966.
7. **Sidhu, G. S., Montgomery, W. A., and Brown, M. A.**, Post mortem changes and spoilage in rock lobster muscle. I, *J. Food Technol.*, 9, 357, 1974.
8. **Love, R. M.**, The post-mortem pH of cod and haddock muscle and its seasonal variation, *J. Sci. Food Agric.*, 30, 433, 1979.
9. **Davie, P. S. and Sparksman, R. I.**, Burnt tuna: an ultrastructural study of postmortem changes in muscle of yellowfin tuna (*Thunnus albacores*) caught on rod and reel and southern bluefin tuna (*Thunnus maccoyii*) caught on handline or longline, *J. Food Sci.*, 51, 1122, 1986.
10. **Biliński, E., Jonas, R. E. E., and Peters, M. D.**, Factors controlling the deterioration of the spiny dogfish *Squalus acanthias* during iced storage, *J. Food Sci.*, 48, 808, 1983.
11. **Stroud, G. D., Early, J. C., and Smith, G. L.**, Chemical and sensory changes in iced *Nephrops norvegicus* as indices of spoilage, *J. Food Technol.*, 17, 541, 1982.
12. **Huxley, H. E. and Hanson, J.**, The molecular basis of contraction in cross-striated muscles, in *The Structure and Function of Muscle*, Vol. 1, Bourne, G. H., Ed., Academic Press, New York, 1960.
13. **Obendorf, P.**, A rotating myosin filament theory of muscular contraction, *J. Theor. Biol.*, 93, 667, 1981.
14. **Bykov, V. P. and Belogurov, A. J.**, Contraction of muscles as an objective test of the quality of trawled fish, in *Tekhnologiya Rybnykh Produktov*, Bykov, V. P., Ed., VNIRO, Moscow, 1984, 101, (in Russian).
15. **Golovkova, G. I.**, Postmortem changes in deep water species of fish at different temperatures, in *Tekhnologiya Rybnykh Produktov*, Bykov, V. P., Ed., VNIRO, Moscow, 1984, 14 (in Russian).
16. **Sidhu, G. S., Montgomery, W. A., and Brown, M. A.**, Post mortem changes and spoilage in rock lobster muscle. II, *J. Food Technol.*, 9, 371, 1974.
17. **Boyd, N. S., Wilson, N. D., Jerrett, A. R., and Hall, B. I.**, Effects of brain destruction on post harvest muscle metabolism in the fish kahawai (*Arripis trutta*), *J. Food Sci.*, 49, 177, 1984.
18. **Trucco, R. E., Lupin, H. M., Giannini, D. H., Crupkin, M., Boeri, R. L., and Barassi, C. A.**, Study on the evolution of *rigor mortis* in batches of fish, *Lebensm. Wiss. Technol.*, 15, 77, 1982.
19. **Kerzhnevskaya, M. M.**, The shelf life of fish in commercial conditions, *Rybn. Khoz.*, (8), 77, 1987, (in Russian).
20. **Curran, C. A., Poulter, R. G., Brueton, A., and Jones, N. S. D.**, Cold shock reactions in iced tropical fish, *J. Food Technol.*, 21, 289, 1986.
21. **Burt, J. R., Jones, N. R., McGill, A. S., and Stroud, G. D.**, Rigor tension and gaping in cod muscle, *J. Food Technol.*, 5, 339, 1970.
22. **Jones, N. R., Burt, J. R., Murray, J., and Stroud, G. D.**, Nucleotides and the analytical approach to the *rigor mortis* problem, in *The Technology of Fish Utilization*, Kreuzer, R., Ed., Fishing News Books, London, 1965, 14.
23. **Stroud, R. G.**, Rigor in Fish. The Effect on Quality, Torry Advisory Note No. 36, Edinburgh, 1969.
24. **Lundstrom, R. C., Correia, F. F., and Wilhelm, K. A.**, Dimethylamine production in fresh red hake (*Urophycis chuss*): the effect of packaging material, oxygen permeability and cellular damage, *J. Food Biochem.*, 6, 229, 1982.
25. **Tokiwa, T. and Matsumiya, H.**, Fragmentation of fish myofibril. Effect of storage conditions and muscle cathepsins, *Bull. Jpn. Soc. Sci. Fish.*, 35, 1099, 1968.
26. **Hjelmeland, K. and Raa, J.**, Fish tissue degradation by trypsin type enzymes, in *Advances in Fish Science and Technology*, Connell, J. J., Ed., Fishing News Books, Farnham, 1980, 456.
27. **Karnop, G.**, The role of proteolytic bacteria in fish spoilage. II. The presence and importance of proteolytic bacteria as spoilage indicators, *Arch. Lebensmittelhyg.*, 33, 61, 1982, (in German).
28. **Matthews, A. D.**, Muscle colour deterioration in iced and frozen stored bonito, yellowfin and skipjack tuna caught in Seychelles waters, *J. Food Technol.*, 18, 387, 1983.
29. **Oshima, T., Wada, S., and Koizumi, C.**, Enzymatic hydrolysis of phospholipids in cod flesh during storage in ice, *Bull. Jpn. Soc. Sci. Fish.*, 50, 107, 1984.
30. **Kołakowska, A.**, Changes in lipids during the storage of krill (*Euphausia superba* Dana) at 3°C, *Z. Lebensm. Unters. Forsch.*, 186, 519, 1988.
31. **Geromel, E. J. and Montgomery, M. W.**, Lipase release liposomes of rainbow trout (*Salmo gairdneri*) muscle subjected to low temperatures, *J. Food Sci.*, 45, 412, 1980.
32. **Han, T. and Liston, J.**, Lipid peroxidation and phospholipid hydrolysis in fish muscle microsomes and frozen fish, *J. Food Sci.*, 52, 294, 1987.
33. **Slabyj, B. M. and Hultin, H. O.**, Lipid peroxidation by microsomal fractions isolated from light and dark muscles of herring (*Clupea harengus*), *J. Food Sci.*, 47, 1395, 1982.
34. **Hobbs, G.**, Microbiology of fish, in *Essays in Agricultural and Food Microbiology*, Norris, J. R. and Pettifer, G. L., Eds., John Wiley & Sons, London, 1987.
35. **Zaleski, S. and Lojkiewicz, L.**, Studies on the quantitative composition of microflora in alimentary canals at the various fishes of Gdańsk Bay, *Acta Ichthyol. Piscatoria*, 1, 107, 1970.

36. **Turkiewicz, M., Galas, E., and Kalinowska, H.**, Microflora of Antarctic krill *(Euphausia superba), Acta Microbiol. Pol.,* 31, 175, 1982.
37. **Liston, J.**, Microbiology in fishery science, in *Advances in Fish Science and Technology,* Connell, J., Ed., Fishing News Books, Farnham, England, 1980, 138.
38. **Kochanowski, J. and Maciejowska, M.**, Bacterial flora of seafish from West African fishing ground. II. Strains isolated from fish on board immediately upon catching, *Pr. Morskiego Inst. Rybackiegow Gdyni,* 14, B, 153, 1967, (in Polish).
39. **Garcia-Tello, P. and Zaleski, S.**, Qualitative and quantitative changes in aerobic microflora from intestinal contents of South-Baltic cod during storage at 1—2°C, *J. Food Sci.,* 35, 482, 1970.
40. **DePaola, A.**, *Vibrio cholerae* in marine foods and environmental waters: a literature review, *J. Food Sci.,* 46, 66, 1981.
41. **Abeyta, C. and Wekell, M. M.**, Potential sources of *Aeromonas hydrophila, J. Food Safety,* 9, 11, 1988.
42. **Hackney, C. R. and Dicharry, A.**, Seafood-borne bacterial pathogens of marine origin, *Food Technol.,* 42(3), 104, 1988.
43. **Gerba, Ch. P.**, Viral disease transmission by seafoods, *Food Technol.,* 42(3), 99, 1988.
44. **Boyd, N. S. and Wilson, N. D. C.**, A bacteriological evaluation of snapper *(Chrysophrys auratus)* at the time of unloading off N.Z. fishing boats, *N.Z. J. Sci.,* 19, 205, 1976.
45. **Kruk, M. and Lee, J. S.**, Inhibition of *Escherichia coli* trimethylamine-*N*-oxide reductase by food preservatives, *J. Food Prot.,* 45, 241, 1982.
46. **Herbert, R. A., Hendrie, M. S., Gibson, D. M., and Shewan, J. M.**, Bacteria active in the spoilage of certain sea foods, *J. Appl. Bacteriol.,* 34(1), 41, 1971.
47. **Matches, J. R.**, Effects of temperature on the decomposition of Pacific coast shrimp *Pandalus jordani, J. Food Sci.,* 47, 1044, 1982.
48. Histamine-forming bacteria in tuna and other marine fish, in *Histamine in Marine Products: Production by Bacteria, Measurement and Prediction of Formation,* Pan, B. S. and James, D., Eds., FAO Fish. Technol. Paper (252), Food and Agriculture Organization, Rome, 2.
49. **Okuzumi, M., Okuda, S., and Awano, M.**, Isolation of psychrophilic and halophilic histamine-forming bacteria from *Scomber japonicus, Bull. Jpn. Soc. Sci. Fish.,* 47, 1591, 1981.
50. **Regenstein, J. M. and Regenstein, C. E.**, *Food Protein Chemistry,* Academic Press, London, 1984, chap. 27.
51. **Hamm, R.**, Biochemistry of meat hydration, in *Advances in Food Research,* Vol. 10, Chichester, C. O., Mrak, E. M., and Stewart, G. F., Eds., Academic Press, New York, 1960, 355.
52. **Hamm, R.**, Functional properties of the myofibrillar system and their measurements, in *Muscle as Food,* Bechtel, P. J., Ed., Academic Press, Orlando, FL, 1986, 135.
53. **Nakai, S.**, Structure-function relationships of food proteins with an emphasis on the importance on protein hydrophobicity, *J. Agric. Food Chem.,* 31, 676, 1983.
54. **Kinsella, J. E.**, Functional properties of proteins in foods: a survey, *Crit. Rev. Food Sci. Nutr.,* 8, 219, 1976.
55. **Sikorski, Z. E. and Naczk, M.**, Modification of technological properties of fish protein concentrates, *Crit. Rev. Food Sci. Nutr.,* 14, 201, 1981.
56. **Ogawa, M., Kurotsu, T., Ochiai, J., and Kozima, T.**, Mechanism of black discoloration in spring lobster tails stored in ice, *Bull. Jpn. Soc. Sci. Fish.,* 49, 1065, 1983.
57. **Kanagaya, S.**, Enhanced protease activity in the muscle of chum salmon during spawning migration with reference to softening or lysing phenomenon of the meat, *Bull. Tokai Reg. Fish. Res. Lab.,* 109, 41, 1983.
58. **Hatae, K., Tamari, S., Miyanaga, K., and Matsumoto, J. J.**, Species difference and changes in the physical properties of fish muscle as freshness decreases, *Bull. Jpn. Soc. Sci. Fish.,* 51, 1155, 1985.
59. **Josephson, D. B., Lindsay, R. C., and Olafsdottir, G.**, Measurement of volatile aroma constituents as a means for following sensory deterioration of fresh fish and fishery products, in *Seafood Quality Determination,* Kramer, D. E. and Liston, J., Eds., Elsevier, Amsterdam, 1986, 27.
60. **Shewan, J. M., Intosh, R. G., Tucker, C. G., and Ehrenberg, A. S. C.**, The development of a numerical scoring system for the sensory assessment of the spoilage of wet white fish stored in ice, *J. Sci. Food Agric.,* 4, 283, 1953.
61. **Hogg, M. G. and Scott, D. N.**, Selection and training of a taste panel for the evaluation of fish, *Fish Processing Bull. DSIR Auckland,* 1, 1984.
62. **Connell, J. J.**, *Control of Fish Quality,* Fishing News Books, Farnham, England, 1980.
63. **Burt, J. R., Gibson, D. M., Jason, A. C., and Sanders, H. R.**, Comparison of methods of assessment of wet fish. I. Sensory assessments of boxed experimental fish, *J. Food Technol.,* 10, 645, 1975.
64. **Burt, J. R., Gibson, D. M., Jason, A. C., and Sanders, H. R.**, Comparison of methods of assessment of wet fish. II. Instrumental and chemical assessments of boxed experimental fish, *J. Food Technol.,* 11, 73, 1976.
65. **Burt, J. R., Gibson, D. M., Jason, A. C., and Sanders, H. R.**, Comparison of methods of assessment of wet fish. III. Laboratory assessments of commercial fish, *J. Food Technol.,* 11, 117, 1976.

66. **Connell, J. J., Howgate, P. F., Mackie, I. M., Sanders, H. R., and Smith, G. L.**, Comparison of methods of assessment of wet fish. IV. Assessment of commercial fish at port markets, *J. Food Technol.*, 11, 297, 1976.
67. **Sanders, H. R. and Smith, G. L.**, The construction of grading schemes based on freshness assessment of fish, *J. Food Technol.*, 11, 365, 1976.
68. **Barile, L. E., Milla, A. D., Reilley, A., and Villadsen, A.**, Spoilage patterns of mackerel *Rastrelliger faughni Matsui, in Spoilage of Tropical Fish and Products Development,* FAO Fish. Rep. No. 317, Food and Agriculture Organization, Rome, 1985, 146.
69. **Fatima, R., Faroqui, B., and Qadri, R. B.**, Inosine monophosphate and hypoxanthine as indices of quality of shrimp *(Panaeus merquierisis)*, *J. Food Sci.*, 46, 1125, 1981.
70. **Licciardello, J. J., Ravesi, E. M., Gerow, S. M., and D'Entremont, D.**, Storage Characteristics of Iced Whole Loligo Squid, in Proc. Meet. Storage Lives of Chilled and Frozen Fish and Fish Products, Aberdeen, October 1 to 3, 1985, 197.
71. **Ehira, S. and Uchiyama, H.**, Formation of inosine and hypoxanthine in fish muscle during ice storage, *Bull. Tokai Reg. Fish. Res. Lab.*, 75, 63, 1973.
72. **Ehira, S. A.**, Biochemical study on the freshness of fish, *Bull. Tokai Reg. Fish. Res. Lab.*, 88, 1, 1976.
73. **Tamioka, K. and Endo, K.**, K-value increasing and IMP-degrading activities in various fish muscles, *Bull. Jpn. Soc. Sci. Fish.*, 50, 889, 1984.
74. **Obtake, A., Doi, T., and Ono, T.**, Post mortem degradation of inosinic acid and related enzyme activity in the dark muscle of fish, *Bull. Jpn. Soc. Sci. Fish.*, 54, 283, 1988.
75. **Hebard, C. E., Flick, G. J., and Martin, R. E.**, Occurrence and significance of trimethylamine oxide and its derivatives in fish and shellfish, in *Chemistry and Biochemistry of Marine Food Products,* Martin, R. E., Flick, G. J., Hebard, C. E., and Ward, D. R., Eds., AVI Publishing, Westport, CT, 1982, 149.
76. **Kolakowski, E., Kolakowska, A., and Rózalski, S.**, The Objective Assessment of Freshness of Fish, Report Academy of Agriculture, Szczecin, 1972, 2, (in Polish).
77. **Murata, M. and Sakaguchi, M.**, Changes in contents of free amino acids, trimethylamine and nonprotein nitrogen of oyster during ice storage, *Bull. Jpn. Soc. Sci. Fish.*, 52, 1975, 1986.
78. **Woyewoda, A. D. and Ke, P. J.**, Laboratory Quality Assessment of Canadian Atlantic Squid, Fisheries and Marine Service Tech. Rep. No. 902, Department of Fisheries and Oceans, Halifax, Nova Scotia, 26, 1980.
79. **Pechanek, U., Pfannhauser, W., and Woidich, H.**, Histamine contents of fish with respect to regulatory and recommended limits, *Ernährung/Nutrition,* 7, 683, 1983, (in German).
80. Sweden, Statens Livsmedelsverks Forfattnings-samling SLV FS: 3.2, 1980, (in Swedish).
81. **Taylor, S. L.**, Histamine food poisoning: toxicology and clinical aspects, *Crit. Rev. Toxicol.*, 17(2), 91, 1986.
82. **Chang, O., Cheuk, W. L., Nickelson, R., Martin, R., and Finne, G.**, Indole in shrimp: effect of fresh storage temperature, freezing, and boiling, *J. Food Sci.*, 48, 813, 1983.
83. **Jason, A. C. and Lees, A.**, *Estimation of Fish Freshness by Dielectric Measurement,* Torry Research Station, Aberdeen, 1971.
84. Intellectron Fish Tester VI, Intellectron International Electronics, Hamburg.

Chapter 5

THE PREPARATION OF CATCH FOR PRESERVATION AND MARKETING

Piotr J. Bykowski

TABLE OF CONTENTS

I.	The Purpose of Preliminary Processing		78
II.	Major Preprocessing Operations		78
	A.	Grading	78
	B.	Washing	78
	C.	Scaling	79
	D.	Deheading and Gutting	80
	E.	Filleting	84
	F.	Skinning	86
	G.	Meat Separation	87
III.	Production Line in Fish Processing		92
References			92

I. THE PURPOSE OF PRELIMINARY PROCESSING

The main objective of preliminary processing is the full or partial separation of edible parts from inedible ones. As a result, a semiproduct is obtained of the shape, size, and quality approved by the consumer and meets the needs of further processing. It also allows for efficient utilization of inedible parts, e.g., for animal feed production. Isolating the highly perishable parts extends the life of the parts used in further processing. The decrease in the mass of the raw material affords economy in the transport of the semiproduct or the final product. Preliminary processing of a raw material the meat of which is nutritive and tasty, but looks unattractive or unknown to the consumer, allows it to enter the market.

Figures 1 and 2 present the major products of fish and squid processing, from the least to the most labor intensive. In the case of fish, subsequent operations result in the growing degree of edible/inedible part separation. The choice of a particular form of processing depends on the requirements of the technology, the kind and size of the material, and the technical potential to the producer. The economic and marketing aspects are also of great importance.

In the fish industry of today, the preprocessing is largely mechanized. There are special machines for scaling, gutting, deheading, nobbing, deheading and gutting, filleting, skinning, cutting, and meat separating. The processing of squids and crustaceans is less mechanized.

Other machines are also used in preprocessing, i.e., deicing, grading, and orienting machines as well as automatic feeders.

There are many types of the above-mentioned machinery. They differ in output capacity, the size and species range of the processed material, the way in which the operation is performed, the technological yield, etc. Due to high labor intensity and arduousness of manual work, there is a permanent labor shortage in the fish-processing industry of some countries. The solution to this problem is the introduction and development of mechanization of particular operations as well as the whole technological process.

II. MAJOR PREPROCESSING OPERATIONS

A. GRADING

Preprocessing begins with the grading of raw material according to species and size, as well as isolating the fish which are unfit for consumption or damaged. Grading according to species has not been mechanized so far. However, machine size grading is widely used. It increases the technological efficiency of mechanized fish processing; it is also particularly important in these technological processes where the weight and temperature of the material change in the processing, as in smoking or salting, for it is then possible to adjust the parameters of the process to particular size groups.

Size grading is used extensively for small fish, e.g., herring, sprat, mackerel, and sardine. The material is graded according to the maximum thickness, as this is correlated with the length of the fish. Most frequently, the grading takes place in an opening slit formed by some vibrating elements (Figure 3), or between rotating rollers (Figure 4). The arrangement of the rollers may be parallel or fan shaped. In case of parallel rollers, the opening of the slit is regulated by their diameter. The precision of machine grading is higher than of hand grading. Because of rigor mortis and postrigor fish deformation, machine grading is more accurate in case of the fish just caught; hence, it should be done on board rather than on shore.

B. WASHING

The main purpose of washing is the reduction of fish contamination with bacteria. Effective washing depends on two factors: the kinetic energy of the washing water and the

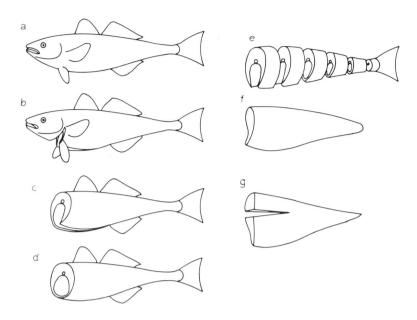

FIGURE 1. Major form of preprocessed fish. (a) Round; (b) gutted; (c) deheaded; (d) after nobbing; (e) chunks; (f) fillet; and (g) V-cut fillet.

water-to-fish proportion. To ensure proper washing, this proportion must be at least as 1:1; in practice, however, twice the amount of water is used. The washing action of water is supported by mechanical rubbing of the fish surface in various types of washers. An effective machine washing reduces the quantity of bacteria by one order of magnitude. In processing plants on shore, tap water is used for washing; on board, clean sea water is used, which should be collected at the bow of the ship.

There are several types of washing machines, such as vertical-axis drum washers (Figure 5), horizontal-axis drum washers (Figure 6), and conveyer washers. Periodic action vertical-axis washers can damage the fish thrown by the spinning bottom of the drum onto its walls; the fish after washing can also be fouled by dirty water while being removed. Washers of this type are often used on board, due to their small dimensions. The most popular type is the horizontal-axis drum washer. The main element of the machine is a rotary perforated drum, with perforations about 10 mm in diameter. Inside the drum, metal or rubber slats are fixed, ensuring the proper stirring of the fish. The revolutions of the drum and its inclination make the material move towards the outlet. The process of washing is continuous under a stream of water from the perforated pipe inside the drum. Dirty water runs off into a waste tank. Horizontal-axis washers are used to wash round fish as well as deheaded and gutted fish of fragile tissue, as they do not cause any damage. Due to their continuous action, they are particularly useful in production lines where constant raw material flow is required.

Conveyer washers can also perform the deicing function. The ice, having lower density than the fish, starts floating and is mechanically removed. The fish drops onto a mesh conveyer which takes it out of the tank. Despite an additional spray of water, the effectiveness of washing in this type of machinery is less than in the other two types.

C. SCALING

For some fish species, hand scaling accounts for nearly 50% of the time of initial processing. Machines used in mechanized scaling should not damage the skin or weaken the texture of the muscular tissue. Two kinds of scaling machines are used in the fish processing industry, i.e., drum machines in which the material is scaled by grazing past the

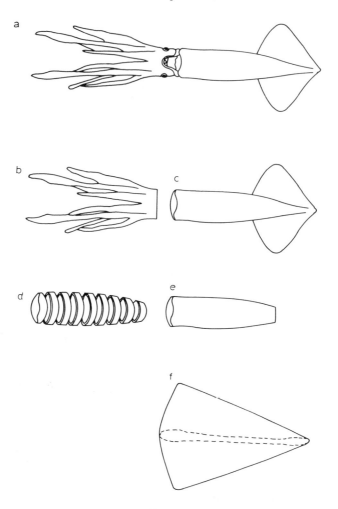

FIGURE 2. Major form of preprocessed squid. (a) Round; (b) arms with corona; (c) tube; (d) rings; and (e) mantle.

rough walls of the rotating drum, and machine scrapers, in which the fish is passed through a system of stationary or moving scrapers (Figure 7). The drum machinery can cause damage to the skin and the weakening of the tissue; their effectiveness amounts to 85 to 90%. The output of machine scrapers reaches 20 to 40 fish per minute with 90 to 95% effectiveness. The actual scaling is done by rotary drums with 2- to 3-mm deep cuts on their surface. Electrical scrapers are also used. The scaling is then done by the repeated drawing of a rotary scraper along the surface of the fish from tail to head.

D. DEHEADING AND GUTTING

The head of the fish accounts for a large proportion of its weight; deheading is thus necessary also from the point of view of reducing the mass of the material, the more so as the head is not fit for human consumption. Deheading is carried out mechanically or by hand.

In modern industry, this operation is largely mechanized. The principal requirement is that deheading should cause the smallest possible loss of muscular tissue. Different kinds of cutting are presented in Figure 8. Cross-cutting (Figure 8c) is used in deheading small fish such as herring, mackerel, or sprat, but slant cutting is more economical (Figure 8d). A V-shaped cut is performed with two angled rotating knives (Figure 8e). The most effective

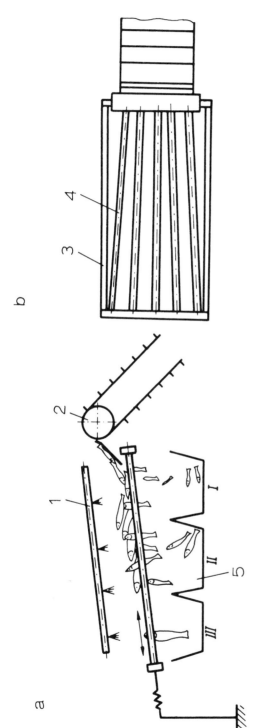

FIGURE 3. Grading on vibrating elements. (a) Side view and (b) top view. (1) Water jet; (2) conveyer; (3) construction frame; (4) vibrator; and (5) output bins.

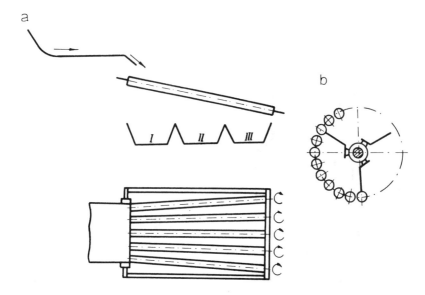

FIGURE 4. Sorting on rotating rollers. (a) Fan shaped arrangement and (b) drum arrangement.

method is the gill cut used in deheading by hand (Figure 8a). In some deheading machines, fashion cutting is used — technically difficult but most economical (Figure 8b). Sometimes the head is incised without severing the viscera connected with it. This type of cutting makes it easy to remove them by pressing out in further deheading. Such operation is called nobbing and is used, for example, preprocessing of herring for salting.

The most widely used means of machine deheading is by cross- or slant cutting. The fixing of the most economical plane of cutting is not mechanically adjustable and depends on the thoroughness and expertise of the person working the machine. Deheading is more economical in machines in which the fish is leaned on or fixed to runners, e.g., by the gills or the pectoral fins, and then taken into the machine, where it is deheaded by rotary knives with an economical V-shaped cut. An operator of these types of machines is able to dehead up to 40 fish per minute. In Poland, a fashion-cutting deheading machine has been devised. It gives raw material economies of 2 to 3% as compared with V-shaped cutting machinery.

Gutting machines are used in fish processing while preparing the material for canning, salting, or smoking and in preprocessing of those fish species for which there is so far no mechanized filleting. The most common type of machine gutting is by cutting the belly open before or after deheading and removing the viscera mechanically. There are also techniques in which the viscera are removed by suction after deheading.

In industrial practice, the gutting-deheading units are of greatest use. They are applied in production lines for machine filleting (Figure 9). The fish are suspended by the pectoral fin in special grippers placed on a rotary mechanism. The first operation is deheading by means of a rotary knife, then the belly is cut open from the anus upward, and finally the belly cavity is gutted and washed. Such units are used in processing 35 to 70 cm long gadoids; with one operator, an output of 35 fish per minute is reached.

In Poland, a gutting-deheading unit of a very simple design and small dimensions and weight is used. Owing to its small dimensions, it can be used on fishing vessels (Figure 10). Its essential elements are two belt conveyers carrying the fish, two slanting knives which dehead the fish and cut off the belly flap, and the mechanism changing the position of the fish during the process (Figure 10a). An incision severing the spine is made on the dorsal side, then the position of the fish is changed (Figure 10b), by which the deheading

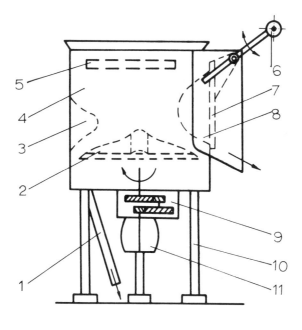

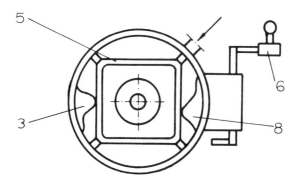

FIGURE 5. Vertical-axis drum washer. (1) Water outlet; (2) spinning bottom; (3) bumper; (4) drum; (5) water jet; (6) counterweight; (7) clean fish outlet; (8) bumper; (9) gear; (10) construction frame; and (11) electric motor.

is completed and the lower part of the belly flap is cut off together with the viscera. The machine is designed for the processing of gadoids, mackerel, carangid, and ocean perch of 24- to 45-cm length; one-man operated, it reaches an output of 60 fish per minute.

Deheaded small fish, such as sprat or capelin can be gutted by suction (Figure 11). The accuracy of the gutting depends on the design of the suction nozzle and the vacuum pressure. When the viscera have been removed, the belly cavity is washed under a stream of water. Vacuum-pressure machines are used in the U.S.S.R. with output capacity of 200 per minute, for the 8- to 12-cm long fish.[2]

Figure 12 presents the work of a nobbing machine. This deheads and removes the alimentary tract, while leaving the gonads in an unopened belly cavity. The blades incising the head operate in slits between fish pockets and do not sever the alimentary tract. A change in the direction of the fish pocket conveyer causes the viscera to be torn out. The residuals are removed by pinions. The machine can be supplemented with a device for cutting the fish into chunks. The fish pockets are changed depending on the size of the fish processed, and the output reached amounts to 145 to 200 fish per minute.

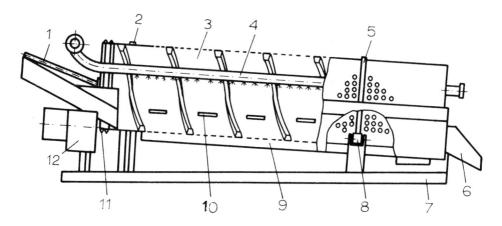

FIGURE 6. Horizontal-axis drum washer. (1) Water jet; (2,5) drum guidance; (3) perforated drum; (4) main water jet; (6) clean fish outlet; (7) construction frame; (8,11) chain wheel; (9) waste water tank; (10) bumper; and (12) electric motor with gear. (From Kawka, T. and Dutkiewicz, D., *Fish and Squid Processing Machinery. An Outline of Design*, Wydawnictwo Morskie, Gdańsk, 1986. With permission.)

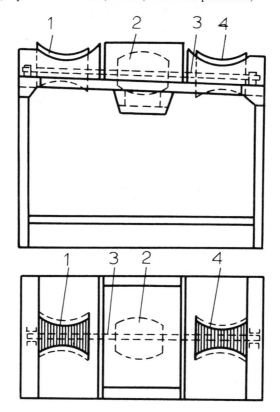

FIGURE 7. Drum scaler. (1,4) Rough surface rotating drum; (2) electric motor; and (3) drive shaft.

E. FILLETING

The filet, i.e., the block of meat composed of the dorsal and abdominal muscles, is now one of the most popular forms of fish-obtained culinary raw material on the market. The technological yield of filleting, e.g., of gutting, depends on the fish species, its sex, size, alimentation, etc. Hand filleting is labor intensive and high productivity requires much

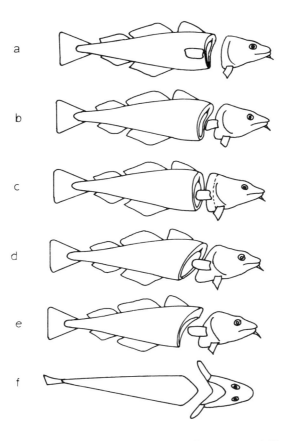

FIGURE 8. Ways of cutting in machine-deheading. (a) Around gills cut; (b) fashion cut; (c) cross-cut; (d) slant cut; and (e, f) V-shape cut.

skill and experience from the workers. It is for this reason that filleting machines have been implemented in fish processing on a wide scale, despite high costs of purchase and maintenance.

Since particular species differ in shape and individual specimens differ in size, filleting machines with nonadjustable processing tools, e.g., knives, would lead to large losses of material. Therefore, the design of machines ensures the adjustability of tools before each fish is processed. In the filleting machines used today this adjustability is achieved by mechanical automated systems, and electronic control is applied in new generation of machines. A filleting machine should be characterized by high output capacity, even surface of cuts, simple, not too laborious operation, as well as easy and effective maintenance. A machine designed for filleting many fish species should be easy to switch from one species to another. Filleting machines are composed of three basic parts: (1) the internal handling system (linear or rotary, holders handling the fish) grippers, saddle-shaped holders, conveyer belts, or chains with holding bite or needles, (2) the control-adjustment system, and (3) filleting tool units, mainly disk knives.

The basic operations of machine filleting are cutting along the upper and lower appendices on the spine and cutting over the ribs and along the vertebrae. As most fish are symmetrically built, each operation is performed by a pair of symmetric knives.

The number of particular cuts and the order in which they are performed depend on the way the fish is handled in the machine, e.g., head or tail first; they also depend on the way in which the fish is held. With smaller fish, such as herring, one pair of blades removes both the ribs and the upper appendices on the spine.

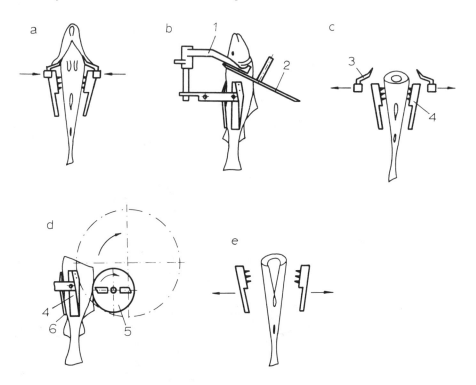

FIGURE 9. Operational scheme of deheading and gutting machine. (1) Hanger; (2) deheading knife; (3) gripper arm; (4) gripper; (5) gutting cutter; and (6) fish back support. (From Kawka, T. and Dutkiewicz, D., *Fish and Squid Processing Machinery. An Outline of Design*, Wydawnictwo Morskie, Gdańsk, 1986. With permission.)

Figures 13 and 14 present the functional diagram of machines filleting herring, cod, and mackerel. The filleting unit (Figure 14) is combined with the deheading unit.

To meet the requirements of some consignees, it is sometimes necessary to produce fillets without intermuscular bones, the so-called V-cut fillet. This operation is usually performed by hand. A certain proportion of meat is then removed together with the appendices, which reduces the yield by as much as 25%. The production of 1 ton of skinned "V" fillet takes 16 to 45 man hours, nearly 25% of which is spent removing the bones.[3] This operation has been mechanized — it can be performed by means of cutting through the skin at the sides of the fish (Figure 15). The essential mechanism contains two pairs of angled disk knives. The length and the depth of cutting can be adjusted to the size of the fish.

F. SKINNING

Following the wide application of filleting machines in fish processing, skinning machines were introduced. Skinned fillet has become the most popular form of culinary semiproduct and is in high demand. Skinning machines must ensure high output and effectiveness of the operation. A correctly skinned fillet must not be damaged on the skinned side, where the silvery pellicle connecting myomers must be left.

Figure 16 presents an older type of a skinning machine. The fillet placed tail first and skin down on a conveyer enters the gap between a roller and the operation drum. At this point, a flat knife approaches the drum in a reciprocating motion. The skinned fillet slides down the knife surface onto the output conveyer. The knife retracts and is ready for the next operation. Output capacity of this type of machine is about 60 fillets per minute. The 2- to 3-cm long fillet tip remains unskinned and is cut off as waste; thus, this type of machine is uneconomical.

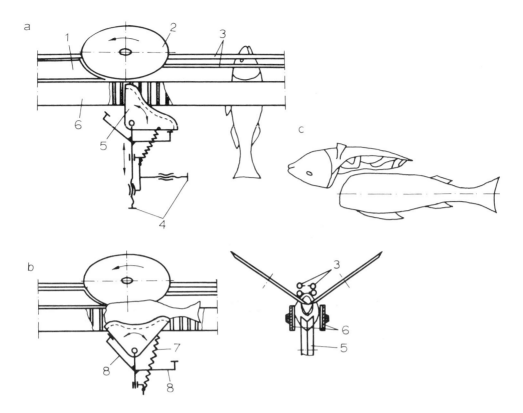

FIGURE 10. Operational scheme of deheading and gutting machine. (1) Eviscerating element; (2) rotating knives; (3) head fastener conveyer; (4) adjustment; (5) mechanism changing the position of the fish; (6) dehead fish conveyer; (7) spring; and (8) stop of element 5.

This drawback has been eliminated from machines using a stationary flat knife (Figure 17). The fillet placed skin down on a conveyer is placed by a feeder on a grooved operation drum. Before meeting the knife, the fillet is pressed down by a roller, after which it gets skinned and slides along the upper side of the blade, while the skin is removed underneath. This type of machine can be used for various fish species and the output capacity is high, e.g., a Baader 51 skins 140 to 150 fillets per minute, thus doing the job of two machines of the old type.

For raw material of weakened texture, such as salted or marinated fish or flounder fillets, skinning machines with a band knife are used, e.g., the Norwegian-made Trio FDS model (Figure 18). The fillets are placed skin up on rubber conveyer belts. The conveyer moves on under a stainless-steel refrigerated drum. The skin freezes onto the drum and is cut off the muscle by the band knife. The fillet is taken away on the conveyer, and the frozen skin is removed by a scraper. The advantage of this machine is that it can be adjusted to cut off the skin thick, together with a layer of the muscle, which in case of, for example, hake gets rancid easily. The output capacity of the Trio FDS skinning machine is 100 to 150 herring or mackerel fillets per minute, and 30 to 150 cod or flounder fillets per minute, with the maximum fillet width of 33 cm.

G. MEAT SEPARATION

In recent years, fish mince has become popular as raw material in fish processing industry. It is obtained from filleting leftovers, deheaded and gutted fish, and parts of the spine. This sort of production has been promoted by economizing on raw materials and became possible with the construction of machinery which separates the meat from the

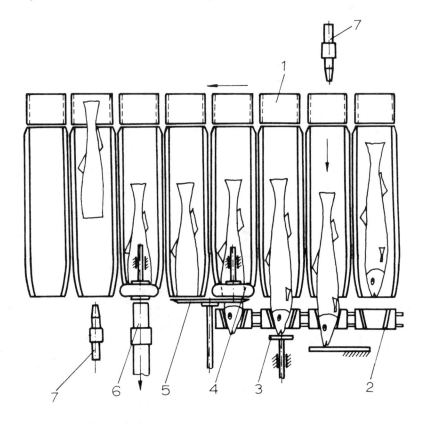

FIGURE 11. Suction gutting and deheading. (1) Fish pocket conveyer; (2) conveyer for the heads; (3) positioning mechanism; (4) pressing pulley; (5) deheading knife; (6) suction nozzle; and (7) water jet.

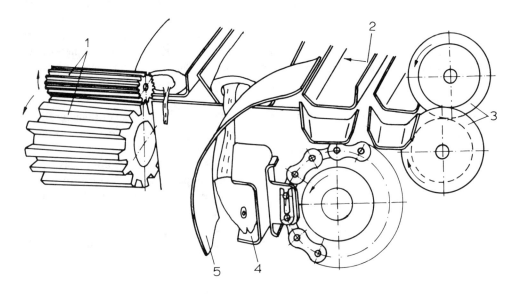

FIGURE 12. Operational scheme of nobbing machine. (1) Pinions; (2) fish pockets; (3) incising knives; (4) head pockets; and (5) tearing off element. (From Kawka, T. and Dutkiewicz, D., *Fish and Squid Processing Machinery. An Outline of Design*, Wydawnictwo Morskie, Gdańsk, 1986. With permission.)

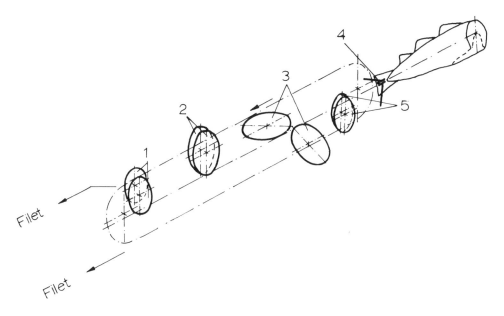

FIGURE 13. Operational diagram of gadoid filleting machine: (1) Knives cutting fillets off; (2) upper filleting knives; (3) knives cutting ribbs off; (4) lower filleting knives; and (5) gripper.

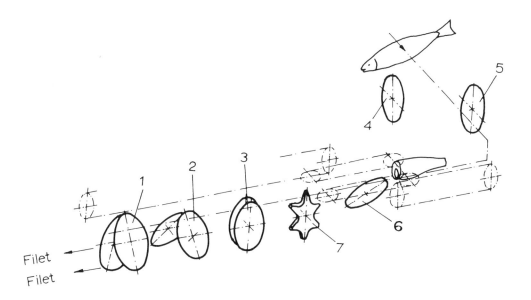

FIGURE 14. Operational scheme of mackerel and herring filleting machine. (1) Upper filleting knives; (2) knives cutting ribs off; (3) lower filleting knives; (4) deheading knife; (5) knife cutting tail off; (6) knife cutting belly open; and (7) cutter for the viscera.

inedible parts, such as bones, fins, and skin. The use of separators enables us obtain 15 to 30% of meat more in the form of fish mince than in the production of boned fillets.

Figure 19 presents the functional diagram of a separator. The raw material is passed from a bin onto the elastic band of a conveyer. The band contacts a section of the perforated drum tightly. The meat is squeezed into the drum through its perforations by the pressure of the band, and removed therefrom. Bones and skin remain outside the drum and are scraped

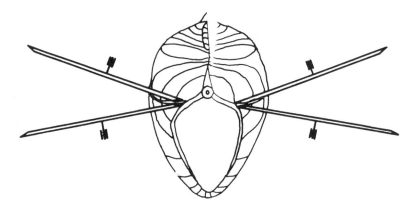

FIGURE 15. Intermuscular bones cutting.

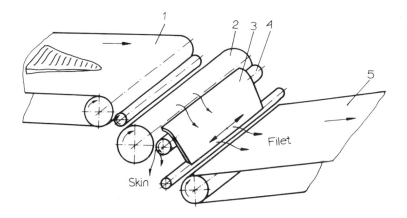

FIGURE 16. Skinning machine with vibrating knife. (1) Feeder; (2) operational drum; (3) flat knife; (4) roller; and (5) skinned fillet conveyer.

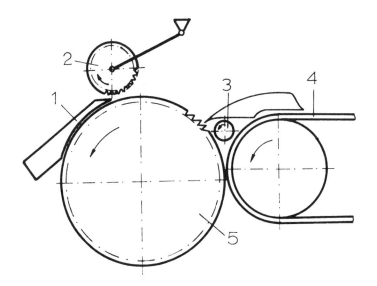

FIGURE 17. Skinning machine with stationary flat knife. (1) Flat knife; (2) press down roller; (3) intermediate roller; (4) feeder; and (5) operational drum. (From Kawka, T. and Dutkiewicz, D., *Fish and Squid Processing Machinery. An Outline of Design,* Wydawnictwo Morskie, Gdańsk, 1986. With permission.)

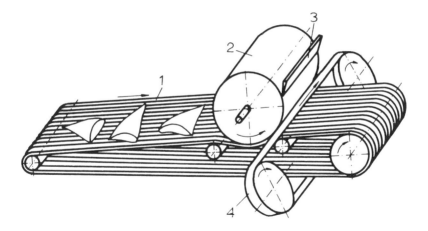

FIGURE 18. Skinning machine with band knife. (1) Feeder; (2) refrigerated drum; (3) scraper; and (4) band knife.

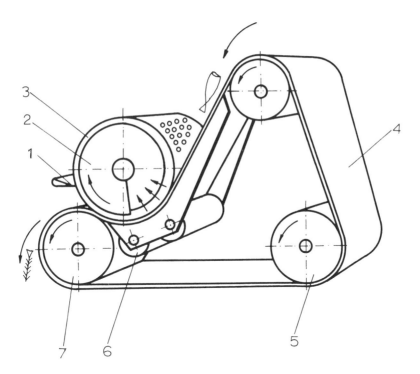

FIGURE 19. Scheme of meat separator. (1) Scraper; (2) screw type meat remover; (3) perforated drum; (4) rubber band; (5) band tension roller; (6) pressing roller; and (7) transmission roller.

away by knife. The thoroughness of the separation is regulated by the band tension and depends on the size of the perforation, 2 to 5 mm in diameter. Separators of this type give a yield of 150 to 2500 kg/h. In technologies requiring more thoroughly minced or cleaned meat, screw conveyer separators are used. The mince is pressed through 1.2- to 2.6-mm holes made in a stationary cylinder. The raw material is fed into the cylinder by a screw conveyer of a variable worm lead and growing diameter, which make the pressure increase. The separated waste is removed through a spring-weighted valve at the end of the cylinder.

III. PRODUCTION LINE IN FISH PROCESSING

In modern fish-processing plants, both land- and ship-based, machinery usually works in production lines. The line comprises, apart from machinery, raw material bins, transport facilities, and manual work stations. The basic parameter bringing the work of machinery and other facilities together is the output capacity required under the given processing conditions. A number of factors have to be accounted for in designing a production line:

- Proper composition of the line, i.e., the type, size, and output capacity of the machinery and equipment that will make particular operations possible
- Proper arrangement of machinery and equipment so that a certain sequence of operations is achieved
- Input/output flow and workforce routes should not intersect
- Raw-material utilization should be as economical as possible
- Transport facilities applied must ensure undisrupted production

An important element which must also be taken into consideration when the production line is designed is making the information on the production process available at every stage. This ensures the proper control of the whole process. One of the characteristics of an advanced production line is the decrease in the amount of manual work. This is difficult to achieve in fish processing due to the properties of the raw material — variability of size, shape, species, etc.

REFERENCES

1. **Kawka, T. and Dutkiewicz, D.**, *Fish and Squid Processing Machinery. An Outline of Design*, Wydawnictwo Morskie, Gdańsk, 1986, chap. 3, 4, and 5, (in Polish).
2. **Terenteev, A. W.**, Preliminary of integrated fish pre-processing, Pishch. Industria, Moscow, 1969, chap. 2 (in Russian).
3. **Bykowski, P., Sikorski, Z., and Zimińska, H.**, *Preservation of Marine Foods by Refrigeration*, Wydawnictwo Morskie, Gdańsk, 1973, chap. 5, (in Polish).

Chapter 6

CHILLING OF FRESH FISH

Zdzisław E. Sikorski

TABLE OF CONTENTS

I. The Effect of Chilling on the Loss of Freshness and Spoilage of Seafood 94

II. Handling and Refrigeration of Fish 94
    A. Handling and Processing of the Catch on Board 94
    B. Chilling in Ice 95
        1. The Use of Different Types of Ice 95
        2. Icing on Board 95
        3. The Storage Life of Iced Fish 96
    C. Chilling at Subzero Temperatures 98
        1. General Considerations 98
        2. Superchilling in Ice 98
        3. Chilling in Ice Slurry 98
        4. Chilling in Refrigerated Sea Water 99

III. Extension of the Shelf Life of Chilled Seafoods 101
    A. General Considerations 101
    B. The Use of Preservatives 101
        1. First Applications and Withdrawals 101
        2. Recent Developments 101
    C. Application of Modified Atmospheres 102
        1. General Considerations 102
        2. CO_2-Enriched Atmosphere Storage 103
            a. The Inhibitory Effect on Microflora 103
            b. The Shelf Life in CO_2-Enriched Atmosphere 104
    D. Radurization 105
        1. Introduction 105
        2. The Effect of Ionizing Radiation on Microflora 105
        3. Sensory Changes in Irradiated Fish 105
        4. Feasibility of Commercial Applications 106

References 107

I. THE EFFECT OF CHILLING ON THE LOSS OF FRESHNESS AND SPOILAGE OF SEAFOODS

The initial loss of the attributes of prime freshness in seafoods is mainly due to the activity of endogenous enzymes, dessication, as well as oxidation of lipids and pigments. Further undesirable quality changes and the final spoilage are caused by bacterial putrefaction. The rate of these processes is controlled mainly by temperature, additional factors being the species and condition of the caught fish, handling and gutting, microbial contamination, humidity and composition of the atmosphere, preservatives, and other antimicrobial treatments.

The effect of chilling and heating on the rate of chemical reactions can be evaluated by using the Arrhenius relationship between the reaction rate constant and the activation energy (see Chapter 7). In food systems, however, the effect of temperature on the rate of the complex deteriorative reactions cannot be adequately described by the Arrhenius equation, as the activation energies of these reactions change significantly close to the freezing point. The same reservation applies also to the empirical formula of van't Hoff:

$$Q_{10} = \frac{k_{T+10}}{k_T}$$

where k_T is the reaction rate constant at temperature T. For many chemical and biochemical reactions, Q_{10} is in the range 2 to 4. However, at low chilling temperatures, it has much higher values.

For predicting the relative spoilage rate of fish, the Spencer and Bains equation can be used:

$$k = k_0(1 + cT)$$

where k is the spoilage rate in spoilage units per day at temperature T, k_0 is the spoilage rate at 0°C, and c is the temperature coefficient.[1] This equation has been found by Olley and Ratkovsky[2] to give reliable results in the temperature range 0 to 6°C when c = 0.24.

The influence of temperature on the rate of bacterial growth and on nucleotide degradation in seafoods, in the range from about −1°C to ambient temperature, can be accurately described by the square root relationship of Ratkovsky et al.,[3,4] presented in Chapter 8.

The existing experimental evidence shows that the effect of temperature on the rate of microbial growth and other deteriorative reactions is especially high close to the freezing point. Thus, rapid chilling to about −1°C is the most effective means of prolonging the period of prime freshness and extending the shelf life of seafoods, as well as of inhibiting the pathogenic mesophiles and retarding the growth of psychrotropic pathogenic microorganisms.

II. HANDLING AND REFRIGERATION OF FISH

A. HANDLING AND PROCESSING OF THE CATCH ON BOARD

The most critical aspect in handling of the catch on deck is generally rapid chilling. Thus, the flow of operations after hauling the catch on board must prevent any delay in decreasing the temperature of fish. There are, however, reports indicating that in some tropical species, aging a few hours on board before chilling could prevent cold-shock reactions and thus a loss in yield of the fillets, without causing a significant reduction in shelf life.[5]

Once on deck, the catch should be immediately sorted to remove fish unsuitable for human food and to avoid damaging of the delicate species by the rough surfaces of thorny specimens. If the processing facilities do not allow for immediate handling of large hauls, the catch should be protected temporarily from the sun and at very low air temperature from freezing. On large enough vessels, the fish should be dumped into a tank with cold sea water.

Stunning the struggling specimens and bleeding large fish is recommended, as it extends the time prior to rigor development. Furthermore, the removal of blood helps to get lighter colored flesh and may contribute to the prevention of oxidative rancidity. Gutting also serves the purpose of bleeding. Removing the stomach and gut reduces the risk of autolysis by digestive enzymes and eliminates the bacterial attack from the gut contents. The removal of the intestines must be complete and no contamination of the catch with the gut content should occur. All these operations are effective only if, under the conditions on board, the time required for such handling does not offset the gain in quality by increasing the temperature of the fish before the chilling commences. Generally bleeding and gutting of small fish on board is impractical if large hauls are taken and no efficient gutting machine is available.

Before stowing away below deck, the fish should be washed with clean sea water in suitable washing equipment or by careful hosing, to remove surface filth as well as contamination resulting from gutting and bleeding. It is recommended by FAO/WHO to add about 10 µg/g of chlorine to the sea water used for washing.[6] Although washing of the catch on board does not remove the slime from the fish surface, it may reduce the number of the total surface bacteria by about one order of magnitude.

B. CHILLING IN ICE
1. The Use of Different Types of Ice

The first use of ice for chilling fish during transport in the European fisheries was apparently made about 200 years ago, although this method of preservation of the catch had been known earlier to the Chinese fishermen.[7] Originally natural ice collected in ponds, rivers, and lakes was used. According to current sanitary requirements, the ice brought in contact with fish should be produced from potable water or clean sea water.

Various types of ice have different suitabilities for being used in fisheries. The block ice (Figure 1) can be easily stored in any insulated or refrigerated shore facility. It has a density of about 720 kg/m^3. As it may be produced in blocks ranging from about 25 to over 100 kg, it must be crushed before loading on the fishing vessel. Crushed ice, because of possible sharp edges of the pieces, may not be best suited for making good contact with the fish and may damage the skin of sensitive species. Other types of ice, produced in continuously operating installations in small pieces, are known under the term small ice. They differ in dimensions and forms and carry different trade names. Flake ice, which is produced by freezing water on the surface of a refrigerated drum and scraping the ice off with a blade, is usually 2 to 3 mm thick. It has the largest surface area per unit weight and a density of 480 kg/m^3. It is easy to handle. Thus, it can be very evenly distributed between the layers of fish. Freezing water on the outer surface of a refrigerated plate or the inner surface of a refrigerated tube, followed by releasing the ice crust by reversing the circulation of the refrigerant, are the principles of producing plate ice and tube ice, respectively. The thickness of plate ice is usually 8 to 15 mm and the diameter of the tube ice about 50 mm, with a wall thickness of 10 to 12 mm. Small ice flows freely and easily lends itself to storage, if dry and well frozen.

2. Icing on Board

The heat transfer takes place mainly between the fish and ice and the cold melt water in direct contact. Thus, to achieve the highest chilling rate, it is necessary to surround each fish completely by ice. Although this is possible in laboratory experiments, the commercial conditions on a fishing vessel do not always allow for such individual treatment of all fish.

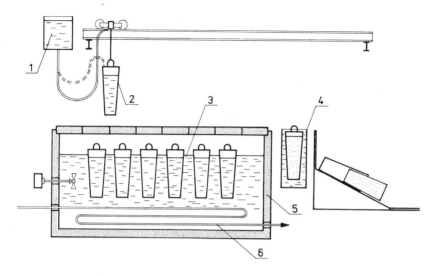

FIGURE 1. The block ice installation. (1) Can filling tank; (2) ice can; (3) refrigerated brine; (4) thawing tank; (5) insulation; and (6) refrigerant.

Icing on board is traditionally carried out manually. On vessels catching small fish such as herring, mackerel, and anchovetta, the individual hauls may be very large, over 50 tons. As there is not much time between the hauls, the fishermen have to stow the fish quickly into the hold to make the deck clear before the next catch. There are, however, developments in mechanized systems of icing and stowing the fish on board of larger vessels.[8]

For bulk stowage of iced fish, the traditional fishroom is divided into pounds by fitting removable boards into vertical stanchions. The boards are presently made mainly of aluminum or plastic. The fish are stored in the pounds between layers of ice and are separated by ice from the shipside and other fishroom structures. To avoid heavy losses due to high pressure in the bottom layers of fish, a second platform is formed at about 50 cm from the bottom of the pound. The quantity of ice to be used depends upon the insulation and refrigeration of the fishroom, on the outside air temperature, and the duration of the trip. It may reach from about 25 to about 100% of the weight of the catch. The practical requirements must be found by experience for the individual vessel and the type of fishery. For unloading the iced fish, baskets or containers are usually used. Much manual labor is required, unless fish pumps or elevators and conveyor systems are employed.

Stowage of iced fish in boxes, stacked one on top of the other, offers a better possibility to separate the fish from different hauls and provides an uninterrupted chilling environment for the fish from deck to the dockside. Furthermore, the icing and unloading operations can be easily mechanized (Figure 2). Currently, plastic boxes are usually used in commercial fisheries, as they are easy to clean, have the required heat insulation properties, are relatively light, resist rough handling, and last several years. They can be molded so as to allow for nesting when empty, stacking when full, and efficient draining of the melt water. Today, insulated containers of different size are also available, which can be supplied with lids. They are usually made of high-density polyethylene and are suitable for being used both on board and in shore transport.

3. The Storage Life of Iced Fish

How long can iced fish be kept in prime freshness or in acceptable quality in commercial conditions of icing? The answer to this question depends upon the species characteristics, the fishing ground and season, the condition of the fish, the method of capture, the care in handling and icing on board, and the system of packaging used in the retail outlets. In

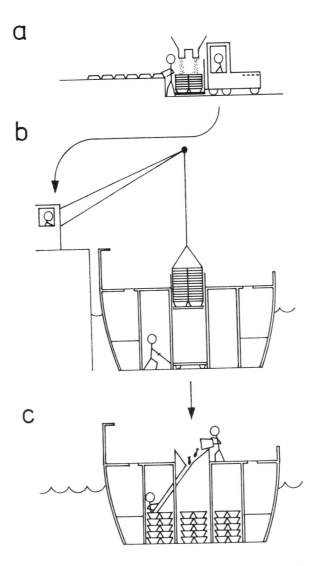

FIGURE 2. A mechanized system of icing fish in boxes. The plastic box has a bottom provided with 25-mm quadratic holes. By vibration, a stack of such boxes may be simultaneously charged with dry flake ice which forms a bottom layer. (a) Ice filling station; (b) quayside crane; and (c) fish hold. (From Hansen, P., *Scandinavian Refrigeration*, Vol. 5, 1977. With permission.)

commercial fisheries, the storage life in acceptable sensory quality is for many small fatty fish such as herring, sardine, and anchovy rather short, about 5 to 8 d, for lean white species such as cod, haddock, and hake up to about 14 d, and for snappers to about 18 d. A few species are especially resistant to spoilage, e.g., the halibuts and flounders, and can be kept in ice about 24 d. Several fish from tropical seas, like some mullets or breams, have a shelf life of up to 29 to 30 d. A large number of published data on the shelf life of commercially important marine and freshwater fish has been presented and commented upon by Lima dos Santos.[9]

Many species of fish, known for their exquisite sensory quality, are especially highly priced on specialized markets, but only in the state of prime freshness. Some of these fish are eaten raw in Japan as sashimi or are used whole for ceremonial dishes. Thus, they must not only be very fresh but should also retain in the market place their best attractive appearance. In such situations, the storage life in acceptable sensory quality is much less important than the high quality life. These species, caught by methods which do not cause exhaustion of the fish or damage to the skin, are individually handled on board. To prevent their long struggling on deck, they may be spiked by piercing the brain to cause immediate death or are stunned and bled. After rapid chilling to 0°C, they are packaged in expanded polystyrene boxes suitable for air freight. If the box has a false bottom and an absorbent pad, the fish are iced. Otherwise the proper amount of ice is added in polyethylene bags. Carefully handled fish can be brought by air to the very demanding market in Japan in the state of prime freshness even from distant areas, e.g., the snapper from New Zealand or the bluefin from the Mediterranean.

C. CHILLING AT SUBZERO TEMPERATURES
1. General Considerations

Extending the shelf life of fresh fish for an additional few days, over that which can be achieved when even optimum parameters of icing are strictly observed, gives a chance of better utilization of resources available in distant fishing grounds. Such extension is possible by lowering the temperature of the fish to near the initial point of freezing of the tissue water, i.e., to about -1.0 to $-1.5°C$. This brings about significant retardation of spoilage, without causing undesirable physicochemical and structural changes in the tissues and texture deterioration. Superchilling at -3 to $-4°C$ increases the shelf life of fish to 4 or 5 weeks by effectively inhibiting the bacterial spoilage. The texture of the muscles, however, deteriorates significantly due to toughening and drip formation. Furthermore, autolytic lipid hydrolysis may induce undesirable changes in the flavor of the fish.

The difficulty in practical application of chilling just below 0°C in commercial conditions lies in securing the required precise control of the level and distribution of temperature in the bulk of stored fish. Many approaches have been suggested, differing in the art of achieving the controlled temperature and in the character of the chilling medium.

2. Superchilling in Ice

The fish stowed in ice in the usual way in pounds can be chilled to the required temperature by refrigerating the whole bulk by cold brine, circulating in heat exchangers fitted into the sides of the pounds. The side walls and the shelves, however, must be constructed of steel plates or aluminum to efficiently conduct the heat from the fish. Such a system was applied in the 1960s on a series of Portuguese trawlers fishing off the West Coast of Africa.[10] In British commercial experiments, the fish were stowed in aluminum boxes in a fishroom that was refrigerated by circulating air at -2 to $-3°C$. The design and stowage arrangement of the boxes were such that gaps necessary for enforced air circulation were created.[11]

Both methods were effective in prolonging the shelf life of the fish by several days, although disadvantages in discharge operations and marketing of the catch were also observed.

Another approach is to chill the fish by using ice of a lower melting point, e.g., prepared from 2% brine or sea water. Careful icing with such ice makes it possible to extend the shelf life of the catch by a few days.

3. Chilling in Ice Slurry

A mixture of sea water and ice, usually 1:2 on a volume basis at the start, forms a slurry that has a temperature of about $-1.5°C$. In such chilled sea water (CSW), the heat transfer between the fish and the cold medium occurs by convection. Thus, the rate of chilling is higher than in ice. Ice and salt should be added to the slurry during chilling to compensate for the loss of ice due to melting and to maintain the salt concentration at about 3%. Agitation

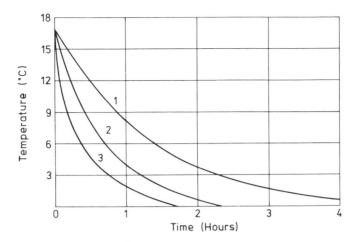

FIGURE 3. The temperature in snapper chilled in CSW. (1) Large fish, 3.8 kg, (2) medium, 1.3 kg, and (3) small, 0.8 kg. (From Harvie, R. E., Importance of Chilling in Producing Top Quality Snapper *Chrysophrys auratus* for the Japanese Market, International Institute of Refrigeration, Commissions C_2, D_1, D_2, D_3, Hamilton, 1982, 127. With permission.)

in the tank prevents accumulation of the ice at the surface and formation of a large temperature difference between the upper and bottom part of the container. Furthermore, forced convection increases the rate of heat transfer.

The rate of chilling of fish in CSW is especially high in the range from ambient temperature to about 5°C, while below 5°C it is not significantly higher than that in crushed ice (Figure 3). Thus, CSW is often used only for rapid initial chilling of highly valued fish on board, e.g., longine snapper, and after at least 2 h the fish is iced in boxes. Another use of CSW is for chilling and holding the catch on board in insulated containers. These same ice (Figure 3). Thus, CSW is often used only for rapid initial chilling of highly valued fish on board, e.g., longline snapper, and after at least 2 h the fish is iced in boxes. Another use container, duration of the trip, air temperature, and the frequency of adding ice.

The shelf life of ungutted fish kept in CSW containers is a few days longer than that of fish carefully chilled with flake ice. Furthermore, no textural damage occurs, except for some loss of scales. In the case of small fatty fish, the CSW treatment offers some protection against rancidity. Substantial modifications of the vessels are, however, necessary to facilitate the handling of large containers, but the operation can be extensively mechanized (Figure 4).

4. Chilling in Refrigerated Sea Water

Similar benefits to those offered by CSW may be achieved by using refrigerated sea water (RSW) or brine for rapid chilling of the catch on board or for chilling and cold storage during the trip. However, larger capital investment is required for the mechanical refrigeration system. Thus, RSW is rather popular on large vessels, while CSW can be applied even on small boats. In order to avoid inefficient, too-slow chilling of the catch, not more than 800 kg of fish should be packed per 1 m^3 of the brine. RSW may be also used to cool the catch by spraying over the top surface of ungutted fish or shrimp in the hold.

Rapid chilling and holding of the catch in RSW is a popular practice on board large prawning vessels. Before being put into the RSW tanks, the prawns should be sorted from the trash, washed with clean sea water, and treated against the development of black spots.

Chilling of the catch in RSW before freezing on board freezer trawlers is a very effective method of preventing rapid quality loss of the fish on subtropical and tropical grounds.[13]

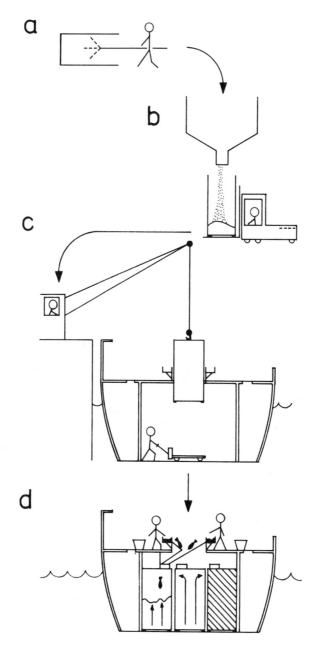

FIGURE 4. A container system for CSW-chilling of fish. (a) Washing station; (b) ice filling station; (c) quayside crane; and (d) fish hold. (From Hansen, P., *Scandinavian Refrigeration*, Vol. 5, 1977. With permission.)

Partial freezing in RSW at 6.5% salt concentration in the brine at −3 to −4°C proved feasible for holding salmon during transportation over long distances from the fishing grounds to canneries. The fish were in satisfactory condition after 15 d from capture, even when kept on the gill netters up to 18 h in open holds without refrigeration at air temperature 7 to 13°C.[14] Commercial trials on two vessels operating in the South China Sea have shown that partial freezing to −2°C of ungutted fish in sea water brine at −5°C, followed by storage in boxes in the hold, maintained at −3°C, was superior to icing. The fish were of acceptable quality after 20 d from catching.[15] Partial freezing of fish was also suggested by Golowkin.[16]

The shelf life and quality of seafoods chilled or stored in CSW or RSW depends upon the species characteristics and the condition of chilling. Generally it is a few days longer than that of iced fish. However, some species are vulnerable to loss of appearance due to bleaching. Furthermore, the uptake of salt may significantly decrease the market value of, for example, the snapper or prawns.

III. EXTENSION OF THE SHELF LIFE OF CHILLED SEAFOODS

A. GENERAL CONSIDERATIONS

Fresh seafoods as landed at the dockside, albeit well chilled, are nevertheless usually several days old. It takes some time, at least a few hours, to prepare them for transportation to inland outlets. Very often chilling is discontinued in the course of handling on shore and the temperature of the fish may rise even above 10°C. First of all, in many markets, the auction system of selling requires a presentation of the catch without ice. Furthermore, gutting, filleting, shucking, etc., if not well organized and mechanized, may cause significant increase in the temperature of the product prepared for shipping. Thus, a large part of the catch, especially from distant fishing grounds or of a very short shelf life due to species characteristics, may not be suitable any more for being sold in remote outlets.

To increase the shelf life of fresh seafoods in the retail chain, many attempts have been made to find suitable chemical preservatives, apply protective atmospheres and packaging, and use ionizing radiation. Low temperature, close to the melting point of ice, which is the main factor retarding spoilage reactions in the fish on board vessel, cannot be relied upon in the supermarket chain, as the temperature in the chilled cabinets is usually in the range 2 to 5°C or even higher.

B. THE USE OF PRESERVATIVES
1. First Applications and Withdrawals

The early investigations, as well as attempts made up to 1958 in search of suitable preservatives for fresh seafoods, have been reviewed by Tarr.[17] Many chemical compounds were tested for their effectiveness, e.g., boric and salicylic acids, benzoic acid and its esters, chloramines and sodium hypochlorite, ethylene dioxide, formaldehyde, glycols, hydrogen peroxide, phosphates, propionates, and sulfur dioxide. They were applied in the form of dips and as additives to ice used for chilling fish. However, the results have not led to commercial applications, either because of low activity of the compounds in concentration causing no objectionable sensory effects or on account of public health implications. Sodium nitrite has been found very effective in suppressing spoilage of iced fish. It was permitted in Canada in amounts not exceeding 200 µg/g of the finished product.[17] It cannot, however, be presently regarded as a safe preservative for fresh fish, as it may lead to the formation of toxic and carcinogenic N-nitrosamines. Public health considerations also prevent commercial application of antibiotics, especially aureomycin (CTC), although extensive investigations in the 1950s have shown very high activity of CTC against spoilage bacteria, resulting in an extension of the shelf life by at least 1 week.[17]

2. Recent Developments

A retardation of spoilage of iced fish fillets by a few days has been achieved by dipping the fillets in a 1% solution of ethylenediaminetetraacetic acid salts (EDTA). The effect is probably caused by inhibition of several groups of psychrotropic bacteria, mainly *Pseudomonas* spp.[18-20]

According to Field et al.,[21] glucose oxidase (GOX) + glucose, used in the form of a dip solution, containing 1 enzyme unit GOX and 4% glucose, in ice, and in an alginate gel cover, was found effective in extending the period of sensory acceptance of flounder fillets at 2 to 4°C by about 6 d. The treatment caused a significant decrease in the pH of the skin and meat of the fillets in the course of storage, in extreme points to 5.2, and retarded the development of ammonia and creatinine. According to the cited authors, the effect was probably caused by the low pH created by the gluconic acid generated in the enzymatic reaction and possibly also due to the metal complexing activity of the gluconic acid. In the experiments of Shaw et al.,[22] however, dipping in glucose oxidase solution, 1 unit per cubic-centimeter or in 0.125% w/v gluconic acid solution, did not effect any extension of the shelf life of cod fillets at 1 to 2°C.

More consistent results were obtained regarding the preservative activity of potassium sorbate (K-sorbate) in fresh seafoods. The antimicrobial properties of sorbic acid were discovered 50 years ago and have been practically utilized for preservation of many food products and feeds.[23,24] Although sorbic acid, $CH_3-CH=CH-CH=CH-COOH$, has a low solubility in water, only about 1% at 25°C and pH 5.9, the K-sorbate is very soluble in a large range of pH. In the U.S., it has the status of a substance generally regarded as safe (GRAS). Sorbates are especially known as growth inhibitors of yeast and molds, but have also been shown to be effective against bacteria, including *Salmonella typhimurium*, *Escherichia coli*, *Pseudomonas* spp., and *Vibrio parahaemolyticus*. The activity of sorbates is highest in low pH foods, as the pK_a of sorbic acid is 4.75 and the undissociated molecule has 10 to 600 times higher antibacterial effect than the dissociated acid. However, at pH 6, about 50% of the growth-inhibiting activity of sorbic acid is due to the dissociated form.[25]

Fresh cod fillets dipped for 10 to 30 s in 3% solution of K-sorbate, stored without ice in covered commercial polyethylene containers, retained the sensory properties of fresh fish 3 d longer than the controls, showed significantly slower growth of total aerobic bacteria, and accumulated trimethylamine (TMA) at a lower rate.[26] A significant retardation of spoilage, by about 5 d, was found in morwong fillets dipped 1 min in 1.2% K-sorbate solution, vacuum packed, and stored at 4°C. Adding 0.1% of K-sorbate to fresh scallop meat, complete with roe packed in plastic bags, increased the high quality shelf life at 4°C from 5 to 21 d, while sorbate treatment and vacuum packing increased the shelf life to 28 d.[27,28] In shucked scallops, inoculated with a mixture of 10 strains of *Clostridium botulinum* types A, B, E, and F, kept at 4, 10, and 27°C, botulinum toxin was found only in vacuum packs at 27°C. All toxins were of the type A. However, all packs containing toxin were inflated, discolored, and slimy, and the scallops would be rejected because of bad appearance and odor.[29]

A very important factor limiting the storage life of chilled prawns is the blackening of the shell. The reactions leading to the formation of black spots can be retarded by dipping the prawns, before ice or RSW chilling, in sodium metabisulfite solution. According to Ruello, immersion of the eastern king prawn *Peaneus plebejus* for 30 s in 0.5% solution of sodium metabisulfite before RSW chilling at $-1.5°C$ completely inhibited the black spot formation for 8 d.[30] The contents of the preservative in the flesh of raw prawns was 15 μg/g wet weight and decreased after cooking or 30-min washing to 0 to 10 μg/g. In American good manufacturing practice (GMP), the treatment of fresh shell-on tails of shrimp involves 1-min dip in 1.25% solution of metabisulfite. After a 15-s rinse, such shrimp contain in the edible part about 80 μg SO_2 per gram wet weight and below 10 μg/g after 6 d in ice.[31]

C. APPLICATION OF MODIFIED ATMOSPHERES
1. General Considerations

The term *modified atmosphere* (MA) storage is being used here in its broad meaning, including not only the system where the concentrations of gases surrounding the product are changed before storage but also controlled atmosphere storage, where optimum composition of gases is constantly controlled; vacuum packing, when the package or container is evacuated and sealed; hypobaric storage, where the rigid container is continuously evacuated and resupplied with water vapor; and hyperbaric storage, when the gas atmospheres are under high pressure.

The effectiveness of these systems depends on the effects of the MA on the microflora and on the chemical changes induced in the stored foods. A composition of the MA which is most effective in retarding the growth of spoilage bacteria may cause undesirable color changes in some muscle foods or even induce health hazards by creating conditions favorable for *C. botulinum*. In order to provide safety with respect to outgrowth and toxin production by *C. botulinum* type E, uninterrupted maintenance of the required low temperature during storage should be secured. Fresh fish stored in a vacuum or packaged in CO_2 atmosphere may contain *C. botulinum* toxins, if stored under abuse temperature conditions, before the fish would be regarded as spoiled on the basis of appearance. This could lead to contamination of other foods after opening of the packaged fish.[32] Therefore, the detailed conditions of MA storage must be worked out individually for different foods. The results of microbiological investigations and storage experiments indicate that vacuum packaging may slightly extend the shelf life of seafoods in refrigerated cabinets. The most promising, however, seems to be the application of CO_2-enriched atmospheres.

2. CO_2-Enriched Atmosphere Storage
a. The Inhibitory Effect on Microflora

The preservative effect of CO_2 on muscle foods has been known since the end of the 19th century. During the following decades, much information regarding the sensitivity of various molds and bacteria towards different concentrations of CO_2 in the atmosphere has been acquired. The results were already utilized commercially in the 1930s for refrigerated shipments of beef from Australia and New Zealand to the U.K. Although during the same decade the first papers on the effectiveness of CO_2 for the preservation of wet fish were published, practical applications of CO_2-enriched atmospheres are still rare in the fishing industry. The early investigations and the developments made up until the beginning of the present decade have been reviewed by Parkin and Brown,[33] Finne,[34] and Wilhelm.[35]

CO_2-enriched atmosphere selectively inhibits the growth of the typical spoilage bacteria, i.e., Gram-negative psychrotropic aerobic organisms such as *Pseudomonas* spp., *Acinetobacter*, and *Moraxella*. The *Pseudomonas* spp. are totally inhibited and some die.[36] Thus, during refrigerated storage in CO_2 atmosphere, eventually Gram-positive organisms predominate in the microflora of the fish, mainly *Lactobacillus* spp., and *Alteromonas*. These organisms do not normally participate significantly in spoiling chilled muscle foods. They grow, however, under refrigeration and MA much more slowly than in air at higher temperatures and produce other metabolites than the typical spoilage microflora, thus changing the sensory characteristics of spoilage.

The optimum concentration of CO_2 in the atmosphere depends upon the properties of the product. For storing red meats, especially beef, the concentration of CO_2 should not exceed 25% to avoid discolorations due to formation of metmyoglobin. There are, however, many reports indicating that the preservative effect increases with higher concentrations of CO_2. As for many fish species the risk of myoglobin oxidation is not essential, it has been recommended to use MA containing more CO_2, even up to 100%.

The inhibitory effect of CO_2 on the spoilage microflora increases generally with decrease in temperature, that is, the extension of the shelf life gained by any given CO_2 concentration is longer at a lower than at a higher temperature. Thus, the best result of MA storage can be achieved at temperatures close to the freezing point. This corresponds to the increase in CO_2 solubility with the decrease in temperature of the medium.[37]

The effect of CO_2 is reflected both by an extension of the lag phase and a reduction in the growth rate of the microorganisms. As to the mechanism of CO_2 inhibition of bacterial growth, the following hypotheses have been proposed:[33]

- Interference in the equilibria of enzymatic decarboxylations in the bacterial cells

- Lowering of the pH of the environment and intracellular acidification of the bacteria by formation of carbonic acid from the absorbed CO_2
- Increase in the permeability of microbial membranes which can lead to leakage of essential ions and thus retard some metabolic processes and growth
- Change in the membrane potential of the bacteria

There is a difference of opinion regarding the residual inhibitory effect of MA storage after exposing the fish to air. Some results lead to the conclusion that the inhibition caused by CO_2 terminates upon contact of the fish with air,[34,38] while other experiments have shown a significant residual effect. According to Wang and Ogrydziak,[36] the residual effect is due to the microbial ecology of the system, i.e., the predominance of *Lactobacillus* spp. and *Alteromonas* spp. in the fish held in MA, as well as to the time required by the typical spoilage microflora to recover in air from the CO_2 exposure before the stage of rapid multiplication.

b. The Shelf Life in CO_2-Enriched Atmosphere

The extension of the shelf life of chilled seafoods held in MA over that in air has been generally recognized as significant. Barnett et al.[39] found that headed and gutted Pacific salmon retained acceptable condition over 21 d at 0°C stored in bulk in MA containing 90% CO_2, while the shelf life of such salmon on ice is usually 12 d. According to Villemure et al.,[40] gutted cod and cod fillets held in bulk at 0 ± 1°C and 25% CO_2 + 75% N_2 were of acceptable sensory quality after 20 d. The surface pH after 20 d in the MA-stored fish was 6.6 against that of 7.5 of the samples held in air. There was a high correlation between the sensory quality and the bacterial count and TVN. Snapper fillets kept at −1°C in 200-g pouches, flashed with CO_2 after evacuation, had a shelf life of 18 d, although at a low level of acceptability.[41] A significant retardation of the growth of psychrotropic aerobic Gram-negative spoilage microflora and of the development of TVN, TMA, and total volatile acids was observed in swordfish steaks in retail packages held at 3.5°C in MA containing 100% CO_2 and 40 and 60% CO_2 in combination with either N_2 or O_2. The effect was proportional to the concentration of CO_2 in the package and was higher in samples held in atmospheres containing N_2 instead of O_2.[42] Shucked scallops stored at 4°C in 250-g lots in Cryovac U barrier bags backflushed, after evacuation, with CO_2 had a shelf life of 22 d, i.e., 12 d longer than the controls held in air.[43] Spotted shrimp *Pandalus platyceros* held in a controlled-atmosphere chamber at 100% CO_2 under ice had after 2 weeks only moderate discolorations and no detectable off-odors, while controls kept in air were unacceptable. The high concentration of CO_2 effectively retarded the black spot formation.[44]

However, there are other published results indicating that only minor effects were obtained by holding fish in CO_2-enriched atmospheres. Woyewoda et al.[45] found that bacterial growth and sensory spoilage in cod fillets were only slightly retarded by 60% CO_2 in the atmosphere at 1°C. The small differences between the MA and control samples were detected mainly towards the end of the storage period. Obviously the preservative effect depends not only on the concentration of CO_2 in the atmosphere and on the temperature of storage, but also on the characteristics of the seafood and the exposure of the fish to the MS, affected by gutting and packaging. Generally the difference in quality between the fish held in air and MA increases with the storage time. In several cases, the MA-treated product had some atypical quality defects, such as dessication in fish stored without ice, especially in continuously flashed containers, metallic odor and flavor, as well as increased toughness and fibrousness,[41] or up to twice as large a weight loss as in the fish stored in air.[40]

Additional slight extension of the shelf life of chilled seafoods is possible by combining CO_2-enriched atmosphere storage with K-sorbate treatment,[46,47] or with hypobaric packaging.[48]

D. RADURIZATION

1. Introduction

The bacterial effect of ionizing radiation on the microflora in muscle foods has been investigated since the early 1940s. Fish have been among the first commodities considered suitable for treatment by radiation. The early investigations dealing with radiation of seafoods were reviewed by Coleby and Shewan in 1965.[49] The prospects presented in that review have been to a large extent confirmed by the progress made during the past 25 years. The results of numerous investigations indicate that it is feasible to apply radurization, i.e., low-dose irradiation, below the level of 10 kGy, recognized by the Joint FAO/IAEA/WHO Expert Committee on Food Irradiation as presenting no toxicological hazard, for extending the shelf life of some refrigerated fishery products.[50]

2. The Effect of Ionizing Radiation on Microflora

The radiation resistance of microorganisms is a characteristic depending on the species and strain. It is also effected by the stage of development of the population as well as by the properties of the medium and by the conditions of irradiation.

Gram-negative nonsporing bacteria have the highest sensitivity to ionizing radiation. The D_{10}-value, i.e., the dose required to reduce the initial bacterial population by 90%, is 0.1 to 0.2 kGy for *Pseudomonas* spp. The resistance of several species of pathogenic nonsporing organisms is considerably higher, although of the same order of magnitude, for example, for *Salmonella* spp. D_{10} is 0.2 to 1.0 and for *Staphylococcus aureus* 0.2 to 0.6. Very much higher is the resistance of many strains of *Moraxella-Acinetobacter*. For 97% of 504 strains isolated from marine fish by Münzner, the D_{10}-values were below 0.7 kGy, but for 13 strains, in the stationary phase of growth, at 22°C, they were in the range 0.95 to 1.90 kGy. For strains irradiated at $-80°C$, the D_{10}-values were 2.20 to 2.90 kGy.[51] Among the vegetative cells, exceptionally resistant is *Micrococcus radiodurans*, with a D_{10}-value above 5 kGy, which is about 2.5 times higher than for bacterial spores. Such high resistance of *M. radiodurans* is the effect of an unusually efficient repair system against ionizing radiation.[52] Generally the sensitivity of bacterial spores is about 1 order of magnitude lower than that of vegetative cells — the *Bacillus subtilis* spores are 10 to 12 times as resistant as their vegetative cells. The following D_{10}-values have been reported for the spores of various strains of *B. subtilis*, *C. botulinum* type A, and *C. botulinum* type E, respectively, irradiated in aqueous conditions: 1.00 to 1.46, 1.00 to 2.53, and 0.8 to 1.6 kGy.[52]

A bacterial population in the phase of logarithmic growth is generally more sensitive than the corresponding bacteria in the stationary phase. Populations growing on foods are less sensitive than in synthetic media or in buffer solutions. The sensitivity of bacteria can be increased in the presence of some chemical sensitizers, e.g., enzyme inhibitors or dyes. The exposure of the population to oxygen during irradiation and/or subsequent storage increases the radiation effects.[52]

The resistance of bacteria to ionizing radiations is especially high at low temperature. The D_{10}-value for *Streptococcus faecium* alfa 21 in phosphate buffer at pH 7.0, at 5, -30, and $-196°C$ is 0.9, 2.4, and 3.8 kGy, respectively.[53]

3. Sensory Changes in Irradiated Fish

High doses of ionizing radiation, such as required for radiation sterilization, i.e., reduction of the bacterial number by 12 orders of magnitude to achieve antibotulinum security, brings about distinct undesirable sensory changes in foods, especially development of off-flavors. Special precautions must be taken to avoid these changes, e.g., anoxic packaging and irradiation in the frozen state at $-40°C$ or lower or combination treatment by applying thermal pasteurization and irradiation. Fish, especially of fatty species, are exceptionally prone to these changes. A significant deterioration in sensory quality is detectable at 5 to 10 kGy. Furthermore, the sensory changes which take place gradually during cold storage

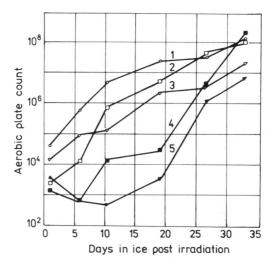

FIGURE 5. The effect of irradiation with 1 kGy and combination treatment on cod fillets sealed in nylon-PVDC-surlyn pouches on the aerobic plate count. (1) Control, (2) irradiated in air atmosphere, (3) irradiated under vacuum, (4) irradiated in an atmosphere of 60% CO_2 and 40% air, and (5) irradiated after dipping 40 s in 5% K-sorbate. All samples were stored in ice. (From Licciardello, J. J., Ravesi, E. M., Tuhkunen, B. E., and Racicot, L. D., *J. Food Sci.*, 49, 1341, 1984. With permission.)

of radurized fish may be atypical, because due to different radioresistance of various species of putrefactive bacteria the composition of the surviving microflora is different from that of the typical population.

4. Feasibility of Commercial Applications

Much effort has been spent in investigating the feasibility of radurization of fresh fish on board, especially in experiments conducted on the American research vessels "Delaware" and "Miller Freemann" and on the West German "Anton Dohrn". The final conclusion of these investigations is that irradiation of whole fish kept on board in open boxes in ice does not result in practical extension of the high-quality shelf life. Although, according to bacteriological and standard chemical tests, the fish irradiated with a dose of 1.5 kGy appeared during storage in ice more fresh than the controls, they were not graded higher by sensory panelists.[54] The high quality life of gutted washed haddock, packed under vacuum in polyethylene pouches, irradiated on board with a maximum dose of 1.8 kGy and kept in ice, did not differ from that of the controls, although it was spoiled after 28 to 35 d, while the vacuum-packed unirradiated fish was unfit for eating after 18 to 21 d.[55]

Radurization of packaged fish fillets with doses of about 1 kGy does not extend the high quality life in ice. It prolongs, however, the period of acceptability by about 1 week to 10 d. In many cases, this could be enough to expand the market for fresh seafood, although it does not help to bring fish of prime freshness into the interior of large continents. Combination treatment by using ionizing radiation and sorbate or CO_2-enriched atmosphere extends the period of acceptability even further (Figure 5).

As the lower dose of ionizing radiation is not effective in reducing the contamination of the fish with *C. botulinum* spores, much effort has been spent to investigate if there is any hazard that the fish become toxic before the onset of spoilage. The conclusion from the available results is that freshly caught seafoods, because of the normally low contamination not exceeding ten spores *C. botulinum* per fish, if held without interruption at temperatures not higher than 5°C, will spoil long before the toxin is detectable, regardless whether radurized or not.[57,58]

Radurization is regarded by some specialists in Europe as an effective means of extending the shelf life of brown shrimp and reducing the hygienic risks in handling such seafoods.[59] The shrimp *Crangon vulgaris*, blanched on board, peeled on shore, and packaged in polyethylene pouches, irradiated after peeling with a minimum dose of 1.3 kGy, had in ice a shelf life of 18 d, while the controls preserved with 1% benzoic acid had a shelf life of 9 d.[60] Irradiation with 1 kGy reduced the number of *Staphylococci*, *Enterococci*, and Enterobacteriaceae by at least two orders of magnitude.[61] For hygienic reasons, radurization is applied in the Netherlands for treatment of imported shrimp.[62]

REFERENCES

1. **Spencer, R. and Baines, C. R.**, The effect of temperature on the spoilage of wet fish. I. Storage at constant temperatures between −1°C and 25°C, *Food Technol.*, 18, 769, 1964.
2. **Olley, J. and Ratkovsky, D. A.**, Temperature function integration and its importance in the storage and distribution of flesh foods above the freezing point, *Food Technol. Aust.*, 25(2), 66, 1973.
3. **Ratkovsky, D. A., Olley, J., McMeekin, T. A., and Ball, A.**, Relationship between temperature and growth rate of bacterial cultures, *J. Bacteriol.*, 149, 1, 1982.
4. **Bremner, H. A., Olley, J., and Vail, A. M. A.**, Estimating time-temperature effects by a rapid systematic sensory method, in *Seafood Quality Determination*, Kramer, D. E. and Liston, J., Eds., Elsevier, Amsterdam, 1986, 413.
5. **Curran, C. A., Poulter, R. G., Brueton, A., and Jones, N. R.**, Effect of handling treatment on fillet yields and quality of tropical fish, *J. Food Technol.*, 21, 301, 1986.
6. **FAO/WHO**, Recommended International Code of Practice for Fresh Fish, CAC/RCP 9-1976, Joint FAO/WHO Food Standards Programme, Codex Alimentarius Commission, World Health Organization, Geneva, 1977.
7. **Cutting, Ch. L.**, *Fish Saving*, Leonard Hill Books, London, 1955, 215.
8. **Hansen, P.**, Improved ice chilling of trawl catches in boxes and containers, *Scandinavian Refrigeration*, 6(5), 262, 1977.
9. **Lima dos Santos, C. A. M.**, The storage of tropical fish in ice — a review, *Trop. Sci.*, 23(2), 97, 1981.
10. **Ranken, M. B. F.**, Superchilling: a new preservation system for wet fishing vessels?, *World Fishing*, 14(2), 60, 1965.
11. **Hopper, A. G. and Merrit, J. H.**, Superchilling — a progress report, *World Fishing*, 15(11), 31, 1966.
12. **Harvie, R. E.**, Importance of Chilling in Producing Top Quality Snapper *Chrysophrys auratus* for the Japanese Market, International Institute of Refrigeration, Commissions C_2, D_1, D_2, D_3, Hamilton, 1982, 127.
13. **Kordyl, E. and Karnicki, Z.**, Factors influencing quality of frozen fish at sea in subtropical and tropical areas, in *Freezing and Irradiation of Fish*, Kreuzer, R., Ed., Fishing News Books, London, 1969, 189.
14. **Gibbard, G., Lee, F., Gibbard, S., and Biliński, E.**, Transport of Salmon over Long Distances by Partial Freezing in RSW Vessels, I.I.F.-I.I.R. Commissions C_2, D_1, D_2, D_3, Boston, 1981, 4.
15. **Ming, Z.**, Application of Partial Freezing Technique on Fishing Vessels Operating in the South China Sea, I.I.F.-I.I.R. Commissions C_2, D_1, D_2, D_3, Boston, 1981, 4.
16. **Golovkin, N. A.**, Storage of food products at temperatures close to the cryoscopic point, in *Proc. 2nd Int. Congr. Food Science and Technology*, Tilgner, D. J. and Borys, A., Eds., Wydawnictwo Przemyslu Lekkiego i Spozywczego, Warsaw, 1967, 161.
17. **Tarr, H. L. A.**, Chemical control of microbiological deterioration, in *Fish as Food*, Vol. 1, Borgstrom, G., Ed., Academic Press, New York, 1961, 639.
18. **Power, H. E., Sinclair, R., and Savagaon, K.**, Use of EDTA compounds for the preservation of haddock fillets, *J. Fish. Res. Board Can.*, 25, 2071, 1968.
19. **Kuusi, T. and Loytomaki, M.**, On the effectiveness of EDTA in prolonging the shelf life of fresh fish, *Z. Lebensm. Unters. Forsch.*, 149, 196, 1972.
20. **Boyd, J. W. and Southcott, B. A.**, Comparative effectiveness of ethylenediaminetetraacetic acid and chlorotetracycline for fish preservation, *J. Fish. Res. Board Can.*, 25, 1753, 1968.
21. **Field, C. E., Pivarnik, L. F., Barnett, S. M., and Rand, A. G.**, Utilization of glucose oxidase for extending the shelf life of fish, *J. Food Sci.*, 51, 66, 1986.
22. **Shaw, S. J., Bligh, E. G., and Woyevoda, A. D.**, Spoilage pattern of Atlantic cod fillets treated with glucose oxidase/gluconic acid, *Can. Inst. Food Sci. Technol. J.*, 19(1), 3, 1986.

23. **Lueck, E.**, *Antimicrobial Food Additives*, Springer-Verlag, Berlin, 1980, chap. 24.
24. **Sofos, J. N. and Busta, F. F.**, Antimicrobial activity of sorbate, *J. Food Prot.*, 44, 614, 1981.
25. **Eklund, T.**, The antimicrobial effect of dissociated and undissociated sorbic acid at different pH levels, *J. Appl. Bacteriol.*, 54, 383, 1983.
26. **Shaw, S. J., Bligh, E. G., and Woyewoda, A. D.**, Effect of potassium sorbate application on shelf life of Atlantic cod *Gadus morhua*, *Can. Inst. Food Sci. Technol. J.*, 16(4), 237, 1983.
27. **Statham, J. A.**, Sorbate extends shelf-life of scallops, *Aust. Fish.*, 42(7), 1983.
28. **Bremner, H. A. and Statham, J. A.**, Effect of potassium sorbate on refrigerated storage of vacuum packed scallops, *J. Food Sci.*, 48, 1042, 1983.
29. **Fletcher, G. C., Murrell, W. G., Statham, J. A., Stewart, B. J., and Bremner, H. A.**, Packaging of scallops with sorbate: as assessment of the hazard from *Clostridium botulinum*, *J. Food Sci.*, 53, 349, 1988.
30. **Ruello, J. H.**, Storage of prawns in refrigerated sea water, *Australian Fisheries*, 33(2), 1, 1974.
31. **Finne, G., Wagner, T., DeWitt, D., and Martin, R.**, Effect of treatment, ice storage and freezing on residual sulfite in shrimp, *J. Food Sci.*, 51, 231, 1986.
32. **Post, L. S., Lee, D. A., Solberg, M., Furgang, D., Specchio, J., and Graham, Ch.**, Development of botulinal toxin and sensory deterioration during storage of vacuum and modified atmosphere packaged fish fillets, *J. Food Sci.*, 50, 990, 1985.
33. **Parkin, K. L. and Brown, W. D.**, Preservation of seafood with modified atmospheres, in *Chemistry and Biochemistry of Marine Food Products*, Martin, R. E., Flick, G. E., Hebard, C. E., and Ward, D. R., Eds., AVI Publishing, Westport, CT, 1982, 453.
34. **Finne, G.**, Modified — and controlled — atmosphere storage of muscle foods, *Food Technol.*, 36(2), 128, 1982.
35. **Wilhelm, K. A.**, Extended fresh storage of fishery products with modified atmospheres: a survey, *Marine Fish. Rev.*, 44(2), 17, 1982.
36. **Wang, M. Y. and Ogrydziak, D. M.**, Residual effect of storage in an elevated carbon dioxide atmosphere on the microbial flora of rock cod *(Sebastes spp.)*, *Appl. Environ. Microbiol.*, 52, 727, 1986.
37. **Ogrydziak, D. M. and Brown, W. D.**, Temperature effects in modified-atmosphere storage of seafoods, *Food Technol.*, 36(5), 86, 1982.
38. **Banks, H., Nickelson, R., and Finne, G.**, Shelf-life studies on carbon dioxide packaged finfish from the Gulf of Mexico, *J. Food Sci.*, 45, 175, 1980.
39. **Barnett, H. J., Stone, F. E., Roberts, G. C., Hunter, P. J., Nelson, R. W., and Kwok, J.**, A study in the use of high concentration of CO_2 in a modified atmosphere to preserve fresh salmon, *Marine Fish. Rev.*, 42(3), 7, 1982.
40. **Villemure, G., Simard, R. E., and Picard, G.**, Bulk storage of cod fillets and gutted cod *(Gadus morhua)* under carbon dioxide atmosphere, *J. Food Sci.*, 51, 317, 1986.
41. **Scott, D. N., Fletcher, G. C., and Hogg, M. G.**, Storage of snapper fillets in modified atmospheres at $-1°C$, *Food Technol. Aust.*, 38, 234, 1986.
42. **Lannelongue, M., Finne, G., Hanna, M. O., Nickelson, R., and Vanderzant, C.**, Microbiological and chemical changes during storage of swordfish *(Xiphias gladius)* steaks in retail packages containing CO_2-enriched atmospheres, *J. Food Prot.*, 45, 1197, 1982.
43. **Bremner, H. A. and Statham, J. A.**, Packaging in CO_2 extends shelf-life of scallops, *Food Technol. Aust.*, 39, 177, 1987.
44. **Matches, J. R. and Layrisse, M. E.**, Controlled atmosphere storage of spotted shrimp *(Pandalus platyceros)*, *J. Food Prot.*, 48, 709, 1985.
45. **Woyewoda, A. D., Bligh, E. G., and Shaw, S. J.**, Controlled and modified atmosphere storage of cod fillets, *Can. Inst. Food Sci. Technol. J.*, 17, 24, 1984.
46. **Fey, M. S. and Regenstein, J. M.**, Extending shelf life of fresh wet red hake and salmon using CO_2-O_2 modified atmosphere and potassium sorbate ice at $-1°C$, *J. Food Sci.*, 47, 1048, 1982.
47. **Statham, J. A., Bremner, H. A., and Quarmby, A. R.**, Storage of morwong *(Nemadactylus macropterus* Bloch and Schneider) in combinations of polyphosphate, potassium sorbate and carbon dioxide at 4°C, *J. Food Sci.*, 50, 1580, 1985.
48. **Haard, N. F. and Lee, Y. Z.**, Hypobaric storage of Atlantic salmon in a carbon dioxide atmosphere, *Can. Inst. Food Sci. Technol. J.*, 15, 68, 1982.
49. **Coleby, B. and Shewan, J. M.**, The radiation preservation of fish, in *Fish as Food*, Vol. 4, Borgstrom, G., Ed., Academic Press, New York, 1965, 419.
50. Wholesomeness of Irradiated Food. Report of a Joint FAO/IAEA/WHO Expert Committee, Tech. Rep. Ser. 659, World Health Organization, Geneva, 1981.
51. **Münzner, R.**, Investigations on radiation resistance strains of *Moraxella-acinetobacter* isolated from sea fish, Archiv für Lebensmittelhygiene, 28, 195, 1977, (German).
52. **Russell, A. D.**, *The Destruction of Bacterial Spores*, Academic Press, London, 1982, chap. 4 and 9.
53. **Annellis, A., Berkowitz, D., and Kemper, D.**, Comparative resistance of nonsporogenic bacteria to low temperature gamma irradiation, *Appl. Microbiol.*, 25, 517, 1973.

54. **Ehlermann, D. A. E. and Reinacher, E.**, Some conclusions from shipboard experiments on the radurization of whole fish in the Federal Republic of Germany, in *Food Preservation by Irradiation*, Vol. 1, International Atomic Energy Agency, Vienna, 1978, 321.
55. **Ehlermann, D., Reinacher, E., and Antonacopoulos, N.**, Shipboard irradiation of haddock, *Chem. Mikrobiol. Technol. Lebensm.*, 5, 81, 1977, (in German).
56. **Licciardello, J. J., Ravesi, E. M., Tuhkunen, B. E., and Racicot, L. D.**, Effect of some potentially synergistic treatments in combination with 100 krad irradiation on the iced shelf life of cod fillets, *J. Food Sci.*, 49, 1341, 1984.
57. **Hobbs, G.**, Clostridium botulinum in irradiated fish, *Food Irradiation Information*, No. 7, 39, 1977.
58. **Giddings, G. G.**, Radiation processing of fishery products, *Food Technol.*, 38, 61, 1984.
59. **Ehlermann, D. and Diehl, J. F.**, Economic aspects of the introduction of radiation preservation of brown shrimp in the Federal Republic of Germany, *Radiat. Phys. Chem.*, 9, 875, 1977.
60. **Ehlermann, D. and Münzner, R.**, Radurization of brown shrimps, *Arch. Lebensmittelhyg.*, 27, 50, 1976, (in German).
61. **Münzner, R.**, Microbiological investigations on irradiated shrimps, *Lebens. Wiss. Technol.*, 7, 288, 1974, (in German).
62. **Grünewald, T.**, Irradiation of foods, *Z. Lebensm. Unters. Forsch.*, 180, 357, 1985, (in German).

Chapter 7

FREEZING OF MARINE FOOD

Zdzisław E. Sikorski and Anna Kołakowska

TABLE OF CONTENTS

I. The Preserving Action of Freezing...112
   A. Formation of Ice Crystals 112
   B. The Effect on Microorganisms 112
   C. The Rate of Chemical Changes..112

II. Deteriorative Changes in Frozen Stored Fish 114
   A. Changes in Proteins 114
      1. Nature of Changes and Effect on Product Quality 114
      2. Causative Factors 114
   B. Changes in Lipids 116
      1. Nature of Changes 116
      2. Lipolysis..116
      3. Lipid Oxidation 117
      4. Interactions 118

III. Commercial Freezing of Marine Food 119
   A. Preparation before Freezing 119
   B. Freezing Methods and Equipment 119
      1. Rate of Freezing 119
      2. Types of Freezers 119
   C. The Storage Life of Frozen Marine Food..............................120
      1. Factors Affecting the Frozen Shelf Life..........................120
      2. Protection against Dehydration and Oxidation 121
      3. Time Temperature Tolerance (TTT) 121

References...122

I. THE PRESERVING ACTION OF FREEZING

A. FORMATION OF ICE CRYSTALS

Freezing food means reducing the temperature below the freezing point so that most of the water contained in the material turns into ice. The freezing point depends upon the concentration of different solutes in the tissue fluids. For cod and haddock it is in the range -0.8 to $-1°C$, for halibut -1 to $-1.2°C$, and for herring about $1.4°C$.

The rate of temperature decrease in the product, at constant outer temperature, changes in time (Figure 1). This is due to the fact that most of the latent heat of crystallization is removed in the range between -1 and $-5°C$ and that the thermal diffusivity of the material increases due to formation of ice crystals. Below $-10°C$, the increase in the amount of ice is very slow (Table 1). Complete solidification of the liquid phase in cod muscle takes place at about $-70°C$.

The rate of freezing, that is, of the movement of the ice front, effects the histological changes in the frozen tissues, as it controls the size and distribution of the ice crystals. During slow freezing, at about 0.2 cm/h, the rate of nucleation is lower than that of water migration from within the cells, where the concentration of the solutes is initially higher, into the intracellular spaces, where the initial salt concentration is lower but increases in the course of freezing due to crystallization. Thus, in slowly frozen muscle, large ice crystals are formed in the intercellular spaces, while at high freezing rates, e.g., 5 cm/h, a large number of small crystals is evenly distributed throughout the whole cross-section of the tissue. Large ice crystals in the intercellular spaces may cause some damage to the histological structure of the muscle.

B. THE EFFECT ON MICROORGANISMS

Low water activity of the liquid phase in frozen fish, caused by concentration of the solutes due to formation of ice, as well as the low temperature of storage, are at least inhibitory for bacterial activity and have a lethal effect on some microorganisms. Some psychrotropic bacteria are able to grow even at temperatures below the freezing point, albeit at a much lower rate than in unfrozen tissue. The lowest recorded growth temperature for these bacteria is about $-10°C$. Some molds and yeasts are able to multiply very slowly at temperatures as low as -15 to $-18°C$.

The lethal effect of freezing and frozen storage is higher between -4 and $-10°C$ than at lower temperatures. Most sensitive are the vegetative forms of yeasts, molds, and Gram-negative bacteria, while Gram-positive bacteria and spores are more resistant. The lethal effect is higher in water and buffer solutions than in foods and increases due to repeated thawing/freezing. The reduction in the number of viable cells may be as high as two orders of magnitude. It is accompanied by a change in the composition of the microflora, as mainly sensitive types are affected. After defrosting, however, the surviving microorganisms find often better conditions for proliferation than in unfrozen fish due to the availability of the thaw drip and to freezing/thawing-induced textural changes in the product.

C. THE RATE OF CHEMICAL CHANGES

Preservation of foods by freezing involves not only the microbial aspects but also retards the chemical and biochemical deteriorative changes. Low temperature decreases the rate of reactions according to the Arrhenius equation:

$$\ln k = \ln A - \frac{E}{RT}$$

where k is the reaction rate constant, A is the frequency factor, E is the activation energy, R is the gas constant, and T is the temperature. However, as the reaction rate depends not

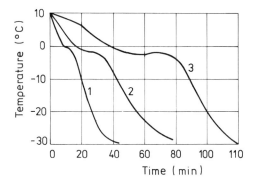

FIGURE 1. The temperature in a block of fish fillets, 75 mm thick, frozen in a plate freezer at −33°C. (1) Surface; (2) 10 mm deep; and (3) center of the block.

TABLE 1
Amount of Ice in Frozen Muscle Formed at Different Temperatures

Temperature °C	Ice %[a]	Temperature °C	Ice %[a]
0	0	−8	82
−1	8	−9	83
−2	52	−10	84
−3	66	−12	86
−4	73	−15	87
−5	77	−20	89
−6	79	−30	90
−7	81	−40	90

[a] Percent of total water content.

Data from Riedel, L., *Kältetechnik*, 8, 374, 1956.

only on the temperature, significant deviations from the above relationship occur in higher freezing temperatures. In the critical zone −1 to −5°C, the rate-enhancing effect of freeze concentration of different solutes, including catalysts and enzyme systems, overrides in some tissues the pure temperature effect to such a degree that the rate of many reactions is higher than above the freezing point. The enzymatic degradation of glycogen in haddock muscle was found by Sharp to proceed at −2°C at least twice as fast as at 0°C.[2] A substantial increase in the degradation rate of glycogen and organic phosphates in cod muscle in the range of temperatures −1 to −5°C, over that in unfrozen fish, was described by Nowlan and Dyer.[3]

Even low storage temperatures do not prevent very slow chemical and enzymatic changes in frozen fish. Generally freezing does not completely inactivate most of the enzymes, although at very low temperatures the activity may decrease significantly. In swordfish muscles, the accumulation of Hy, in micromoles per gram, proceeds at −18°C and −26°C according to the following equations:

$$Hy_{-18} = 0.46 + 0.0316\ t$$

and

$$Hy_{-26} = 0.30 + 0.0007\ t$$

where t is the time of storage in weeks.[4] Although the deteriorative reactions are very slow at $-30°C$, their results, nevertheless, cause changes in sensory properties of frozen fish over many months of storage. The tissue components mostly involved in these changes are proteins and lipids.

II. DETERIORATIVE CHANGES IN FROZEN STORED FISH

A. CHANGES IN PROTEINS
1. Nature of Changes and Effect on Product Quality

Frozen storage may lead to extensive alterations in the proteins of fish meat known as freeze denaturation. These changes involve both denaturation proper, i.e., unfolding of the molecules, and secondary reactions between the reactive groups of different proteins and other components of the fish muscles, leading to cross-linking and formation of aggregates. The proteins lose at least part of their solubility and may have lower enzyme activity. As the result of these changes, a significant deterioration of the functional properties of the fish meat may occur. It is manifested by a decrease in water retention, gel-forming ability, and lipid-emulsifying capacity, as well as by worsening of the texture and increased dryness of the fish meat. The texture of fish kept very long at about $-18°C$ is often described as tough, chewy, rubbery, stringy, crumbly, and fibrous.

2. Causative Factors

Freeze denaturation of fish proteins has been reviewed by several authors, including Connell,[5] Sikorski et al.,[6] Matsumoto,[7] and Shenouda.[8] The factors involved mainly comprise the denaturing and catalytic effect of ice and inorganic salts, the binding of fatty acids and lipid oxidation products, cross-linking induced by formaldehyde generated in the muscles of some fish, and other possible reactions leading to the formation of new covalent bonds in denatured proteins.

Ice crystallization may disturb the water structures surrounding the areas of hydrophobic interactions in proteins. It may also disrupt the water-mediated hydrophobic-hydrophilic interactions, which participate in buttressing the native conformation of protein molecules.[9] By increasing the concentration of salts in the unfrozen pools of water, it may decrease the hydration of proteins, as the concentrated inorganic ions compete for the water molecules. Divalent cations are able to form cross-links by reacting with ionized acid side chains in proteins. The slight shifts in pH in frozen stored fish may favor such interactions.[10] Furthermore, inorganic salts may participate in the freeze denaturation of proteins by catalyzing the hydrolysis and autooxidation of lipids.[11]

Free fatty acids significantly decrease the solubility of myofibrillar proteins in model systems. In frozen fish they accumulate during storage (see Section II.B) and may contribute to the formation of aggregates by binding to proteins due to hydrophobic interactions. Their role is more pronounced in lean fish than in fish flesh containing a few percent lipids. In fish muscles with intramuscular fat deposits, the free fatty acids may be less available for interactions with proteins, as they preferentially associate with the lipid phase. Oxidized fatty acids and secondary products of autoxidation, especially aldehydes, are much more damaging to protein solubility than the acids themselves, as they are able to form covalent bonds with reactive protein groups (Figure 2).

In frozen muscles of some species of fish, the trimethylamine oxide (TMAO) undergoes degradation to trimethylamine (TMA) and formaldehyde. The aldehyde accumulating during frozen storage, being a very reactive compound known to interact with different functional groups in proteins, may bind to some groups in protein side chains and form intra- and intermolecular methylene bridges, e.g.,

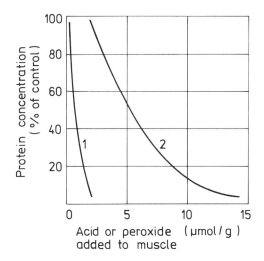

FIGURE 2. Protein concentration in centrifuged KCl extracts of cod muscle myofibrils after incubation for 2.5 h at 2°C with (1) linoleic acid hydroperoxide and (2) linoleic acid. (Data from Jahrenbäck, L. and Liljemark, A., *J. Food Technol.*, 10, 437, 1975.)

$RNH_2 + CH_2O \rightarrow RNHCH_2OH$

$RCONH_2 + CH_2O \rightarrow RCONHCH_2OH$

$RCONH_2 + RCONHCH_2OH \rightarrow RCONHCH_2NHCOR + H_2O$

$ROH + CH_2O \rightarrow ROCH_2OH$

$2\ ROH + CH_2O \rightarrow ROCH_2OH + H_2O$

$2\ RSH + CH_2O \rightarrow RSCH_2SR + H_2O$

These reactions may be involved in the formation of protein aggregates and may decrease the protein solubility. Formaldehyde is especially important in the freeze denaturation of proteins in some Gadidae. Its role is more evident in fish minces than in whole fish or fillets. By removing the water-soluble substrate and the enzyme system responsible for the degradation of TMAO, the undesirable protein changes can be effectively reduced. On the other hand, the decrease in the concentration of TMAO in fish meat may by itself contribute to freeze denaturation, as the TMAO may serve in the fish muscle as a protective osmolyte.[13]

Other covalent bonds which could contribute to protein aggregation are the disulfide bridges. Although significant changes in the number of -SH groups in fish proteins due to freezing and prolonged frozen storage have not been reported, some cross-linking could take place without net change in the total -SH groups. This has been shown by Buttkus[14] in oxidation and SH-disulfide exchange reactions.

The deteriorative protein changes in frozen fish are caused by several factors and interactions with other tissue components (Table 2). The importance of these factors depends in each case upon the species characteristics of the fish, i.e., the composition of the flesh and on the parameters of processing and storage. Mincing of the meat before freezing, conditions that promote the oxidation of the tissue lipids, high frozen storage temperature, and long storage times lead to extensive deteriorative reactions. On the other hand, removing the water-soluble components from the minced meat, protecting against oxidation, and adding suitable cryoprotectors is effective in suppressing freeze denaturation.

TABLE 2
Protein Changes in Frozen Fish

Native Proteins — Water — Ions
↓
Partial damage to histological structure by ice crystals, release of enzymes
Changes in water structures due to crystallization, alterations in hydrogen bonding, and hydrophobic interactions
Concentration of salts and competition for hydration water
Hydrolysis of lipids and hydrophobic interactions of free fatty acids
↓
Denatured Proteins — Water — Ions
↓
Oxidation of lipids and reactions of oxidation products with proteins
Demethylation of TMAO and reactions of formaldehyde with protein functional groups
Oxidation and −SH-disulfide exchange reactions
↓
Denatured and Aggregated Proteins

B. CHANGES IN LIPIDS
1. The Nature of Changes

The changes in lipids are directly and indirectly responsible for the quality deterioration in frozen seafoods. They involve lipolysis, lipid oxidation, and interactions of the products of these processes with nonlipid components.

The endogenous fish lipases are relatively resistant to low temperatures and retain much of their activity in the frozen tissues. Some of them may even be activated in the freezing process, e.g., by release from lysosomes.[15] The free fatty acids, accumulating in the meat during frozen storage, in extreme cases up to about 500 mg/g wet weight, have no effect on the sensory quality of the product. However, they may contribute to texture deterioration by reacting with proteins (see Section II.A.2) and affect oxidative lipid changes.

Lipid oxidation in frozen stored seafoods is primarily nonenzymic in nature, although recently the involvement of microsomal enzymes and lipoxygenase has been reported. In fish containing more than 2% lipids, the oxidation products significantly decrease the sensory odor and flavor scores. On the other hand, in lean fish and shellfish, they have no direct effect on these sensory properties, although they can participate in protein aggregation and in undesirable discolorations in the meat.

2. Lipolysis

In frozen stored seafoods, lipolysis begins with degradation of phospholipids:

$$
\begin{array}{c}
CH_2OR_1 \\
| \\
CHOR_2 \\
| \\
CHOPOX
\end{array}
\xrightarrow{\text{phospholipase } A_2}
\begin{array}{c}
CH_2OR_1 \\
| \\
CHOH \\
| \\
CHOPOX
\end{array}
\xrightarrow{\text{lysophospholipase}}
\begin{array}{c}
CHOH \\
| \\
CHOH \\
| \\
CHOPOX
\end{array}
$$

where X is choline, ethanolamine, serine, etc. Lysophospholipases are usually most active; hence, some fish such as horse mackerel, herring, flounder, and cod contain low amounts of lysophospholipids which are, on the other hand, accumulated preferentially by certain other species, e.g., sardine and skipjack.[16]

Phospholipid hydrolysis is the main cause of rapid accumulation of free fatty acids in the frozen flesh of many species of fish.[17] The rate of decomposition is such that after 1 year of storing lean fish at −20°C, the phospholipid content decreases to 20 to 40% of its initial value.[18] Higher temperatures, e.g., −10°C, may result in decomposition of most phospholipids already during the first month of storage.

Triacylglycerols are hydrolyzed in frozen fish less easily, while the cholesterol esters and waxes change to a slight degree only. The lipases in dark muscle are more active than in white muscle. On the other hand, phospholipases have a similar activity in both types of muscles.[18]

The free fatty acid content is the most popular measure of lipolysis in fish. It correlates closely with time and temperature of storage and depends on fish species; e.g., the rates (micromoles per day per 100 g) of free fatty acid formation in minced flesh stored at $-20°C$ for about 100 d were 12.0 in Alaska pollack, 8.0 in mackerel, 3.1 in yellowtail, and 2.0 in squids.[19] In a given species, the rate of lipolysis depends on the time of harvest, sex, gonad maturity, and also on numerous factors related to processing techniques. Mincing, blending, and prefreezing storage accelerate lipolysis in frozen fish.[20] Storing krill for 12 h prior to freezing accelerates phospholipid hydrolysis and activates triacylglycerol hydrolysis in the frozen product.[21] Free fatty acids may amount even to about 30% of total lipids in lean fish and shellfish and as little as a few percent of lipids in fatty fish.

3. Lipid Oxidation

Lipid oxidation is assumed to proceed along the classical free radical route:

$$\text{initiation} \quad RH \rightarrow R^\bullet + H^\bullet$$

$$RH + O_2 \rightarrow R^\bullet + {}^\bullet OOH$$

$$\text{propagation} \quad R^\bullet + O_2 \rightarrow RO_2^\bullet$$

$$RO_2^\bullet + RH \rightarrow RO_2H + R^\bullet$$

$$\text{termination} \quad R^\bullet + R^\bullet \rightarrow R-R$$

$$RO_2^\bullet + R^\bullet \rightarrow RO_2R$$

and the photooxidation route:

$${}^1O_2^\bullet + RH \rightarrow ROOH$$

where RH = unsaturated lipid; $R^\bullet$ = lipid radical; $RO_2^\bullet$ = lipid peroxyradical; and ${}^1O_2^\bullet$ = excited singlet oxygen. The rate of photooxidation is about three orders of magnitude higher than that of autoxidation.

The hydroperoxides are very unstable and break down to aldehydes, ketones, alcohols, short-chain fatty acids, and hydrocarbons. Volatile carbonyl compounds are thought to be responsible for the rancid odor and flavor. It is mainly cis-4-heptenal in frozen-stored cod and 2,4,7-decatrienals in oxidized mackerel oil, although none of these compounds has a typical rancid odor.[22,23]

The oxidation products are very reactive and decrease the sensory attractiveness, functional properties, and nutritional value of the frozen fish. They may also be toxic — the LD_{50} of the hydroperoxide of highly unsaturated fatty acids is between 280 and 550 mg active hydroperoxide oxygen per kilogram body weight of rat.[24] Symptoms of rancid fat toxicity observed in experimental animals are poor growth rate, cardiomyopathy, hepatomegaly, steatitis, hemolytic anemia, and secondary deficiencies of vitamins E and A. The oxidation products may also be atherogenic and carcinogenic.

In lean fish and shellfish, the products of phospholipid hydrolysis are thought to function as antioxidants. Cod lipid oxidation during frozen storage is extremely slow and sensorily

TABLE 3
Peroxide Value[a] as a Quality Criterion of Frozen Fish

| | Mackerel Dressed fish and fillet | | Herring | | | |
| | | | Whole fish | | Fillet | |
Grade	Lipid	Tissue	Lipid	Tissue	Lipid	Tissue
I	<6	<0.6	<12	0.8	<22	—
II	6—40	0.6—1.7	12—50	—	>22	0.8—3.8
Unfit	>40	>1.7	>60	—	—	>5.5

Note: Peroxide value, mg O per 100 g. [a] Thiocyanate technique.

After Kolakowska, A. and Szybowicz, Z., *Chlodnictwo*, 16(7—8), 37, 1981, (in Polish). With permission.

nondetectable. Effects of lipid oxidation are indirectly observable as brown pigmentation on the surface of a frozen fish fillet block and as deteriorated texture of the fillets.

Lipid oxidation in shellfish is presumably retarded also by nonproteinaceous nitrogen compounds. Regardless, however, of the absence of direct sensory signals of rancidity, lipid oxidation is evidenced, for example, in prawns by a 70% decrease in the contents of $C_{22:6}$ and $C_{20:5}$ acids after 6 months of storage at $-18°C$.[25]

Lipid oxidation in frozen fish is a net result of interactions of numerous factors such as lipid composition, i.e., contents and composition of unsaturated fatty acids, molecular species of the phospholipids and triacylglycerols, contents of pro- and antioxidants, pH, and the amount of unfrozen water. Because of these factors and their interactions, the control of storage conditions does not suffice to predict rancidity rate in frozen seafoods. The rancidity rate varies even in the same species. The periods elapsing before various batches of fish attain the same lipid oxidation level may differ even by as much as 4 months. In herring and mackerel, whose lipid contents vary considerably throughout the year, the fastest lipid oxidation during frozen storage was revealed in muscles of emaciated specimens. However, even individuals of the same species and of similar lipid contents may differ in their lipid oxidation level by a factor of three after several months of storage. The rancidity rate depends on the degree of processing before freezing. In Baltic herring, the rate of lipid oxidation increases in the following order: whole fish, fillets with skin, mince, headed fish, skinned fillets.[20] Skin forms a barrier to oxidation; the barrier is less efficient if the skin lacks scales and black pigments. On the other hand, the presence of lipoxygenase in the skin accelerates oxidation, which is particularly evident in frozen minces contaminated with skin fragments.

Short-term storage of lean fish before freezing retards lipid oxidation in Baltic herring. This treatment, applied to Antarctic krill, inhibits carotenoid oxidation. It is presumably the result of antioxidation by products of autolysis.

The results of sensory assessment of rancidity correlate poorly with the storage time of frozen fish. For the most widespread tests, best correlations are recorded for peroxide value (PV) and TBA, e.g., for horse mackerel stored and $-28°C$ the PV (mgO per 100 g lipids) = $4.22x + 26.17$ where x is the time of storage in months.[26] The PV is proposed as a quality criterion for frozen fish (Table 3).

4. Interactions

Lipolysis and lipid peroxidation effect each other, but the nature of this interaction is not quite straightforward. Hydrolysis may accelerate the oxidation of triacylglycerols. On the other hand, oxidation of phospholipids may be inhibited by hydrolysis.[28] Lipid peroxidation may modulate the susceptibility of phospholipids to specific phospholipases. There are numerous interactions of fish lipids and their oxidation products with proteins (see Section II.A). These interactions may result in various lipid-protein complexes as well as different low-molecular products. Among others, reddish-brown subtances are formed whose *in vivo* equivalents are lipofuscine aging pigments, used to assess the age of marine shellfish. They are formed by reaction of conjugated carbonyl compounds of eicosapentaenoate with amino acids or with taurine in squids.[29,30] Lipid-protein interaction retards lipid oxidation during storage.

III. COMMERCIAL FREEZING OF MARINE FOOD

A. PREPARATION BEFORE FREEZING

In the contemporary fishing industry, freezing is applied for preserving marine fish and invertebrates both on board vessel and on shore. Depending on the characteristics and the intended use of the product, as well as on the availability of space, time, and facilities, the catch is frozen in different forms of preparation. Mollusks may be frozen in shell, e.g., cockles, or after shucking, e.g., oysters. Crustaceans are mainly prepared by cooking, peeling, and grading of the meats. However, raw crustaceans are also frozen, e.g., headed or headed and shelled shrimp, whole raw lobster, or spiny lobster tails. Squid are frozen in blocks, whole or after heading and gutting. Many species of fish are not processed before freezing, e.g., tuna intended for canning, or small fish like herring and sprats to be used off-season for smoking, canning, etc. The most widespread form of preparation of fish for freezing, however, is filleting and mincing. The fillets to be frozen on board are usually formed in standardized blocks, suitable for further mechanical cutting and processing to fish fingers, while in shore facilities they are prepared in retail packages. The fish minces are usually leached with fresh water and cryoprotectors are added (see Chapter 12). For freezing seafood in different forms of preparation, specialized equipment is available.

B. FREEZING METHODS AND EQUIPMENT

1. Rate of Freezing

Generally the methods and facilities employed in the modern fishing industry promote quick freezing due to high heat transfer rates, low temperature of the freezing medium, and small dimensions of the product, at least in one direction of the heat flow.

For most practical purposes, the time required for freezing fish of a shape resembling that of a slab or a cylinder can be predicted on the basis of formulas developed by Plank,[31] provided that the following simplifying assumptions are made

- The product has been previously chilled to the freezing point.
- The total amount of heat during freezing is removed at the freezing point.
- The material is homogenous and isotropic.
- The thermal conductivity and specific heat of the fish are constant during freezing.

These assumptions, however, lead to underestimation of the freezing time when compared with experimental results. Other numerous equations developed by various investigators take into consideration total enthalpy changes from the initial temperature of the fish to that in the frozen product leaving the freezer, phase changes that occur over a wide range of temperatures, as well as changing properties of the fish.[32-35] A comprehensive review on prediction of freezing and thawing times for foods was recently prepared by Cleland et al.[36]

2. Types of Freezers

The choice of the freezing system to be used on board vessel or on shore for the given marine food is made with respect to quality of the final product, the capital requirements and cost of operation, as well as convenience, maintenance problems, and space limitations.

Different types of air-blast freezers have had widespread application because of their high versatility. They are suitable for freezing whole fish of various shapes and sizes, in hanging position, on trays stacked on trolleys or in cabinets as well as on conveyor belts, for individual or block freezing, for products wrapped or packed as well as for unpacked large round fish, in batch system or in continuous operation. Because of such flexibility, blast freezers have been installed not only in shore plants but also on large freezer trawlers. The air at -30 to $-40°C$ is recirculated in a blast freezer at a velocity of 4 to 6 m/s, causing fairly rapid freezing. The time required for lowering the internal temperature from 5 to $-20°C$ in a cod fillet block, 5 cm thick, on a metal tray, is about 2 h. Unpackaged fish may lose several percent of weight in a blast freezer due to evaporation and sublimation and may develop freezer burn (see below).

Fluidized-bed blast freezers are used in the fishing industry for individual quick freezing of small mollusks and shrimp as well as fish fingers. These installations are very compact, freeze unpacked small products in less than 20 min, and work continuously.

Brine freezing was valued in the first half of this century as an inexpensive way of quick freezing. It was used in the fishing industry as the Ottesen method involving direct immersion of the fish in eutectic solution of NaCl at $-21°C$ or by spraying the product with recirculating refrigerated brine.[37] In tuna fisheries, such brine has been used for quick freezing of fish on board directly in the wells. With the development of other equipment, brine freezing lost its importance, as the direct contact of fish with salt accelerates lipid oxidation and for freezing of packed products other methods are more suitable.

Plate freezers are mainly employed for freezing fillets in consumer packs or marine products in blocks, as tight contact with the frozen material is the prerequisite for efficient utilization of the high rate of heat transfer by conduction to the plates at $-40°C$. A large variety of available facilities, comprising installations with vertical or horizontal series of plates, working batchwise or continuously, of different capacities, for manual or automatic operation including loading/unloading, makes it possible to select the most suitable type for the specific purpose. A common characteristic for all types is minimum dehydration of the product and high rate of freezing. A fillet block, 5.7 cm thick in a waxed carton is usually frozen to $-20°C$ in less than 90 min. A plate freezer generally needs less space and energy than an air-blast installation with the same output.

Cryogenic freezers are used mainly for individual rapid freezing of oysters, shrimp, small fillets, etc. The equipment is suitable for being seasonally installed, e.g., during the oyster harvest in remote fishing areas lacking many other industrial premises. The freezing rate is very high due to direct contact of liquid nitrogen at $-196°C$, carbon dioxide at $-78.5°C$, or dichlorodifluoromethane at $-29.8°C$ with the food. To avoid quality defects caused by excessively rapid freezing in liquid nitrogen, the material is first exposed on the conveyor belt to cold circulating nitrogen gas and only before the exit from the tunnel meets a liquid nitrogen spray. Cryogenic freezing of unpackaged food causes minor losses of weight of about 0.5%.

C. THE STORAGE LIFE OF FROZEN MARINE FOOD
1. Factors Affecting the Frozen Shelf Life

The factors involved comprise the properties of the fish, the protection of the product against oxidation, loss of moisture, and protein changes, as well as the rate of freezing, temperature, and stability during storage. The properties inherent to the product comprise the contents and distribution of lipids, the ability to generate large amounts of formaldehyde, the initial freshness, and the preparation before freezing by bleeding, gutting, filleting, skinning, peeling, mincing, leaching, and cooking.

The biochemical and chemical changes leading to quality loss of frozen fish during storage have been treated in Section II. Practical measures aimed at prolonging the shelf life of different frozen marine food products comprise adding of various stabilizers and extenders (see Chapter 12), glazing, use of protecting coatings, proper packaging, and control of storage temperature.

2. Protection against Dehydration and Oxidation

Dehydration of frozen fish, which causes a dry and wrinkled appearance on the surface and toughening of the outer layers of the pack, is known as freezer burn. These quality defects are detectable in consumer packs of frozen fillets, when the weight loss due to dehydration is about 0.5% or higher.[38] Freezer burn may be inhibited or prevented by glazing or impervious wrapping.

Glazing is an old, effective, and inexpensive technique which has been in use since the beginnings of commercial freezing of fish.[39] By sliding the frozen fish through cold tap water, a glaze of ice is formed on the surface. The thickness of the glaze depends on the number of passes through the water. Usually several percent weight is added to the product. The glazing should be repeated after 4 to 5 months of storage to renew the protective layer of ice.

By using a dip of alginate solution, a coating of gel can be formed on the fish frozen in blocks. This coating not only protects the product against dehydration, but also facilitates taking the block apart prior to final thawing of the fish.

For consumer packs of frozen seafood, the most effective means of preventing dessication is proper packaging. The water vapor transfer rate through the packaging should not exceed 0.4 g/m² 24 h at $-20°C$ at 75% relative humidity to protect frozen marine foods from freezer burn during 9 months of storage.[38]

3. Time Temperature Tolerance (TTT)

The quality of frozen fish declines gradually during storage at a rate depending on the product, process, and packaging characteristics (PPP), and on the temperature. The storage life of the given product can be presented as:

- The high quality life (HQL), defined as the time of storage of the initially high quality product to the moment, when the first statistically significant ($p < 0.01$) difference in quality appears
- The practical storage life (PSL), defined as the period of storage, during which the product retains its characteristic properties and suitability for human consumption or intended process.

In order to provide for long storage life of frozen seafood, generally cold stores are kept at temperatures between -30 and $-35°C$. Fish destined for the sashimi market are even stored at temperatures as low as -55 to $-60°C$. Most of the available data on storage life of frozen marine food products regard, however, -18, -23, and $-29°C$. There is a substantial scatter in the reported values, as various investigators used different quality criteria and assessment procedures. Furthermore, very often important PPP characteristics have not been described.[41] Thus, the published figures should be regarded as approximations. Generally PSL/HQL for different frozen products is 2 to 5.

On the basis of many experimental results, the relation between the storage life and storage temperature, known as the TTT diagram, has been developed for various food products. As the quality losses due to abuse temperature are irreversible and additive, regardless of their sequence, the TTT diagrams (Figure 3) can be used for evaluating the effect of fluctuating temperature of storage on the quality of the frozen product (Table 4). The precision of such predictions depends on how much the TTT data reflect the effects of

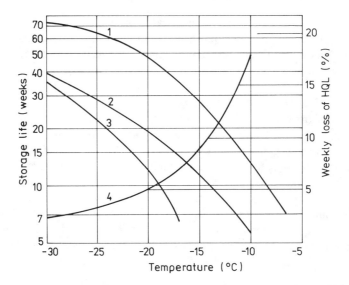

FIGURE 3. Time temperature tolerance of frozen fish. (1) Haddock, PSL: (2) haddock, HQL; (3) herring, PSL; and (4) loss of HQL of haddock.

TABLE 4
Example of Calculating the Total Loss of HQL in Frozen Cod

Stage	Average temperature (°C)	Storage time (weeks)	Weekly[a] loss of HQL (%)	Total loss of HQL (%)
Producer	−20	0.4	4.9	2.0
	−30	4.0	2.5	10.0
Transport	−18	0.3	6.0	1.8
Cold store	−30	20.0	2.5	50.0
Transport	−22	0.4	4.5	1.8
Wholesaler	−20	2.0	4.9	9.8
Transport	−20	0.1	4.9	0.5
Display cabinet	−15	1.0	8.9	8.9
Total loss of HQL				84.8

[a] From Figure 3.

PPP on the storage life and on the reliability of the records of time and temperature during production, storage, and distribution. Many types of temperature indicators and time-temperature integrators are available which can supply the data necessary for predicting the remaining shelf life of frozen marine products.[37,42,43]

REFERENCES

1. **Riedel, L.**, Calorimetric investigations on the freezing of sea fish, *Kältetechnik*, 8, 374, 1956, (in German).
2. **Sharp, J.**, Post-mortem breakdown of glycogen and accumulation of lactic acid in fish muscle, *Proc. R. Soc. London Ser. B*, 114, 506, 1934.
3. **Nowlan, S. S. and Dyer, W. J.**, Glycolytic and nucleotide changes in the critical freezing zone −0.8 to −5°C, in prerigor cod muscle at various rates, *J. Fish. Res. Board Can.*, 26, 2625, 1969.

4. **Dyer, W. J. and Hiltz, D. I.**, Nucleotide degradation in frozen swordfish muscle, *J. Fish. Res. Board Can.*, 26, 1597, 1969.
5. **Connell, J. J.**, Effect of freezing and frozen storage on the proteins of fish muscle, in *Low Temperature Biology of Foodstuffs*, Hawthorn, J. and Rolfe, E. J., Eds., Pergamon Press, Oxford, 1968, 333.
6. **Sikorski, E. E., Olley, J., and Kostuch, S.**, Protein changes in frozen fish, *Crit. Rev. Food Sci. Nutr.*, 8, 97, 1976.
7. **Matsumoto, J. J.**, Denaturation of fish muscle proteins during frozen storage, in *Proteins at Low Temperatures*, (Adv. Chem. Ser., No. 180), Fennema, O., Ed., American Chemical Society, Washington, D.C., 1979, 205.
8. **Shenouda, S. V.**, Theories of protein denaturation during frozen storage of fish flesh, in *Advances in Food Research*, Vol. 26, Chichester, C. O., Mrak, E. M., and Stewart, G. F., Eds., Academic Press, New York, 1980, 275.
9. **Lewin, S.**, *Displacement of Water and its Control of Biochemical Reactions*, Academic Press, London, 1974, chap. 1 to 5.
10. **Powrie, W. D.**, Characteristics of food myosystems and their behavior during freeze-preservation, in *Low Temperature Preservation of Foods and Living Matter*, Fennema, O. R., Powrie, W. D., and Marth, E. H., Eds., Marcel Dekker, New York, 1973, 332.
11. **Kolodziejska, I. and Sikorski, Z. E.**, Inorganic salts and extractability of fresh and frozen fish proteins, *Int. J. Refrig.*, 3, 151, 1980.
12. **Jahrenbäck, L. and Liljemark, A.**, Ultrastructural changes during frozen storage of cod (*Gadus morhua* L.). III. Effects of linoleic acid and linoleic acid hydroperoxides on myofibrillar proteins, *J. Food Technol.*, 10, 437, 1975.
13. **Owusu-Ansah, Y. J. and Hultin, H. O.**, Trimethylamine oxide prevents insolubilization of red hake muscle proteins during frozen storage, *J. Agric. Food Chem.*, 32, 1032, 1984.
14. **Buttkus, H.**, Accelerated denaturation of myosin in frozen solution, *J. Food Sci.*, 35, 558, 1970.
15. **Geromel, E. J. and Montgomery, M. W.**, Lipase release lyposomes of rainbow trout (*Salmo gairdneri*) muscle subject to low temperatures, *J. Food Sci.*, 45, 412, 1980.
16. **Oshima, T., Wada, S., and Koizumi, C.**, Accumulation of lyso-form phospholipids in several species of fish flesh during storage at $-5°C$, *Bull. Jpn. Soc. Sci. Fish.*, 51, 965, 1985.
17. **Olley, J., Pirie, R., and Watson, H.**, Lipase and phospholipase activity in fish skeletal muscle and its relationship to protein denaturation, *J. Sci. Food Agric.*, 13, 501, 1962.
18. **Tsukuda, N.**, Changes in the lipids of frozen fish. II. Changes in the lipids of chum salmon and cod muscle during frozen storage, *Bull. Tokai Reg. Fish. Res. Lab.*, 87, 1, 1976.
19. **Takama, K., Zama, K., and Igarashi, H.**, Changes in the flesh lipids of fish during frozen storage. II. Flesh lipids of several species of fish, *Bull. Fac. Fish. Hokkaido Univ.*, 22, 290, 1972.
20. **Kolakowska, A.**, Effect of initial processing on fat rancidity dynamics during storage of frozen fish, Proc. 15th Int. Congr. Refrigeration, *Bull. Int. Inst. Refrig.*, 4, 1184, C2-54, 1978.
21. **Kolakowska, A.**, Krill lipids after frozen storage of about 1 year in relation to storage time before freezing, *Nahrung*, 33(3), 241, 1989.
22. **McGill, A. S., Hardy, R., and Gunstone, F. D.**, Further analysis of the volatile components of frozen cold stored cod and the influence of these on flavour, *J. Sci. Food Agric.*, 28, 200, 1977.
23. **Ke, P. J., Ackman, R. G., and Linke, B. A.**, Autoxidation of polyunsaturated fatty compounds in mackerel oil: formation of 2,4,7-decatrienals, *J. Am. Oil Chem. Soc.*, 52, 349, 1975.
24. **Arai, K. and Kinumaki, T.**, Lethal doses of fatty acid ester hydroperoxides in oral administration, *Bull. Tokai Reg. Fish. Res. Lab.*, 102, 7, 1980.
25. **Reddy, S. K., Nip, W. K., and Tang, C. S.**, Changes in fatty acids and sensory quality of fresh water prawn (*Macrobrachium rosenbergii*) stored under frozen conditions, *J. Food Sci.*, 46, 353, 1981.
26. **Kolakowska, A., Czerniejewska-Surma, B., and Deutry, J.**, Assessment of Rancidity in Frozen Stored Horse Mackerel, Proc. Symp. Fat Chemistry and Technology, Gdańsk, 1985, 203.
27. **Kolakowska, A. and Szybowicz, Z.** An attempt to fix criteria of rancidity of frozen fish on a basis of colorimetric determination of peroxide value of fat, *Chlodnictwo* , 16(7—8), 37, 1981, (in Polish).
28. **Shewfelt, R. L.**, Fish muscle lipolysis — a review, *J. Food Biochem.*, 5, 79, 1981.
29. **Nakamura, T. and Hama, Y.**, Conjugated carbonyls with a prostaglandin-like structure formed by autoxidation of eikosapentanoate, *Bull. Jpn. Soc. Sci. Fish.*, 54, 271, 1988.
30. **Haard, N. F. and Arcilla, R.**, Precursors of Maillard browning in Atlantic short finned squid, *Can. Inst. Food Technol. J.*, 18, 326, 1985.
31. **Plank, R.**, The maintenance of freshness of foods by cold, in *Handbuch der Kältetechnik*, Vol. 10, Plank, R., Ed., Springer-Verlag, Berlin, 1960, 1, (in German).
32. **Golowkin, N. A. and Czizow, G. B.**, *Chilling and Freezing of Foods*, Państwowe Wydawnictwo Techniczne, Warsaw, 1953, chap. 6, (in Polish).
33. **Cleyland, A. C. and Earle, R. L.**, Freezing of Irregular Shapes under Time-Variable Conditions, International Institute of Refrigeration, C2, D1, D2, D3, Hamilton, 1982, 447.

34. **Fellows, P.**, *Food Processing Technology*, Ellis Horwood, Chichester, England, 1988, 379.
35. **Postolski, J. and Gruda, Z.**, *Freezing of Foods*, 2nd ed., Wydawnictwa Naukowo-Techniczne, Warsaw, 1985, chap. 2, (in Polish).
36. **Cleland, D. J., Cleland, A. C., and Earle, R. L.**, Prediction of freezing and thawing times for foods — a review, *Int. J. Refrig.*, 9, 182, 1986.
37. **Sikorski, Z. E.**, *Marine Food Technology*, 2nd ed., Wydawnictwa Naukowo-Techniczne, Warsaw, 1980, chap. 6, (in Polish).
38. **Heiss, R.**, State of the art and problems of frozen fish packaging, in *Freezing and Irradiation of Fish*, Kreuzer, R., Ed., Fishing News Books, London, 1969, 409.
39. **Clark, E. D. and Almy, L. H.**, *The Commercial Freezing and Storing of Fish*, U.S.D.A. Bull. No. 635, U.S. Department of Agriculture, Washington, D.C., 1918.
40. *Recommendations for Processing and Handling of Frozen Foods*, 3rd ed., International Institute of Refrigeration, Paris, 1986, 40.
41. **Learson, R. J. and Licciardello, J. J.**, Literature reporting of shelf life data. What does it all mean?, *Int. J. Refrig.*, 9, 179, 1986.
42. **Olley, J. and Lisac, H.**, Time/temperature monitors, *Infofish Marketing Digest*, (3), 45, 1985.
43. **Schubert, H.**, Indicators for measuring the time-temperature effect on frozen foods, *Int. Z. Lebensmittel Technol. Verfahrenstechnik*, 31, 137, 1980, (in German).

Chapter 8

DRYING AND DRIED FISH PRODUCTS

Peter Doe and June Olley

TABLE OF CONTENTS

I. Fish Drying 126
    A. Drying Methods 126
        1. Relevant Factors 126
        2. Sun Drying 126
        3. Curing and Drying 126
        4. Solar Drying 128
        5. Agrowaste as Fuel for Drying 128
        6. Mechanical Drying 129
        7. Other Methods 130
    B. Principles of Drying 130
        1. General Considerations 130
        2. Constant Rate Drying 130
        3. Falling Rate Drying 130
        4. Effect of Salt and Fat 131
    C. Sorption Isotherms 131
        1. Introduction 131
        2. Moisture Content 131
        3. Water Activity 133
            a. Definition 133
            b. Measurement 133
            c. Significance 133
        4. Temperature Dependence 133
        5. Effects of Salt and Fat 134
    D. Control of Spoilage 134
        1. Physical Spoilage 134
        2. Autolytic Spoilage 134
        3. Chemical Spoilage 134
        4. Microbial Spoilage 135
        5. Insect Spoilage 136
    E. Dried Fish Products 137
    F. Quality of Dried Fish 137
        1. Sensory Evaluation 137
        2. Score Sheet Evaluation 138
        3. Chemical Indicators 138
            a. Flavor 138
            b. Spoilage 138
        4. Nutritional Quality 139

II. Production of Fish Protein Concentrates and Preparations 139
    A. History 139
    B. Production Methods 140
    C. Functional and Nutritional Properties 140

D. Future Prospects 141

References 142

I. FISH DRYING

A. DRYING METHODS
1. Relevant Factors

Drying is one of the earliest known means of preserving foods. Fish have been dried by traditional methods everywhere fish are caught. In high latitudes, a combination of cold, dry air and low humidity allows fish to be dried very simply with a minimum of wastage. However, in some tropical countries, particularly in the wet season, much of the catch spoils before it can be eaten.

Methods of drying fish cover the spectrum from traditional sundrying to high-technology computer-controlled industrial processes. Figure 1 depicts the relationship between the degree of technology of a drying process and its relative cost. Which method may be preferred by a community depends on many factors, not the least important of which is the profit to the fish processor. However, other factors are relevant such as climate, consumer preference for a particular product, availability of alternative energy sources, or the introduction of improved technology. The effect of the drying method on the nutritive value of the product should also be considered.

The assessment of the cost/benefit of introducing new technology is not simple; the benefit to a community through the introduction of a fish-drying method which gives a more stable and wholesome product and creates employment in other industries might outweigh the additional cost of the process.

2. Sun Drying

By far the most widely used method of drying fish is direct exposure to sunlight. The method of sun drying varies from fishery to fishery; larger varieties of fish may be split; the fish may be brined or salted before being spread out to dry. In the tropics it is common for the fish to be placed on trays woven from bamboo, rattan, or similar materials; the trays are supported on racks at a convenient height above the ground. Fish may be hung vertically as is the case for "bombay duck". A less hygienic method is to place the fish directly on the ground.

It is usual for fish to be moved under cover during the night and when it rains. Also, trays of fish are sometimes stacked during the hottest part of the day to avoid overheating which might cook the flesh.

Infestation by fly larvae is the greatest source of loss of fish during sun drying. There may also be losses due to birds and other scavenging animals. During periods of high humidity and clouds, fish may spoil through bacterial or mold growth during drying. Fatty fish may become rancid during drying, but in some traditional products, e.g., sun-dried anchovies and sardines used as condiments in many tropical countries, a rancid flavor and odor are expected.

3. Curing and Drying

Many traditional dried fish products rely on factors additional to the removal of water. The fish may be salted before drying (Figure 2); antioxidants and antimicrobial agents may be added; the fish may be cooked or smoked or fermented.[1] Such products are listed by

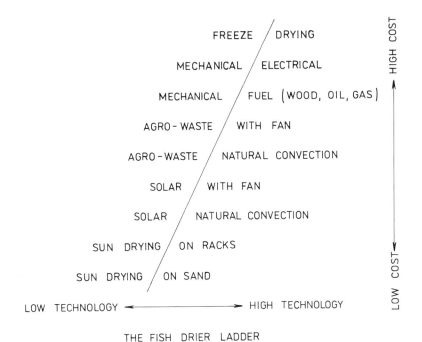

FIGURE 1. Relative cost of fish driers vs. degree of technology.

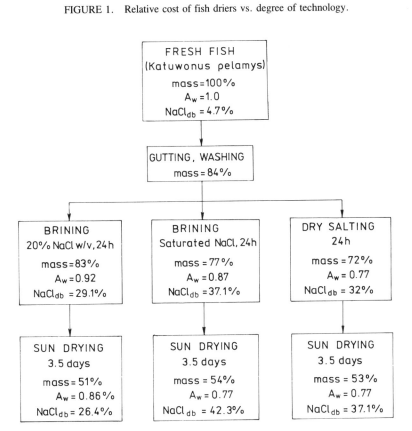

FIGURE 2. Flowchart for brining and sun drying.

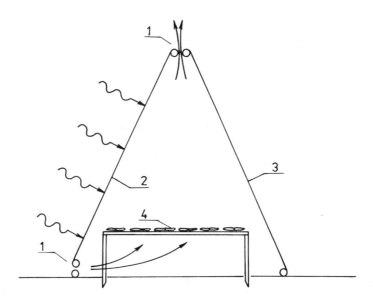

FIGURE 3. Solar tent drier in Bangladesh. 1, Vent; 2, clear polyethylene sheeting; 3, black sheeting; and 4, fish.

Tanikawa et al.[2] and are generally described as cured-dried. They were originally developed to solve the problem of increasing the keeping time to suit particular fresh fish availability and patterns of distribution of the cured-dried product, and to provide definitive flavors. Motohiro[3] gives detailed descriptions of how a wide variety of products has been developed in Japan.

In some communities, improvements in transportation and storage facilities (e.g., refrigerated trucks and home refrigerators) have meant that the keeping attributes of the cured products are no longer relevant. Consumers, however, maintain a demand for the traditional products even when some of the products — e.g., heavily smoked products — are potentially hazardous to the health of the consumer.

4. Solar Drying

Since the mid-1970s, there has been much activity aimed at improving traditional drying methods. The term ''solar drier'' is used to describe devices that collect or concentrate solar energy so that the drying is faster or the product quality is improved.

Solar driers made from bamboo or other locally available materials with glass or plastic sheeting have been tested in many parts of the world including Bangladesh,[4] (Figure 3), Papua New Guinea,[5] the Philippines, Malaysia, Thailand, India, Sri Lanka, Ecuador, Rwanda, Indonesia, Senegal, Mali, Ghana, Gambia, and Yemen.[6]

The driers are designed so that an airflow is induced through natural convection. At the same time, the air temperature is increased and the relative humidity is reduced.

One notable development of a solar fish drier was the manufacture and successful operation in Yemen and Gambia of solar dome driers with a capacity of 1 t of fish (Figure 4). A study comparing the cost and effectiveness of several designs of solar driers and traditional sun drying was undertaken on the Galapagos Islands in Ecuador.[7] The study concluded that fish dried on racks were a better product than those dried by the placing on black rocks (the local traditional method); all the solar driers tested gave a better product and dried the fish at a rate higher than that of the sun-drying methods.

5. Agrowaste as Fuel for Drying

Rice hull, methane gas obtained from bioconversion, animal dung, and other agricultural

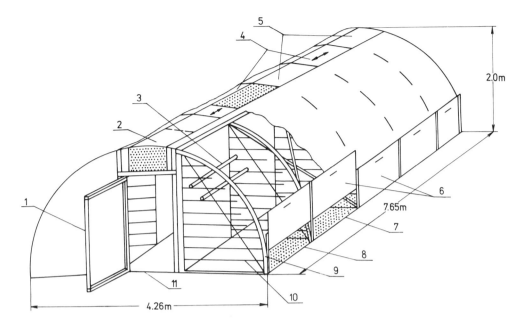

FIGURE 4. Solar drier with 1-t capacity. The drier is modeled on a horticultural green house. Clear plastic (UV-stabilized polyethylene) covers most of the surface except for screened vents at the sides and top to allow air to flow through. Fish are hung from beams. 1, Door frame with netting and removable plastic cover; 2, fixed roof vent; 3, fish-drying beam; 4, sliding roof vent with netting underneath; 5, fixed roof vent; 6, sliding side vents with netting underneath; 7, solar collector bay; 8, fish drying bay; 9, tubular steel external frame; and 10, internal metal frame. (From Sachithanathan, K., Trim, D. S., and Speirs, C. I., Proc. FAO Expert Consultation on Fish Technology in Africa, Lusaka, Zambia, FAO Fish. Rep. No. 329, Food and Agriculture Organization, Rome, 1986, 161. With permission.)

wastes are used in a variety of ways to dry fish. For example, the process for smoking the product "tinapa" in the Philippines[8] uses coconut husk, bagasse, peanut husk, or corn cobs when sawdust is not readily available. Agrowaste driers[9] which rely on natural convection have the inherent difficulty of maintaining a sufficiently high air flow while keeping the air temperature below that which would cook the fish.

6. Mechanical Drying

The prospect of food shortages in Europe and difficulties with transporting frozen fish in the 1940s prompted an intensive study into mechanical fish dehydration.[10] This work produced excellent examples of minced dried cod, smoked herring, and other products; the questions arise as to why there has been no commercial development since,[11] and why mechanical fish dehydration is not more widely employed in developing countries.

Mechanical driers are now widely used for the production of dried and smoked products in parts of the world where sun drying is not effective. Fish are either supported on trays or hung vertically. The air can be fully or partially recirculated by an electric fan; electrical heating and wood fires (with or without smoke) are used. Because air temperature, humidity, and speed can be controlled closely and adjusted automatically during the drying, a high level of quality control can be maintained.[12]

Early designs of mechanical driers suffered from problems when operated in climates with high ambient humidities. In order to reduce the air humidity to a level at which the fish would dry, the air temperature in the drier needed to be increased to a level which adversely affected product quality. Recent developments have been to use heat pumps instead of wood or electrical heaters in mechanical driers so as to operate independently of ambient conditions. A further refinement is continuous as distinct from batch operation.[13]

7. Other Methods

The methodologies of freeze drying and accelerated freeze drying (AFD) of fish products are well established. The process is expensive and the quality of the product is inferior to that of good quality frozen fish.[14] Commercial application is limited to "instant" meals and fish soups.

Drying fish (herring) in hot oil was found to give a protein utilization as high as that from the freeze-dried product.[15] Synthetic antioxidants in the cooking oil acted synergistically with the natural antioxidants in the fish to improve the stability of the oil and the dried product. This method has not been commercially exploited.

Other drying methods include drying on heated drums and solvent extraction/drying. These methods are mainly used for the production of fish protein concentrates, which are discussed in Section II below.

B. PRINCIPLES OF DRYING

1. General Considerations

Fish dry by the evaporation of water which has diffused through the fish muscle and skin to an exposed surface. Initially the rate of drying is governed by the rate of evaporation from the exposed surfaces; after a time, depending on the evaporation rate and the rate at which the water can diffuse to the surface, the surfaces start to dry and the drying rate falls. These distinct phases of drying are termed "constant rate" and "falling rate" drying according to whether external convection or internal diffusion processes govern the drying rate. The latter phase is further divided into stages corresponding to the availability of water bound to the protein substrate in different ways.[16]

2. Constant Rate Drying

The initial rate of drying is governed by heat and mass transfer processes external to the fish. Air temperature, air humidity, the shape and orientation of the fish relative to the air stream, and the air speed all have a direct effect on the drying rate. The drying rate can be calculated using the equation

$$e = h_m A (p_s - p_a) \tag{1}$$

where e is the drying rate (kg/s), h_m is the mass transfer coefficient (kg/s m^2 Pa), A is the surface area of the fish (m^2), and p_s and p_a are, respectively, the partial pressures of water vapor in the air at the fish surface and in the air stream (Pa).

Thus, in the early stages of drying, the rate can be increased by increasing the air speed and temperature and by reducing the air relative humidity. There is a limit; if dried too fast, a relatively impermeable layer can develop on the surface of the fish (case hardening) and, at temperatures above about 40°C (depending on the fish species), the fish will start to cook.

3. Falling Rate Drying

The end of the constant rate period occurs when the surface of the fish starts to dry and the rate at which moisture can diffuse to the surface limits its drying rate.

The drying rate during the falling rate drying period can be predicted with the unsteady-state diffusion equation

$$\frac{dC}{dt} = D_x \frac{d^2C}{dx^2} + D_y \frac{d^2C}{dy^2} + D_z \frac{d^2C}{dz^2} \tag{2}$$

where C is the moisture concentration (kg H$_2$O/m^3 of fish), D_x, D_y, D_z are the diffusivities of water vapor in fish in three directions x, y, and z (m^2/s), and t is time (s).

Equation 2 can be integrated either numerically or analytically to give the drying rate, subject to some approximations for the shape of the fish, the change in diffusivity with moisture concentration, and the effects of skin and shrinkage, etc. However, a good approximation to the solution is the relationship

$$M - M_e = (M_c - M_e)\exp(-t/T_i) \tag{3}$$

where M is the mass of the fish (kg), M_c is the mass at the end of the constant rate period, M_e is the equilibrium mass of the fish corresponding to the temperature and humidity of the surrounding air, and T_i is a time constant related to the diffusivity of the water in the fish muscle.

Thus, as the mass of the fish approaches its equilibrium value exponentially, the process can be speeded up by reducing the ambient air humidity, and by increasing the drying temperature which increases the rate at which water diffuses through the fish.

4. Effect of Salt and Fat

Adding salt to fish alters its drying characteristics. The constant rate period becomes shorter and the drying rate is reduced because of the lowering of the water vapor pressure at the fish surface. The drying rate is also reduced during falling rate drying as the diffusivity of water in the fish muscle is lowered by addition of salt.[17]

Fatty fish dry slower than nonfatty fish; the diffusivity decreases with increasing fat content.

C. SORPTION ISOTHERMS
1. Introduction

A sorption isotherm of a food is the relationship between the moisture content of the food and its water activity (defined below) at a particular temperature. This relationship is sometimes known as an "equilibrium moisture content curve" which relates moisture content to the relative humidity of air in equilibrium with the food. Some foods exhibit different sorption characteristics when dried to those when hydrated; these are known as desorption and adsorption isotherms, respectively.

The manner in which water is held within the food influences the form of the sorption relationship and the shape of the sorption isotherm curve (Figure 5). At a low moisture content, water is bound strongly to the fish protein as a monolayer of molecules adsorbed onto specific sites in the food — the BET isotherm.[18] At higher values of moisture content, the water molecules form additional layers over this monolayer; at a higher moisture content, the water is present in liquid form as a solution of various solutes present in the food.[19]

2. Moisture Content

The moisture content of fish is usually expressed on a wet-weight basis—i.e., is the mass of water in a unit mass of the fish. The moisture content of fish is usually determined by oven drying at 100 to 102°C for 16 to 18 h; the loss of mass in that time being equated to the mass of water in the original sample. There are several other ways of expressing moisture content, some of which have application in the mathematical modeling of drying and sorption behavior, e.g., a salt-free, fat-free dry basis (SFFFDB). The conversion between moisture contents expressed in different ways can be accomplished using the following formulas:

- Mass of fish

$$M = M_w + M_s + M_f + M_b \tag{4}$$

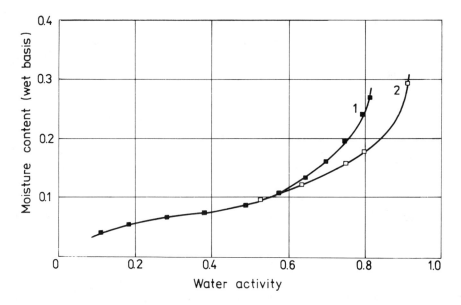

FIGURE 5. Sorption isotherms for FPC Types A and B. 1, FPC type B and 2, FPC type A.

where M_w is mass of water, M_s is mass of salt, M_f is mass of fat, and M_b is the salt-free, fat-free, dry mass of the fish obtained by subtracting the masses of salt and fat from the mass remaining after oven drying.

- Definitions

Moisture content:	wet basis: mc = M_w/M;	SFFFDB:	md = M_w/M_b
Salt content:	wet basis: sc = M_s/M;	SFFFDB:	sd = M_s/M_b
Fat content:	wet basis: fc = M_f/M;	SFFFDB:	fd = M_f/M_b

- Conversions

  SFFFDB to wet basis:

  $$mc = md/(1 + md + sd + fd) \qquad (5)$$

  $$sc = sd/(1 + md + sd + fd) \qquad (6)$$

  $$fc = fd/(1 + md + sd + fd) \qquad (7)$$

- Wet basis to SFFFDB

  Wet basis to SFFFDB:

  $$md = mc/(1 - mc - sc - fc) \qquad (8)$$

  $$sd = sc/(1 - mc - sc - fc) \qquad (9)$$

  $$fd = fc/(1 - mc - sc - fc) \qquad (10)$$

- Useful relationships

  $$M_b = M(1 - mc - sc - fc) \qquad (11)$$

  $$M = M_b(1 + md + sd + fd) \qquad (12)$$

3. Water Activity
a. Definition

The formal definition of water activity, a_w, is in terms of a water vapor pressure ratio — that of the partial pressure of water vapor in air to the partial pressure of water vapor in saturated air at the same temperature. This definition equates the water activity of a food to the relative humidity (expressed as a fraction rather than a percentage) of air in equilibrium with the food. Water activity is a measure of the availability of water within a food for microbial growth. It can be thought of as the relative humidity of air in equilibrium with a food, e.g., the humidity of the air in the headspace of a sealed container containing the food. Put another way; if dried fish is exposed to air at a relative humidity of, for example, 85%, it will absorb or desorb water until it reaches equilibrium with the air. The water activity of the dried fish when it reaches equilibrium will be 0.85.

b. Measurement

Water activity can be measured by any of the many methods of measuring relative humidity in air.[20] In addition, there are methods which rely on allowing the food to equilibrate with a material with an accurately known sorption isotherm.[21] The most widely used method for routine determination of water activity is the measurement of the relative humidity of air in the headspace of a sealed container.

c. Significance

Most of the factors which influence the acceptability and stability of foods can be related to water activity.[22,23] In particular, the growth of microorganisms in dried fish is strongly dependent on water activity. If the water activity is reduced below about 0.62, no bacteria or mold will grow. The growth of pathogenic and putrefactive bacteria in fish can be suppressed by reducing the water activity below 0.91.[24] No mycotoxins are produced when the water activity is reduced below 0.81.[25] Other deteriorative processes such as lipid oxidation, Maillard reactions, enzymic and nonenzymic browning, hydrolytic reaction, and enzyme activity in fish vary with water activity.[26] All these deteriorative processes with the exception of lipid oxidation and Maillard reactions decrease as the water activity is reduced by drying.[27] Lipid oxidation decreases with decreasing water activity to $a_w = 0.2$; at lower values of water activity, lipid oxidation increases due to the removal of a protective water shell.[28]

The main rationale for drying, therefore, is to lower the water activity of the fish and so reduce microbial and other deteriorative changes to an acceptable level.

4. Temperature Dependence

The sorption isotherms of a wide variety of foods have a temperature dependence which, from theoretical thermodynamic considerations, can be expressed by the equation,

$$\ln[\ln(1/a_w)] = a/RT + r \ln(mc/mc_m) \qquad (13)$$

where a and r are parameters determined experimentally for a particular food, mc is the moisture content, R is the universal gas constant, and T is temperature (K). The moisture content mc_m is that corresponding to the B.E.T. monolayer.[18] Many alternative expressions have been proposed, each with application to particular foods or groups of foods.[29] Put simply, the effect of an increase in temperature is to shift the sorption isotherm downwards. This has the effect of increasing the water activity at the same moisture content.

The deteriorative processes are also affected by temperature (see Chapter 4).

Chemical reactions such as lipid oxidation are claimed to obey the Arrhenius equation, but lipids, when heated to a higher temperature, do not return to their slower reaction rate when cooled to a lower temperature due, it is supposed, to an accumulation of free radicals.[30]

Besides the traditional use of reduced temperature for control of bacterial growth, use can also be made of higher temperatures. There is an upper limit to the temperature at which biological activity can occur; mesophilic bacteria commonly associated with the spoilage of tropical fish will not multiply at temperatures above about 45 to 50°C.[31] However, increasing temperatures to above 40°C in the early stages of drying is not an option for many products because the fish become cooked.

5. Effects of Salt and Fat

The addition of salt to preserve fish has its origins in antiquity. Numerous methods are used ranging from boiling in saturated brine to pressing the fish with dry salt. Salt uptake can range up to 20% on a wet weight basis. The addition of salt to fish has a direct and marked effect on its water activity and drying characteristics.

The effect on water activity is due to the ability of a salt solution to lower the partial pressure of water vapor. Air in the head space in a closed container of a saturated solution of common salt has a humidity of close to 75%. Consequently, salted fish which have been dried sufficiently to saturate unbound water will have a water activity of 0.75 or less. Sorption isotherms for salted dried fish (isohalic sorption isotherms) have been determined by measurement and theory.[32] A simple relationship can be used to calculate the water activity of dried fish from measured values of moisture content, fat, and salt contents.[24] For dried cod containing natural salt, the expression

$$a_w = 1.084 - 0.077(M_b/M_w) \tag{14}$$

is valid ($r = 0.998$) over the range $1.5 < (M_b/M_w) < 10$.

Fat content has no direct effect on the sorption isotherm.[33] There is an indirect effect as fat does not contain much water, but adds to the total mass of the fish; thus, if moisture content is expressed on a wet-weight basis, the sorption isotherms will vary with fat content, but by expressing moisture contents on a salt-free, fat-free, dry-matter basis the sorption isotherms are not fat dependent.

D. CONTROL OF SPOILAGE

1. Physical Spoilage

Fish with a low moisture content is fragile and may be damaged through rough handling. Birds and small animals eat dried fish. Exposure of the fish to contaminants such as diesel fuel or dust/dirt can render it unfit for human consumption. Good handling and packaging practice can prevent much of the losses of dried fish due to physical damage.[34]

2. Autolytic Spoilage

The effect of drying on autolytic changes such as nucleotide and phospholipid breakdown are best understood by studying the classical work of Acker[35] on the effects of water activity on enzyme activity in cereals. As water activity is lowered, enzyme activity is slowed and the asymptote of the reaction decreases. In other words, the reactions do not proceed to completion. If the water activity is raised, then the reaction proceeds once more at the rate for the higher water activity. The Japanese are aware of this and know that the flavor enhancer, inosinic acid,[36] accumulates in dried fish because the dephosphorylatory enzyme is inhibited at lower water activities.[3] Phospholipase activity is another example of the same phenomenon.

3. Chemical Spoilage

Oxidation of fish fats can produce unacceptable levels of rancid and off-flavors in dried fish products. However, in some traditional products, a degree of rancidity is esteemed.[37]

The nutritional value of fat is lowered by oxidation and some lipid peroxides are toxic. Oxidation is accelerated at low water activities and by exposure to sunlight.[26] The effect of temperature on the rate of lipid oxidation is largely independent of water activity at temperatures above 45°C. Temperature has a greater influence than water activity on lipid oxidation during storage of sun-dried filefish;[38] shelf life at 35 and 55°C was 58 and 8 d, respectively, while at 25°C shelf life ranged from 125 to 106 d with a change of water activity from 0.44 to 0.75.

Smoking fish reduces the rate of oxidation because of the antioxidant activity of smoke components.[28,39] Food antioxidants are not generally used in dried fish production.

Chemical contamination may be caused by the indiscriminate use of insecticides. There are reported instances of substances with high residual levels of toxicity (e.g., DDT) being applied directly to dried fish. There is now available an organophosphorous insecticide ("Actellic®" ICI) approved by the World Health Organization for use with fish. Insecticides made from pyrethroids have a low residual toxicity.[40]

4. Microbial Spoilage

Microbial spoilage of fish can be prevented by drying and storing the fish under conditions unfavorable to microbial growth. In fresh fish, the water activity is close to unity; bacteria will grow on fresh fish at temperatures above about $-5°C$ at a rate described by the expression,[41]

$$\sqrt{r} = b(T - T_{min}) \tag{15}$$

where r is the rate of reaction which includes microbial growth, nucleotide breakdown, or the (reciprocal of the) time to reach a specified chemical concentration or number of organisms, b is the slope of the regression line, T is temperature, and T_{min} is the intercept of the ensuing straight line on the temperature axis.

Equation 15 has been extended to cover the higher temperatures where microbial organisms and their enzymes are destroyed by heat.[42] Thus,

$$\sqrt{r} = b(T - T_{min})\{1 - \exp[c(T - T_{max})]\} \tag{16}$$

where c and T_{max} describe the region of the growth curve where the growth rate reduces due to temperature stress.

As the fish dries, the water activity drops, putting additional stress on the bacteria; the growth of a species of bacteria (*Staphylococcus xylosus*) isolated from Indonesian dried fish is described by the equation

$$\sqrt{r} = 0.0205\sqrt{(a_w - 0.838)}\,(T - 275.9) \tag{17}$$

for which the temperature $T_{min} = 275.9$ K was found not to vary as the water activity was lowered.[43] Thus, a combination of high or low temperature and reduced water activity can limit the bacterial growth rate and so prevent spoilage during drying.

A mathematical model has been developed which simulates sun drying of tropical low-fat fish species, salted or unsalted prior to drying; the model is based on the principles of drying (described above) from which the temperature and water activity during drying are computed, together with measured growth rates of bacteria implicated in the spoilage of dried salted fish. The model can be used to predict the effects on drying and bacterial growth of the different factors involved in sun drying of fish such as salt content, fish thickness, air temperature, and relative humidity.[44]

Halophilic "pink" bacteria grow on salted dried fish at a water activity of 0.75. The bacteria originate in the salt used for salting the fish and multiply in brines and on the surfaces of brine tanks. Levels of halophilic bacteria can be minimized by the use of uncontaminated salt and by renewing brines regularly.

Washing equipment with fresh water is an effective method of reducing the numbers of halophilic bacteria. Minerals in salt, particularly iron and copper, also are deleterious to quality; calcium and magnesium salts should be within the limits 0.15 to 0.3% and 0.05 to 0.15%, respectively.[45]

Molds and yeasts germinate and grow on dried fish at water activities above 0.62. The mold, *Polypaecilum pisce*, which has an optimum growth at 30°C between water activity values 0.90 to 0.96 on media containing salt, has favorable conditions for growth on dried fish obtained from fish markets in Indonesia.[46] The occurrence of the brown "dun" mold *Wallemia sebi* (*Sporondonema*), traditionally regarded as the principle cause of spoilage of salt fish in temperate climates, is rare in Indonesia, probably due to higher ambient storage temperatures. Growth of *W. sebi* is poor at 30°C (radial growth rate of 6.3 μm h^{-1} at a_w = 0.85) and almost inhibited at 34°C especially in the presence of NaCl.[47] These and other molds do not necessarily spoil dried fish — for example, fish with visible mold growth are sold for human consumption in Indonesia. The toxin-producing mold *Aspergillus flavus* has been isolated from dried fish as a contaminant. Aflatoxin was not detected.[48] It is highly unlikely that aflatoxin is a health hazard in salted dried tropical fish as *A. flavus* grows very slowly at 30°C in the presence of salt (radial growth rate 10 μm h^{-1} at a_w = 0.86) and is likely to be outcompeted by other molds, e.g., *P. pisce* (radial growth rate 45 μm h^{-1} at a_w = 0.85).

Mold growth during the storage of dried fish can be controlled by control of temperature or air humidity or a combination of these factors. Fish that are dried so that their water activity is below about 0.65 can be packaged to prevent rehydration and kept at low temperature. Molds germinate and grow particularly rapidly on fish stored under damp, poorly ventilated conditions in climates with high ambient relative humidity and temperature. For example, at 30°C and 90% relative humidity (a_w = 0.9), the mold *P. pisce* can germinate and grow to a colony 2 mm in diameter in 26 h.

5. Insect Spoilage

Insects are reported as causing greater damage to cured fish than bacteria, fungi, or mites in tropical countries.[49] In the early stages of drying, fish are susceptible to attack by flies. The flies lay eggs which hatch within a few hours; the larvae feed on the fish flesh — moving into wetter fish or into the soil or other moist places as the fish dry out. The life cycle of the house fly *Musca domestica* can be as short as 10 d from egg to adult; 90 to 120 eggs in a single batch can hatch within 1 d under ideal conditions (28 to 32°C). A female *Chrysomyia* can lay 200 to 300 eggs at once.

A significant reduction in fly populations at fish markets and drying yards can be achieved by eliminating places where flies breed and by reducing their supply of food. Floors of fish markets should be paved and sloped to prevent pools from forming and facilitate cleaning; drains should be cleaned out regularly; fish waste should be collected and disposed of by burying or ensilation; facilities for personal hygiene should be provided.

Flies are less attracted to fish which has been brined before drying. Damage from flies can be reduced by screening during brining and drying. Dipping fish in 0.003% pyrethroid insecticide (Fastac) solution was found to be an effective method of preventing blowfly larvae infestation in salted/dried marine catfish.[50]

Dermestid and other species of beetles can live and breed in dry salted fish;[51] dried fish can also be infested by mites. The beetle *Dermestes maculatus* has a life cycle of 32 to 45 d; it can increase its numbers 30-fold in a 4-week period. Adult *D. maculatus* beetles can fly. Fish become infested both from direct egg laying or by migration of larvae.

Control of beetles and mites requires good housekeeping in dried fish stores to break the pattern of successive infestation. Dried fish containers should be raised above the floor; stores should be well ventilated; adequate packaging can prevent access of the beetles to the dried fish; first in-first out warehousing practice can be adopted; scraps of dried fish and badly infested fish should be removed.

Beetles do not survive in fish which have a water activity of 0.75 or less and a salt content (wet basis) in excess of 8%. The table below gives salt and moisture contents required to give a water activity of 0.75 in fish with a low fat content:

Moisture content (% wet basis)	Salt content (% wet basis)
21	8.0
25	9.4
30	11.2
35	13.1
40	14.9

Dried fish stores can be emptied and chemically disinfested. Pirimphos-methyl and chlorpyriphos-methyl are suggested for use as surface sprays at an application rate of 0.5 to 1.0 g/m^2; methyl bromide for carefully controlled commercial use and phosphine for small-scale operations have been suggested at dosage rates of 80 g/m^3 for 2 h and 0.1 g/m^3 for 72 h.[52] However, this is pointless if poor housekeeping practices permit reinfestation.

Fish can be disinfested by heating — a solar tent drier has been used to raise the fish temperature to above 45°C for several hours to remove fly larvae.[4] *D. maculatus* larvae are killed by exposure to a temperature of 50°C for more than 15 min.

Keeping dried fish refrigerated is also an effective method of insect control. For example, it is known that three of the four dermestes species which infest dried tropical fish cannot breed at temperatures below 20°C.[53]

E. DRIED FISH PRODUCTS

In tropical countries where the fish caught cannot be eaten fresh or otherwise processed, the surplus may be converted to fermented products. Some of the processes retain the form of the original fish; in some, the original form is lost. There is a wide variety of products ranging from whole fermented fish (e.g., *Pindang* in Indonesia) and squid[54] to fish pastes or sauces and silage for animal feed.[1] Thus, low-priced fish, or species that are disliked, may be utilized.

The products rely for their stability on reduced water activity (from added salts and sugars or drying) and in some products, the pH is also lowered. Perhaps the widest range of dried and cured fish products is in Japan where eight classifications of dried marine products can be identified;[2] plain dried products, fish dried after being boiled, fish dried after being broiled, salt-dried products, frozen and dried products, boiled, dried and roasted products, seasoned and dried products, and smoked products.

F. QUALITY OF DRIED FISH
1. Sensory Evaluation

Dried fish is often used as a flavoring agent rather than as a meal. The remarkable flavor-enhancing properties of inosine monophosphate[36] (IMP) were discovered from the Japanese fully dried product "bonito". The flavor requirements of different communities are so diverse that few categorical statements can be made concerning acceptability (Table 1).

TABLE 1
Recommended Quality Control Standards for Dried Fish[55]

Factors of quality	Grade A Normal (no defects)	Grade A Tolerance[a]	Grade B Tolerance[b]	Grade C
Discoloration of cut surfaces (white, yellow, brown, green)	Normal (yellowish brown)	Slight	Significant	Excessive
Brittleness	None	Moderate	Moderate	Significant
Cleaning defects (residuals of blood viscera, other objects foreign to the products)	Normal (slight residuals)	Moderate	Significant	Excessive
Insect infestation	None	None	Slight	Significant
Mold contamination	None	None	Slight	Significant
Odor defects (rancid, ammoniacal, smoky)	Normal (moderately rancid)	Slightly ammoniacal, smoky	Significant rancidity, ammoniacal, smoky	Excessive rancidity, ammoniacal, smoky
Water and salt content				
Form A (nonsalted)	Water maximum 35%, salt under 1%	—	Water 35 to 50%, salt under 1%	Water over 50%, salt under 1%
Form B (salted)	Water maximum 45%, salt 8 to 15%	—	Water 45 to 55%, salt 5 to 8% or 15 to 20%	Water over 55%, salt under 5% or over 20%
pH	6.0 to 6.9	—	6.9 to 7.2	<6.0 and >7.2

[a] Four or more defects under Grade A reduce product to Grade B.
[b] Five or more defects under Grade B reduce product to Grade C.

From FAO, FAO Fish. Tech. Paper 219, Food and Agriculture Organization, Rome, 1981, 67.

2. Score Sheet Evaluation

For consumer acceptability trials, various hedonic scales are available. There is a recommended number of tasters required for each test which is taken as the "magic number" required to give validity to the results.[56] Defects in a dried fish product are probably best summarized by a demerit point scoring system such as that developed for fresh fish by Bremner et al.[57] An example of such a system for salted dried fish is given in Table 2. Any community can make its own list of undesirable characteristics and develop a score sheet accordingly.

3. Chemical Indicators
a. Flavor

Nucleotide breakdown products, such as IMP which enhance flavor[58] can be readily determined by high performance liquid chromatography. Glutamic acid, which is also a potent flavor enhancer can be determined enzymically by the method of Skurray and Pucar.[59] The Japanese, when artificially enhancing flavor in dried fish, add glutamic acid and IMP in the ratio 10:1.[3]

b. Spoilage

The chemical indicators for assessing the quality of fresh fish can also be applied to dried fish. However, care should be exercised in interpreting the results. Trimethylamine (TMA) is a common end product of the metabolism of psychrotrophic bacteria; some mesophilic bacteria, likely to be implicated in the spoilage of fish during drying, have a different metabolic pathway and do not reduce triethylamine oxide (TMAO) to produce TMA.

TABLE 2
Score Sheet for Dried Fish Quality

		\multicolumn{3}{c}{Sample number}	
		poor	fair	good	
Appearance					
Physical damage	absent/moderate/extreme 0 / 1 / 2	0	1	2	
Sheen	bright/dull 0 / 1	0	0	1	
Discoloration	absent/present 0 / 1	0	0	1	
Texture	tender/too soft or too firm/brittle 0 / 1 / 2	0	1	2	
Infestation					
Mold	absent/present/excessive 0 / 1 / 2	0	1	2	
Pink bacterial spoilage	absent/present/excessive 0 / 1 / 2	0	1	2	
Insects eggs, larvae, etc. (check gills)	absent/present/excessive 0 / 1 / 2	0	1	2	
Score		0	5	12	

After Gorczyca, E., unpublished.

Histamine and other biogenic amines may be found in cured fish.[54,60] The toxic effects of histamine are greatly increased by the presence of other diamines and polyamines such as cadaverine and putrescine[61] for which methods for simultaneous determination are available.[62]

4. Nutritional Quality

The nutritional quality of dried fish has been extensively reviewed recently.[63] In summary, the nutritional value of the original material is maintained with respect to the individual nutrients (proteins, amino acids, vitamins, polyunsaturated fatty acids, minerals, and individual elements) if there is the minimum of temperature abuse and oxidation during drying. Natural antioxidants are sometimes present in the fish, but these vary considerably with the seasons.[64] Smoke also provides antioxidant activity to protect polyunsaturated fatty acids.[39] Vitamins may be destroyed in the presence of oxidizing fat. Cooking of the fish prior to drying leads to considerable losses of vitamins and amino acids in the cooking liquor. On the other hand, cooking prior to drying may destroy endogenous enzymes which hydrolyze lipids to free fatty acids, leading to a destruction of polyunsaturated fatty acids during drying and storage.[65]

II. PRODUCTION OF FISH PROTEIN CONCENTRATES AND PREPARATIONS

A. HISTORY

Concentrated forms of fish protein for human consumption were produced commercially in the 1890s.[66] An egg-white substitute *Wiking Eiweiss* was produced in Germany in the 1930s. Fish protein concentrate (FPC) factories were built at the same time in Norway and South Africa, but neither was a commercial success. Further trials in the 1950s in South

Africa and Iceland were likewise discontinued. Work begun in the early 1950s in Canada continued through the 1960s to culminate in the construction of a plant with a design annual production capacity of 7900 t of FPC. Because of financial and industrial difficulties, the plant was never commissioned.[66]

In Morocco and Chile, two FPC plants with capacities of up to 145 t per annum were in production in the early 1960s. These plants attracted much interest from the international aid organizations as it was hoped that the production of FPC would alleviate the nutritional problems being experienced by the developing countries. Human feeding trials were conducted but the product was not generally accepted.

In the 20-year period from the early 1960s, there were many attempts worldwide to establish a viable FPC industry. Most of the attempts paralleled those in Morocco and Chile — the early expectations were never realized. There were, however, some notable exceptions; FPC plants established in Sweden, Norway, and Peru still produce quantities of human quality FPC for domestic consumption and for emergency famine relief.

The problem of acceptance of FPC for human consumption remains. For many years, FPC was not permitted as an additive for manufactured foods by the U.S. Food and Drug Administration (FDA); there is now a product made from the flesh of edible fish which is accepted.[67] Unless special production methods are employed, the functional properties of FPC detract from its usefulness as a substitute for other high grade proteins such as meat, egg, and soya bean.

The worldwide production of fish meal for animal feed is estimated at 20 million t annually or nearly 30% of the landed catch.[68] The conversion rate from animal feed protein to edible protein is variously estimated at between 6:1 and 10:1.[69]

B. PRODUCTION METHODS

FPC is classified as follows:[68]

- FPC Type A — a deodorized and tasteless product containing less than 0.75% fat and a minimum of 67.5% protein.
- FPC Type B — a hygenically prepared fish meal with a maximum of 3% fat.
- FPC Type C — fish meal.

The principal method of producing FPC is by solvent extraction from comminuted whole fish or fish by-products (Figure 6). Isopropyl and ethyl alcohols are the extractants most commonly used. Other suggested methods include acid or alkaline treatment and biological processes.[69] Following recovery of the solvent, the extract is dried, milled, and screened for bone particles.

Fish are very liable to spoilage due to bacterial action and highly active proteolytic enzymes in the gut; fish fats oxidize very rapidly. Because of this, taints develop rapidly. Efficient handling of the raw material and hygienic design and operation of processing plant together with effective control of the process are essential for the assurance of product quality.

C. FUNCTIONAL AND NUTRITIONAL PROPERTIES

The term "functional properties" is used to describe those physical and chemical characteristics of a food which contribute to their performance during manufacture, processing, storage, and consumption. Attributes such as color, flavor, solubility, wettability, foaming behavior, and inertness as well as the rheological properties of the solutions and gels form a profile of properties which contribute to the acceptance of the product.[70] The failure of FPC to be accepted as a food additive is attributed in part to its poor functional properties. Unmodified FPC has an extremely low water affinity and imparts a gritty, powdery texture

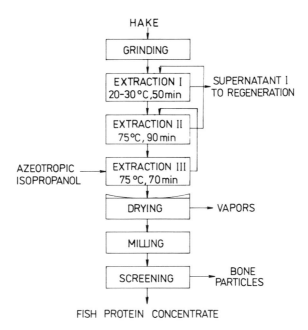

FIGURE 6. Flowchart for fish protein concentrate. (From Sikorski, Z. E. and Naczk, M., *Crit. Rev. Food Sci. Nutr.*, 14, 201, 1981. With permission.)

to foods. However, the functional properties of FPC can be improved by using chemical modifications or partially controlled proteolysis.[71]

In the manufacture of FPC Type B, concentrated fish solubles are added back to the press cake before entering the drier. The added salts, amino acids, and other solutes added back to the press cake lower the water activity of the product. The sorption isotherms (Figure 5) of solvent extracted "joy fish" prepared by Norsildmel A/L show that the FPC Type B product is inherently more stable than the Type A product.[72]

FPC is not intended to be used as a complete diet; rather, its use is as a high quality protein supplement. It has an excellent amino acid balance and is particularly effective as a supplement to cereals, which are low in lysine. The averaged protein efficiency ratios of nine FPC preparations ranged from 102 to 113%.[69]

Residual "fishy" flavor levels and its poor functional properties limit its proportion in foods to around 10%, depending on the quality of the product.

D. FUTURE PROSPECTS

The hope that FPC would be the solution to the nutritional problems of the world has largely disappeared with the lack of acceptance and the failure of most of the commercial scale ventures. Also in question is the assumption that the food resource of the oceans is unlimited.[73] Recent research has been towards improving the functional properties of fish protein concentrates with the aim of overcoming the acceptance difficulty. Any future commercial developments are likely to involve new products such as fish protein hydrolysates (Figure 7) and the other preparations.

Proteolytic enzymes can be used to produce fish hydrolysates which have functional properties greatly superior to those of unmodified FPC.[71] Plastein gels can be synthesized to give a range of rheological properties ranging from elastic to plastic, depending on the concentration of hydrolysate. Different chemical methods are available, including alkaline hydrolysis, acylation, and partial hydrolysis prior to extraction. Feasibility studies have been done on the preparation of concentrates from krill.[68]

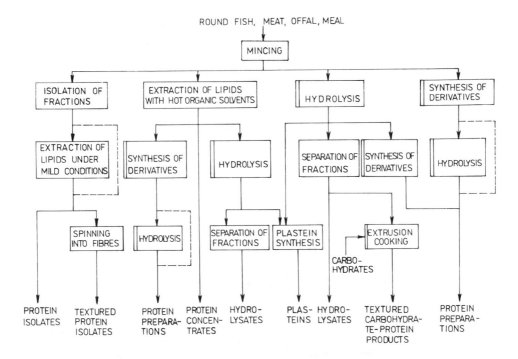

FIGURE 7. Main routes for manufacturing different concentrated fish protein products. (From Sikorski, Z. E. and Naczk, M., *Crit. Rev. Food Sci. Nutr.*, 14, 201, 1981. With permission.)

REFERENCES

1. **Burt, J. R., Ed.,** The effect of smoking and drying on the nutritional properties of fish, in *Fish Smoking and Drying,* Elsevier, London, 1988, chap. 9.
2. **Tanikawa, E., Motohiro, T., and Akiba, M.,** *Marine Products in Japan,* Koseisha Koseikaku, Tokyo, 1985, 193.
3. **Motohiro, T.,** Dried and smoked fish products: preparation and composition, in *Fish Smoking and Drying, The Effect of Smoking and Drying on the Nutritional Properties of Fish,* Burt, J. R., Ed., Elsevier, London, 1988, chap. 8.
4. **Doe, P. E., Ahmed, M., Musselmuddin, M., and Sachithananthan, K.,** A polythene tent drier for improved sun drying of fish, *Food Technol. Aust.,* 29, 437, 1977.
5. **Richards, A. H.,** A fish drier for the salt fish industry, *Harvest,* 5, 104, 1979.
6. **Sachithananthan, K., Trim, D. S., and Speirs, C. I.,** A solar-dome dryer for drying fish, in *FAO Fish Processing in Africa,* Proc. FAO Expert Consultation on Fish Technology in Africa, Lusaka, Zambia, FAO Fish. Rep. No. 329, Food and Agriculture Organization, Rome, 1986, 161.
7. **Trim, D. S. and Curran, C. A.,** A comparative study of solar and sun drying of fish in Ecuador, Report of the Tropical Products Institute, London, L60, 1983.
8. **Mendoza, L. S.,** Traditional methods of smoking fish in the Philippines, in *Cured Fish Production in the Tropics,* Proc. Workshop on the Production of Cured Fish, Reilly, A. and Barile, L. E., Eds., University of the Philippines in the Visayas, Diliman, Quezon City, 1986, 146.
9. **Roberts, S. F.,** Agrowaste fish driers, in *Cured Fish Production in the Tropics,* Proc. Workshop on the Production of Cured Fish, Reilly, A. and Barile, L. E., Eds., University of the Philippines in the Visayas, Diliman, Quezon City, 1986, 108.
10. **Cutting, C. L., Reay, G. A., and Shewan, J. M.,** Dehydration of Fish. Department of Scientific and Industrial Research, Food Investigation Special Report No. 62, Her Majesty's Stationery Office, London, 1956.
11. **Jason, A. C.,** quoted by Olley, J. N., Structure and proteins of fish and shellfish. I, in *Advances in Fish Science and Technology,* Connell, J. J., Ed., Table 2, Fishing News, Farnham, England, 1980, 72.

12. **Maddocks, K., Jason, A. C., and Slater, R. W.,** Improvements in and relating to the drying of fish, The Patents Office London, patent number 1056844, 1967.
13. **Anon.,** A continuously operated drying tunnel, *INFOFISH Marketing Dig.*, 2/83, 40, 1983.
14. **Burgess, G. H. O., Cutting, C. L., Lovern, J. A., and Waterman, J. J.,** in *Fish Handling and Processing,* Her Majesty's Stationery Office, London, 1965, 125.
15. **Abrahami, N. and Naismith, D. J.,** The dehydration of foods in edible oil in vacuo, *J. Food Technol.*, 3, 55, 1968.
16. **Jason, A. C.,** Fundamental aspects of the dehydration of foodstuffs, Society of Chemical Industry, London, 1958, 103.
17. **Jason, A. C. and Peters, G. R.,** Analysis of bimodal diffusion of water in fish muscle, *J. Phys. D: Appl. Phys.*, 6, 512, 1983.
18. **Brunauer, S., Emmett, P. H., and Teller, E.,** Adsorption of gases in monomolecular layers, *J. Am. Chem. Soc.*, 60, 309, 1938.
19. **Labuza, T. P.,** Sorption phenomena in foods, *Food Technol. (Champaign)*, 22, 263, 1968.
20. **Labuza, T. P., Acott, K., Tatini, S. R., Lee, R. Y., Flink, J., and McCall, W.,** Water activity determination: a collaborative study of different methods, *J. Food Sci.*, 41, 910, 1976.
21. **Voss, P. T. and Labuza, T. P.,** Technique for measurement of water activity in the high a_w range, *J. Agric. Food Chem.*, 22, 326, 1974.
22. **Olley, J., Doe, P. E., and Heruwati, E. S.,** The influence of drying and smoking on the nutritional properties of fish: an introductory overview, in *Fish Smoking and Drying,* Burt, J. R., Ed., Elsevier, London, 1988, chap. 1.
23. **Troller, J. A. and Christian, J. H. B.,** *Water Activity and Food,* Academic Press, New York, 1978.
24. **Lupin, H. M.,** Water activity in preserved fish products, in *Cured Fish Production in the Tropics.* Proc. Workshop on the Production of Cured Fish, Reilly, A. and Barile, L. E., Eds., University of the Philippines in the Visayas, Diliman, Quezon City, 1986, 16.
25. **Troller, J. A.,** Influence of water activity on microorganisms in foods, *Food Technol. (Chicago)*, 34, 76, 1980.
26. **Labuza, T. P.,** Kinetics of lipid oxidation in foods, *Crit. Rev. Food Technol.*, 2, 355, 1971.
27. **Ledward, D. A.,** Intermediate Moisture Meats, in *Current Developments in Meat Science,* Lawrie, R. A., Ed., Applied Science Publishers, London, 1981, 174.
28. **Bligh, E. G., Shaw, S. J., and Woyewoda, A. D.,** Effects of smoking on lipids of fish, in *Fish Smoking and Drying, The Effect of Smoking and Drying on the Nutritional Properties of Fish,* Burt, J. R., Ed., Elsevier, London, 1988, chap. 3.
29. **Chirife, J. and Iglesias, H. A.,** Equations for fitting water sorption isotherms of foods. I. A review, *J. Food Technol.*, 13, 159, 1978.
30. **Labuza, T. P. and Ragnarsson, J. O.,** Kinetic history effect on lipid oxidation of methyl linoleate in a model system, *J. Food Sci.*, 50, 145, 1985.
31. **Olson, J. C., Jr. and Nottingham, P. M.,** Temperature, in *Microbial Ecology of Foods,* Vol. 1, Silliker, J. H., Ed., Academic Press, New York, 1980, 1.
32. **Doe, P. E., Hashmi, R., Poulter, R. G., and Olley, J.,** Isohalic sorption isotherms I. Determination for dried salted cod (*Gadus morrhua*), *J. Food Technol.*, 17, 125, 1982.
33. **Leistner, L.,** in *Intermediate Moisture Foods,* Davis, R., Birch, G. G., and Parker, K. L., Eds., Applied Science Publishers, London, 1976, 135.
34. **FAO,** The prevention of losses in cured fish, FAO Fish. Tech. Paper 219, Food and Agriculture Organization, Rome, 1981, 14.
35. **Acker, L.,** Enzymic reactions in dried foodstuffs of plant and animal origin, in *The Technology of Fish Utilisation. Contributions from Research,* Kreuzer, R., Ed., Fishing News Books, London, 1965, 252.
36. **Kuninaka, A., Kiki, M., and Sakaguchi, K.,** History and development of flavour nucleotides, *Food Technol. (Champaign)*, 18, 287, 1964.
37. **Waterman, J. J.,** The production of dried fish, FAO Fish. Tech. Pap. No. 160, Food and Agriculture Organization, Rome, 1976, 28.
38. **You, B. J. and Lee, K. H.,** Kinetics of lipid oxidation in dried fish meat stored under different conditions of water activity and temperature, *Bull. Korean Fish. Soc.*, 15, 83, 1982.
39. **Loayza-Salazar, E.,** quoted by Olley, J., Unconventional sources of fish protein, *CSIRO Food Res. Q.*, 32, 27, 1972.
40. **Taylor, R. W. D.,** Insecticides for the protection of dried fish, in *FAO, Proc. FAO Expert Consultation on Fish Technology in Africa,* FAO Fish. Rep. No. 268, Food and Agriculture Organization, Rome, 1982, 181.
41. **McMeekin, T. A., Olley, J., and Ratkowsky, D. A.,** Temperature effects on bacterial growth rates, in *Physiological Models in Microbiology,* Vol. 1, CRC Ser. Mathematical Models in Microbiology, Bazin, M. J., Ed., CRC Press, Boca Raton, FL, 1988, chap 4.
42. **Ratkowsky, D. A., Lowry, R. K., McMeekin, T. A., Stokes, A. N., and Chandler, R. E.,** Model for bacterial growth rate throughout the entire biokinetic temperature range, *J. Bacteriol.*, 154, 1222, 1983.

43. **McMeekin, T. A., Chandler, R. E., Doe, P. E., Garland, C. D., Olley, J., Putro, S., and Ratkowsky, D. A.**, Model for combined effect of temperature and salt concentration/water activity on the growth rate of *Staphylococcus xylosus*, *J. Appl. Bacteriol.*, 62, 543, 1987.
44. **Doe, P. E. and Heruwati, E. S.**, A model for the prediction of microbial spoilage of sundried tropical fish, *J. Food Eng.*, in press.
45. **van Klaveren, F. W. and Legendre, R.**, Salted cod, in *Fish as Food*, Vol. 3, Borgstrom, G., Ed., Academic Press, London, 1965, chap. 4.
46. **Pitt, J. I. and Hocking, A. D.**, New species of fungi from Indonesian dried fish, *Mycotaxon*, 22, 197, 1985.
47. **Wheeler, K. A., Hocking, A. D., and Pitt, J. I.**, Effects of temperature and water activity on germination and growth of *Wallemia sebi*, *Trans. Br. Mycol. Soc.*, 90, 365, 1988.
48. **Wheeler, K. A., Hocking, A. D., Pitt, J. I., and Anggawati, A. M.**, Fungi associated with Indonesian dried fish, *Food Microbiol.*, 3, 351, 1986.
49. **Daniel, D. J. E. and Etoh, S.**, Insect infestation of dry fish in Sri Lanka, in *The Production and Storage of Dried Fish*, Proc. Workshop on the Production and Storage of Dried Fish, Universiti Pertanian Malaysia, James, D., Ed., FAO Fish. Rep. No. 279, Food and Agriculture Organization, Rome, 1983, 162.
50. **Esser, J. R., Hanson, S. W., and Taylor, K. D. A.**, Loss reduction techniques for salted/dried marine catfish, in *Spoilage of Tropical Fish and Product Development*, Proc. Symp. held in conjunction with the Sixth Session of the Indo-Pacific Fishery Commission Working Party on fish technology and marketing. Reilly, A., Ed., Melbourne, FAO Fish. Rep. No. 317, Food and Agriculture Organization, Rome, 1985, 315.
51. **FAO**, The prevention of losses in cured fish, FAO Fish. Tech. Paper 219, Food and Agriculture Organization, Rome, 1981, 21.
52. **FAO**, The prevention of losses in cured fish, FAO Fish. Tech. Paper 219, Food and Agriculture Organization, Rome, 1981, 56.
53. **FAO**, The prevention of losses in cured fish, FAO Fish. Tech. Paper 219, Food and Agriculture Organization, Rome, 1981, 35.
54. **Kreuzer, R.**, Cephalopods: handling, processing and products, FAO Fish. Tech. Paper No. 254, Food and Agriculture Organization, Rome, 1984.
55. **FAO**, The prevention of losses in cured fish, FAO Fish. Tech. Paper 219, Food and Agriculture Organization, Rome, 1981, 67.
56. **IFT**, Sensory evaluation guide for testing food and beverage products, *Food Technol. (Chicago)*, 35, 1981, 50.
57. **Bremner, H. A., Olley, J., and Vail, A. M. A.**, Estimating time-temperature effects by a rapid systematic sensory method, in *Seafood Quality Determination*, Kramer, D. E. and Liston, J., Eds., Proc. Int. Symp. coordinated by the University of Alaska Sea Grant College Program, Anchorage, November, 1986, 413.
58. **O'Mahoney, M. and Ishii, R.**, in *Umami: A Basic Taste*, Kawamura, Y. and Kare, R. M., Eds., Marcel Dekker, New York, 1987, 86.
59. **Skurray, G. R. and Pucar, N.**, L-Glutamic acid content of fresh and processed fish, *Food Chem.*, 27, 177, 1988.
60. **Pan, B. S.**, Undesirable factors in dried fish products, in *Fish Smoking and Drying, The Effect of Smoking and Drying on the Nutritional Properties of Fish*, Burt, J. R., Ed., Elsevier, London, 1988, chap. 5.
61. **James, D. and Olley, J.**, Summary and future research needs, in *Histamine and Marine Products: Production by Bacteria, Measurement and Prediction of Formation*, Sun Pan, B. and James, D., Eds., FAO Fish. Tech. Paper. No. 252, Food and Agriculture Organization, Rome, 1985, 47.
62. **Ritchie, A. H. and Mackie, I. M.**, The formation of diamines and polyamines during the storage of mackerel (*Scomber scombrus*), in *Advances in Fish Science and Technology*, Connell, J. J., Ed., Fishing News, London, 1980, 489.
63. **Burt, J. R., Ed.**, *Fish Smoking and Drying*, The effect of smoking and drying on the nutritional properties of fish, Elsevier, London, 1988.
64. **Astrup, H.**, Oxidation of highly unsaturated herring oil, *J. Chem. Ind. (London)*, 1964, 107.
65. **Takiguchi, A.**, Lipid oxidation and hydrolysis in dried anchovy products during drying and storage, *Bull. Soc. Jpn. Sci. Fish.*, 53, 1463, 1987.
66. **Pariser, E. R., Wallerstein, M. B., Corkery, C. J., and Brown, N. L.**, *Fish Protein Concentrate: Panacea for Protein Malnutrition?*, MIT Press, Cambridge, 1978, 11.
67. **Hannigan, K. J.**, Fish protein isolate okayed by FDA, *Food Eng.*, 54, 92, 1982.
68. **Mackie, I. M.**, New approaches in the use of fish protein, in *Developments in Food Protein — 2*, Hudson, B. J. F., Ed., Applied Science Publishers, Barking, Essex, 1983, chap. 6.
69. **Finch, R.**, Fish protein for human foods, *Crit. Rev. Food Technol.*, 1, 519, 1970.
70. **Kinsella, J. E.**, Functional properties of proteins in foods: a survey, *Crit. Rev. Food Technol.*, 7, 219, 1976.

71. **Sikorski, Z. E. and Naczk, M.**, Modification of technological properties of fish protein concentrates, *Crit. Rev. Food Sci. Nutr.*, 14, 201, 1981.
72. **Norsildmel A/L,** Norse Fish Powder. Fish protein concentrate for human consumption, Norsidmel A/L, Bergen, Norway, 1975.
73. **Harris, G. P.**, *Phytoplankton Ecology, Structure, Function and Fluctuation,* Chapman Hall, New York, 1986, 287.

Chapter 9

SALTING AND MARINATING OF FISH

Vladimir I. Shenderyuk and Piotr J. Bykowski

TABLE OF CONTENTS

I. Preservation of Fish by Salting 148
    A. Evolution of Fish Salting Technique 148
    B. Physical and Chemical Bases of Salting 149
    C. Ripening of Salted Fish 151
    D. Technology of Producing Salted Fish 152
    E. Techniques for Producing Preserves in Large Metal Cans 153
    F. Techniques for Producing Preserves in Small Cans 153
    G. Caviar Production Technology 155
    H. Storage of Salted and Pickled Fish and Preserves 155

II. Marinating 156
    A. Introduction 156
    B. Cold Marinades 156
        1. Maturing 156
        2. Factors Affecting the Quality and Shelf Life of Cold Marinades 156
        3. Manufacturing Procedures and Products 157
    C. Cooked Marinades 159
    D. Fried Marinades 160

References 162

I. PRESERVATION OF FISH BY SALTING

A. EVOLUTION OF FISH SALTING TECHNIQUE

Preservation of fish by salting is one of the most ancient techniques, which can be traced back to 3500 to 4000 B.C., having reached the peak in the 18th and 19th centuries. The development of other methods of fish preservation since the second half of the 19th century has resulted in a certain reduction of salted-fish production. With broadened production of the frozen and smoked fish and canning, the fish species composition for salting has been undergoing certain selection. Among the fish species designed for preparing the salted product, those which, when salted, acquire a peculiar flavor and taste of "ripened" product (Clupeidae and Salmonidae) have become popular. This practice is typical of many European and U.S. countries as well as of the U.S.S.R. and Japan. In the developing countries of Africa and Latin America, salting of fish combined with artificial or natural drying has been widely in use until now for preparing salted-dried product, which can be stored at ambient temperature. The latter point is of special importance, since these countries suffer from acute deficiencies in freezing and cold storage facilities.

The joint studies carried out by the Soviet scientists together with the scientists from the Fisheries Investigation Center in Angola, have suggested wide opportunities for developing a technique for salting fish in African countries, with a "European" model of this preservation method as an analogue. It is meant to allow consumption of salted fish without additional thermal processing, provided that the salt content is considerably reduced in the final product, which acquires the properties characteristic of the "ripened" fish, or that new flavor additives are introduced during the fish processing. Nevertheless, the task of constructing refrigeration facilities in developing countries remains indispensable, as its realization could promote the use of more advanced methods for salting fish. In this context, attention is focused on a description of technology for producing the salted product with lowered salt content which is practiced on a large scale in most countries throughout the world and may be applied in the developing African and Latin American countries in prospect.

Technology of salted fish production is undergoing significant changes in the process of evolutionary development under the influence of the scientific technological progress in the field of technology and storage of food commodities. The Clupeoid and Salmon species, main items in production of salted fish until recently, have now been supplemented by mackerel, horse mackerel, sardine, and other fish species, the process of ripening of which markedly differs from that observed, for instance, for salted herring. Special processing regimes permit preparing high quality products of these fish species. The developed processes also make use of actually nonripening fish species — cod, grenadier, and the other lean fish — for production of the high quality salted food. This has become possible due to introduction of smoking and use of oil fillings in the salted-fish technology. Thus, the natural process of ripening of the salted fish, influenced by a complex of biochemical changes taking place in the constituents of the raw fish resources, is being replaced by new regulated processes for producing the salted fish with better taste-flavor properties ensuring high organoleptic indices of the final product. This has become possible due to intensive investigations into the chemistry of ripening of salted fish, the improvement of traditional and development of essentially new techniques for salting fish. Salted-fish packages have also changed considerably. From the early barrels, the industry has progressed to containers made of metal, aluminum, and polymeric materials of small capacities, mainly 50 to 200 cm^3. It can be expected that the traditional packing for salted fish — barrels — will be eliminated in some countries by the end of the current millenium.

Sodium chloride is one of the most important components that determine the taste of salted fish, direction, and intensity of chemical processes during its ripening. The sodium chloride content is essential not only for the rate of the above-stated processes, but also for the product stability during storage. In this connection, the data on optimum amounts of salt in salted fish ensuring a high-quality and stable product are of interest. Sociological inquiry of a group of the Soviet fish consumers has shown that most demanded for products prepared of the same fish species were those where the salt content did not exceed 4 to 5%. About 70% of consumers gave preference to the salted fish having the above salt concentrations while only 15% preferred the salted fish product with the salt amount exceeding 6%. It is worth noting that the salted fishery products with reduced salt quantities enjoyed wide popularity in all times and in many countries throughout the world. However, such fishery products could be only produced in cold seasons. Progress in freezing technology and construction of a network of cold stores for fish has enabled expansion of producing the salted fish with reduced salt content, as low storage temperatures play the role of a preservative while the salt is mostly assigned the part of flavor additive.

In the first half of the 1980s, about 14% of the world fish catch was used on annual basis for production of salted, smoked, and dried commodities, which is indicative of the high importance of these preservation methods for producing fish products.

A long history of producing the salted-fish products suggests that this preservation technique will continue to occupy a prominent place in the future. Efforts of technologists will be aimed at producing the salted product with high hygienic and taste properties.

Prospective lines of development of this technique for producing the fish food are as follows:

- Reduction of sodium chloride dose in final product
- Substitution of sodium chloride by other, less harmful substances which could imitate the taste of the salted product
- Search for new preserving additions which could increase stability and safety of the salted product during storage
- Improvement of regimes for producing fish products with high rheological properties
- Improvement of flavors and odors due to directed process of the salted fish ripening, addition of flavorings and ferment preparations
- Use of modern packages and materials for packaging the salted fish
- Development and mastering technology of the analogue salted product imitating the taste of valuable fish species (salmon, sturgeon, trout, etc.)

B. PHYSICAL AND CHEMICAL BASES OF SALTING

The process of producing salted fish is known to be divided into three stages:[1]

- Salting for bringing fish into contact with salt or salt solution
- Proper salting, during which salt and moisture are transported within fish-salt-brine system
- Ripening of salted fish, when flavor, taste, and consistency of product are established

The above succession of the process of producing salted fish may be considered conventional to a certain degree, as ripening of the product begins since the fish is brought into contact with salt, which leads to intensive interaction of sodium chloride and water in the system. On completion of salt and water transport, the process of ripening of salted fish proceeds throughout storage of the product.

Formation of sodium chloride solution is an indispensable condition for sodium chloride and water transport within the fish-salt system. As the fish is brought into contact with sodium chloride crystals, hydration of chlorine and sodium ions by dipoles of the water covering the surface of the fish takes place. Forces of interaction of water dipoles with chlorine and sodium ions exceed those acting in crystal lattice of sodium chloride, thus ensuring separation of hydrated ions and dilution of salt. Rate of salt dilution depends on salt crystal size — the larger crystals the lower their dilution rate. The temperature of the system, in fact, exerts no considerable influence on the rate of salt dilution. To speed up the process of transport of sodium chloride and water in the fish-salt system, the sodium chloride solution is added which results in formation of fish-salt-brine system and intensified transport of sodium chloride and water dipole ions responsible for salting of the fish. In this case, salt dilution occurs due to reduced sodium chloride concentration in brine at the expense of transport of water from fish. When processes of salt dilution and transport of water from fish are balanced, concentration of sodium chloride in brine may remain unchanged until salt is completely dissolved. However, if the process of water transport from fish forestalls that of salt dilution and transport in fish, sodium chloride concentration in brine tends to decrease.

At the stage of salting of fish, sodium and chlorine ions are transported from brine into fish and water dipoles from fish to brine. The majority of investigators believe that transport of sodium and chlorine ions during the process of thorough salting results from diffusion.[1-6] Regarding water transport, the views of investigators of the nature of this process differ. Most are apt to relate the nature of this process to osmosis, but some adhere to the opinion that it takes place due to diffusion. In our opinion, transport of sodium chloride and chlorine ions and of water dipoles is of a more complex character, and its rate and direction are governed by unbalanced state of chemical potential of two systems: organic matter-fish water dipoles and sodium chloride solution surrounding the fish. This assumption is confirmed by the fact that the process of sodium chloride and water transport in fish-brine system continues throughout storage of the salted fish, which can be explained by variation of chemical potential of organic system of the fish and its water dipoles during ripening process as a result of continuous hydrolysis of proteic substances. It should be stressed, however, that sodium chloride and water transport proceeds with differing intensities during salting and ripening, and depends on the value of chemical potential of organic system in the fish and brine. Most intensive transport takes place during salting and slackens during ripening, the rates of transport of sodium and chlorine ions and water dipoles differing in both processes.

For use of scientific evidence on sodium chloride and water transport during the salting-in process in practice, the knowledge of factors influencing the rate of this process is of great importance. Concentration of sodium chloride in fish muscle tissue and brine is the most important factor determining the rate of transport of constituents under consideration in the salting-in process. In practice, sodium chloride concentration gradient can be increased by changing quantities of salt relative to fish mass. By increasing amounts of salt, conditions are established when higher salt concentration in brine promotes a more intensive sodium chloride and water transport. Therefore, for instance, with the increase of the salt amount from 9 to 21% relative to fish mass in salting horse mackerel, salting-in rate increases 2.5 times, and that of mackerel 1.5 times. Size of fish and its thickness, in particular, are very important factors influencing the rates of sodium chloride and water transport. Rate of fish salting is proportionate to its squared specific surface. To make practical use of this factor, the fish is dressed — beheaded and gutted — then split or filleted before salting. Therefore, for example, rate of salting-in the horse mackerel fillets increases 50- to 100-fold compared with the salting-in rate for whole horse mackerel. Thus, dressing the fish is a major factor to speed up salt and water transport while salting. Chemical composition and structure of fish muscle tissues and peculiarities of its skin are of no less importance. Skin and scales on fish body reduce salting-in rate by 1.6 and the skin only by 1.6. Hypodermic fat also impedes sodium chloride and water transport. Rate of salting-in the Atlantic herring with 15 to 20% fat content is twice as low as that of herring having 2 to 5% fat content. Hypodermic fat functions as a peculiar hydrophobic barrier for sodium chloride transport during salting-in. Removal of scales and skin from the fish body may help considerably to intensify the transport process. However, it should be remembered that skin removal may lead to a changing of the exterior of the finished product from some fish species to the worse and to rapid oxidation of hypodermic fat. In this connection, the question of whether the fish has to be skinned or not before salting is decided with regard for species composition of the raw material, structure of fish muscle tissue, and expediency of intensification of sodium chloride and water transport. Salting-in rate in fish in the state of rigor mortis is lower than at the final stage of rigor mortis. Freezing and defrosting of fish favors acceleration of salting-in 1.2 to 1.3 times, as penetrability of fish muscle tissue changes after freezing and subsequent defrosting.[7] Salting temperature is not ranked as important for salting-in rate as the above-stated factors. Therefore, the rise of the temperature in salting by 10° would increase salting-in rate by as low as 14 to 18%. However, it is accompanied by accelerated post-mortem changes and growth of microorganisms in fish which is intolerable at salting. The rate of sodium chloride transport depends on chemical composition of salt. The presence of calcium and magnesium ions slackens the sodium chloride transport.

Chemical composition and weight of the salted fish undergo considerable changes during the salting-in process, subsequent ripening, and storage. During the salting-in process, the changes in chemical fish composition are mainly caused by increasing amounts of sodium chloride and reduced water content. On completion of the salting-in process, the salt content in muscle tissue actually becomes stable. Water and sodium chloride transport from the brine into the fish occurring during ripening and storage of the salted product affects the weight and chemical composition of the salted fish. Changes of the fish weight during salting-in and ripening process result from sodium chloride and water transport within the fish-salt-brine system. The knowledge of regularities of these processes will enable the foundation of technological regimes and standard expense of the raw material, salt and packs, to produce the salted fish.

C. RIPENING OF SALTED FISH

Ripening of salted fish is the second important phase that forms their structural, plastic, flavor, and odor properties which add to their quality and make the fish ready-to-use product without any additional processing. Ripening is a complex physical and chemical process of transforming proteins, lipids, and carbohydrates brought about by functioning of enzymic systems which results in the formation of peculiar taste, flavor, and consistency of salted fish.

The changes of proteic substances during ripening of salted fish have been studied most thoroughly. These changes are based on hydrolysis of proteins under the influence of the peptide hydrolase complex. In ripening salted product from dressed fish, the hydrolysis of proteic substances is called forth by the action of peptide hydrolases of cathepsin A, B, and C types as there exists a close agreement between their optimum pH values and those in fish muscle tissues. In ripening salted whole fish, the role of ripening agents is played by the peptide hydrolase complex in viscera, particularly in pyloric appendages containing a highly active complex of peptide hydrolases of trypsin and peptidase types. Having gained in activity as a result of partial hydrolysis, the complex of these peptide hydrolases penetrates into fish muscle tissues and, having combined with muscle enzymic system, promotes hydrolysis of proteins. The resultant free amino acids and peptides undergo complex reactions with lipid and carbohydrate transformation products. The higher the activity of visceral and muscle peptide hydrolase complex, the more intensive the hydrolysis of proteins and the faster the ripening process in salted fish. The fish lipids also undergo complex changes during ripening. Lipid hydrolysis is well described by experimental data on accumulation of free fatty acids. Changes of fish muscle tissue structure influenced by enzymes involve redistribution of lipids. The ripened salted fish seems to be enveloped with oil. Favorable conditions arise for interaction of protein and lipid hydrolysis products. The released organoid oil and products of its hydrolysis become oxidized, especially when largely exposed to the air. The content of carbonyl compounds and volatile fatty acids increases. There is every reason to admit that carbohydrates also undergo transformation as the common salt does not ensure inhibition or interruption of chemical reactions. However, the data on carbohydrate transformation in the phase of ripening of salted fish are not so extensive in the literature as those on lipid and protein transformation.

Marked differences exist in consistency, flavor, and odor of the salted fish prepared from various kinds of raw material. A high-quality salted product is prepared from salmon, sturgeon, and herring. The final product from lean fish species, fish species noted for low peptide hydrolase activity and inadequate extent of hydrolyzation of proteins (horse mackerel, cod, grenadier), lacks the consistency, flavor, and odor peculiar to ripened fish. For a long time differences in the salted-fish ripening pattern have been attributed to varying activity and composition of muscle and visceral peptide hydrolase complexes. The latter caused peculiarities of composition of the protein hydrolysis products and, as a result, differences in organoleptic properties of the salted fish prepared from various fish species.[8-10] Extensive investigation into characteristics of muscle and visceral peptide hydrolase complexes carried out during 2 recent decades showed that major peptide hydrolase characteristics are identical in different fish species. The validity of this conclusion is confirmed by the evidence that the active center of main proteolytic enzymes has an identical composition irrespective of fish species.[5] At the same time, some data are indicative of a considerable importance of peculiarities in proteic substance composition by species for the pattern and rate of accumulation of hydrolysis products generated by peptide hydrolases.[5] The new data underlie a substrate hypothesis of ripening of salted fish.[5] This hypothesis suggests that ripening of salted fish is a complex of enzymic transformations of main components of raw material and subsequent changes of products of their hydrolysis which is responsible for organoleptic properties of the product. Quantitative composition of ripening-induced products depends on specifity of structure and composition of the substrate (protein, lipids, carbohydrates) in each fish species, and the rate of ripening is highly dependent on enzymic activity and number of links being hydrolyzed in original substrates. The substrate hypothesis allows finding practical ways to improve the quality of the salted product. The most important among these are the increase of enzyme peptide hydrolase activity by addition of enzymic preparations while salting and the use of wide assortment of aromatizers to achieve the preset properties in the salted product.

In developing methods for regulating rates of proteic substance hydrolysis during ripening of salted fish, the following factors which govern the rate of this process should be considered: peptide hydrolase concentration in raw material, peculiarities of structure of muscle tissues and their proteic substance composition succession of amino acids in primary structure of proteic molecules in fish, temperature at proteic substance hydrolysis, hydrogen ion concentration in the medium where proteic substance hydrolysis occurs, and presence of activators and inhibitors of peptide hydrolases in raw material.[5]

D. TECHNOLOGY OF PRODUCING SALTED FISH

Salted and pickled fish are produced from fresh fish on ships and ashore or from defrosted fish. Whole or dressed fish with heads and viscera removed are used for salting.

In producing salted fish aboard ship, mixed completed salting in nonsaturated salt solution is the most suitable method. Barrels and vats made of polymeric materials of maximum 50 dm^3 capacity serve as containers for the salted fish. The fish are uniformly mixed with the required amount of salt (2.5 to 10.0% to fish weight). Before packing the containers with fish-salt mixture, they are filled with saturated salt solution, precooled at most to 5°C, which takes 2 to 6% of the capacity of the container. Salted fish are packed into barrels 3 to 5 cm above chime on the basis of 43 kg of fish per 50 dm^3. Packed fish are slightly pressed, the barrel sealed and transported to a cool room for salting and subsequent storage. Of the total amount of dry salt, 80% is used for rolling fish in salt, adding it in between layers of fish packed into a barrel, and the remaining 20% is used to cover the upper fish layer. In a room for salting and storage of the salted fish, the barrels are opened and filled with saturated salt solution cooled to +5°C to −5°C. After 24 to 72 h, containers are opened once again and filled up with salt solution. The total amount of saturated salt solution for filling a container varies from 13 to 20% of the total container capacity.

The ambient temperature in the storeroom is maintained within the range of +2 to −5°C. On completion of salting the last lot of fish, the temperature in room for salting and storing is decreased to −5 to −8°C.

E. TECHNIQUES FOR PRODUCING PRESERVES IN LARGE METAL CANS

In the U.S.S.R., preserves are produced in cans of 860-cm^3 to 5-dm^3 capacity depending on fish species and available facilities. This product occupies intermediate position between the fish salted in barrels and preserves in cans of 50- to 250-cm^3 capacity. In terms of technology, production of preserves in larger cans is approximately that of salted fish in barrels, the only difference being the kind of package and recipe ingredients, which permit producing the fish product with lower sodium chloride content and better flavor pattern.

For producing preserves, both dressed and whole fish chilled to 5°C is used. After dressing and washing, the fish is mixed on salting tables with certain amounts of salt, sugar, and spices, when spicy preserves are produced. In cans with packed salted fish, the saturated salt solution amounting to 7% of can capacity and a preservative — in the order of 1 g per 1 kg of can content — are added. Cans packed with fish are sealed and dried. Storage time for perserves depends on fish species and varies from 1.5 to 6 months from production at −2 to −8°C. To accelerate maturation and to ensure better taste and flavor properties of the end product from dressed fish, the Soviet preparation "Ocean" made of viscera of oceanic fishes in proportion of 1 to 2% of the fish weight could be added as well as 100 mg of proteinase B-500 of microbiological origin (France) per 1 kg of the product and 20 mg of neutral proteinase NOVO of microbiological origin (Denmark) per 1 kg of the product. Comparative studies on the use of these preparations to speed up maturation of salted herring and horse mackerel fillets have demonstrated that the preparation Ocean is most advantageous for this purpose, as its peptide hydrolases provide for more uniform maturation of the product and add natural taste and flavor of mature product. This evidently can be attributed to the fact that in addition to peptide hydrolases, the preparation contains flavor substances characteristic of mature product. Availability of high molecular peptide hydrolase fractions in fermented preparations of microbiological origin prevents even penetration of these into fish muscle tissue, thus resulting in increased softening of upper layers of the fillet. In addition, the presence of accompanying products of microbiological origin in preparations adds a flavor and taste unusual for the salted fillet. The recipe for spicy preserves from the oceanic fish includes the following ingredients (grams per can of 1300-cm^3 capacity): fish, 1126; common salt, 82.6; sugar, 1.3; black pepper, 3.9; sweet pepper, 7.8; ginger, 0.39; nutmeg, 0.334; nutmeg bloom, 0.316; clove, 0.39; cardamon, 0.130; coriander, 0.480; cinnamon, 0.13; sodium salt of benzoic acid, 1.22; and saturated sodium chloride solution, 74.3. A combination of spices may vary within a wide range in both ingredient composition and their amounts depending on eating habits of the consumers.

Preserves contained in large metal cans are promising products that could be realized through the network of public eating places, this type of package being particularly convenient for short-term storage and preparing snack food.

F. TECHNIQUES FOR PRODUCING PRESERVES IN SMALL CANS

Production of preserves from fillet, sliced fillet, small pieces of fillet, and fillet rolls in small cans of 50- to 200-cm^3 capacity in various flavored fillings is the most progressive way of preparing top-quality salted products. The use of ferment preparations and flavor additions in fillings yields a wide range of high-quality salted products from diverse raw materials, which may actually meet all food requirements of the consumers. At present, at the majority of plants for producing preserves from the filleted fish in small packs, the salted half-ready product of special or spicy salting after partial maturation is used. Fillets, fillet slices, and fillet pieces made of the salted half-product are packed into cans which are then filled with flavored fillings and kept for maturation and subsequent marketing. Among the disadvantages of this technological technique are intermittent and too long processing times, labor and energy intensity, large expenses of raw material and salt, need for additional working areas for producing the salted half-product, and the lack of facilities for technological process preventing the product from being prepared with preset proportions of salt and required maturation stages. Additionally, the problem is aggravated by the fact that much salted waste is left after dressing the salted fish, which cannot be converted into good-quality fishmeal to be fed to livestock.

To eliminate these disadvantages, Soviet technology scientists have developed a technique for producing preserves from fish fillet slices in different flavored fillings without preliminary salting. The salt and flavored fillings are subsequently added to the content of a can. All ingredients are introduced and the cans are vacuum sealed and kept for salting-in and maturing. The following technological scheme can be formulated for producing preserves: chilling or defrosting the frozen fish; sorting out; filleting; portioning and packing; adding the salt, flavored fillings, and ferment preparation; sealing; washing; drying and wiping of cans; labeling; piling; maturating; and storing.

To produce preserves from fillet pieces, the fresh or frozen fish is used. Before dressing, the fresh fish is chilled to 5 to 0°C. Defrosted or chilled raw material is then sorted out and dressed. The fish is filleted, fillet skinned, and mashed. The salt, after preliminary drying and seiving through the seive with 0.8 × 0.8 mm mesh, is applied to packed fillet. Then the cans are filled with ferment preparation solution, flavored additions, garnishes, and preservative solution. Flavored fillings can be made of vegetable oil and mayonnaise, with addition of spices, tomato paste, mustard, etc. Sodium salt of benzoic acid, acetic, or muriatic acids are used as conservatives. The temperature of cans prior to packing into boxes must not exceed 10°C. Chilling time for cans to the temperature of −2°C is about 24 h. To salt-in fillet pieces in fillings such as solutions and suspensions will require 24 to 26 h, and in oil and emulsions (mayonnaise) 15 d. After partial maturation at the given temperature, the salted-in preserves can be frozen to −18°C to ensure longer storage time. Freezing kills larval nematodes[12] and large numbers of microorganisms thus increasing the stability of preserves on occassions when they happen to be stored for some time at above-zero temperatures.

Paste-like salted products, normally packed in small cans, are in public demand in many countries. Paste-like salted products are produced from the salted fish or muscle tissues of defrosted fish. For mildly salted paste, various fish species of marine raw resources are used. The fish is dressed, washed, and brought to special separators for mince production. The mince is seasoned with salt, sugar, butter or margarine, spices and other flavor additives, and ferment preparations. The mixture is thoroughly stirred and ground in a mincer-and-blender-type device for 5 to 10 min. To accelerate maturing, the ferment preparation Ocean is added at 1% of fish mince weight. The ground paste is packed into small cans and kept at the temperature ranging from 0 to −5°C for maturation. Mildly salted fish pastes become ready-to-eat products after 10 to 15 d.

There obviously is an increasing market for the salted, smoked sliced fillets packed in attractive multicolored film made of combined polymeric materials.[11] The product is vacuum sealed. Packing in modified air consisting of a mixture of carbon dioxide, oxygen, and air is also practiced. The technique used for producing this kind of product involves filleting the fish, salting the fillet in sodium chloride solution in the ratio of 1:1 until the salt content in the fillet is 4 to 5% and curing at 25 to 35°C for as long as 0.5 to 4 h depending on fillet size. The fillet is cut into slices 1 to 2.5 mm thick, which are placed on polymeric film and vacuum sealed. To give the product unusual flavor, the surfaces of the slices are covered with aromatized vegetable oil. Vegetable oil can be aromatized with various flavor additives or carbon dioxide extracts from natural spices. The storage time for film-packed smoked fillet at -2 to $-5°C$ is 30 d.

G. CAVIAR PRODUCTION TECHNOLOGY

Fish eggs, especially those of sturgeon and of fishes of Salmonidae, are valuable raw materials for delicatessen production.

To produce caviar, the eggs are used immediately after the fish is caught. In sturgeons, the eggs are removed while the fish are alive. Ovaries in their membranes removed from the fish are rubbed through special nets to separate the eggs from the connective tissue. Salting and subsequent pasteurization is a basic technique used for caviar preservation. Pasteurized soft caviar packed in small cans is the most valuable kind of egg product. Common salt is the main preserving substance. Antiseptics are additional preserving substances allowed by health authorities.

Pasteurized soft caviar from sturgeon is produced as follows. The rubbed eggs are washed with pure cold water and placed on the sieve to let the water stream down. The washed eggs are salted with a mixture of dry fine salt and an antiseptic. The salt amount constitutes 3 to 5% of the egg weight. The brine formed during salting is removed after the eggs are salted-in by again placing the eggs on the sieve. The eggs are packed in cans 28, 56, and 112 g by weight, which are then vacuum sealed. Caviar is pasteurized in water at 60°C. The pasteurization process lasts for 3 h. On completion of pasteurization, the cans with caviar are cooled in cold water until the temperature of 20 to 30°C is attained, then they are wiped or dried and kept at 0 to 2°C for 24 h. Cooled cans are packed in cartons.

Pasteurized soft caviar from fishes of Salmonidae is prepared in a similar way. The only exceptions are the salting method and pasteurization regime. The eggs are salted in a boiled, cooled, and settled saturated solution of sodium chloride at the temperature up to 15°C. The eggs to brine ratio must be 1:3. The salting lasts for 8 to 18 min depending on the fish species and egg quality until the salt content in the eggs is 4 to 6%. The eggs must be mixed during salting. On completion of salting, the eggs are placed on a sieve to remove the brine. The eggs are packed in cans with subsequent pasteurization at 69 to 70°C for 2.5 h. The procedures to follow are similar to those applied to pasteurized cans packed with eggs from sturgeon. Pasteurized caviar can be stored for 3 to 4 months at 10 to 18°C and for 6 to 8 months at $-2°C$.

H. STORAGE OF SALTED AND PICKLED FISH AND PRESERVES

Storage temperature for salted and pickled fish and preserves is the main factor governing the rate of fermentative hydrolysis of most important components of the raw material and determining storage times for the products. Variation of storage temperatures for the salted product may permit adjustment of the speed of product maturation. The common practice of storing the salted products is from about 5°C to the cryoscopic temperature for this kind of production. The cryoscopic temperature values for the salted product depend upon the salt amount in the final product:

Salt amount (%)	4	6	8	10	12
Cryoscopic temperature (°C)	-4.3	-5.5	-7.1	8.7	-10.5

For short-term storage, the product is kept at 5 to 6°C, and, for storage over 10 to 15 d, it is placed in chambers with lower temperatures ranging from −6 to −10°C. The higher the peptide hydrolase complex activity in the raw material, the lower the storage temperature (−5 to −10°C). Storage temperatures for the salted products from slowly aging fish ranges from 0 to −5°C. The salted products and preserves may be frozen on completion of maturation if it is found necessary to prolong storage times. On such occasions, freezing temperatures range from −20 to −25°C. Freezing of the salted fish and preserves leads to softening of fish muscles, the extent of which depends on maturation stage of the product: at earlier maturation stages, softening of muscles is more extensive than in mature products, the consistency of which actually does not change. The salted products and preserves can be stored frozen to about 9 months. Before sale, the products are placed in chambers at 5 to 0°C for 5 to 10 d for defrosting.

The technology of production of the salted fish is a rapidly developing branch which, in addition to traditional techniques, involves novel methods permitting a prominent rise in quality of products and broadening their spectrum.[13] Among the tasks facing the modern technology of the salted fish products are putting the analogue salted products into production, developing techniques for producing products with reduced sodium chloride content, and substituting the latter by new harmless substances to promote higher biological value of this commodity for human consumption popular in many countries of the world.

II. MARINATING

A. INTRODUCTION

Marinating is preserving fish by means of sodium chloride and acetic acid solutions. It is one of the oldest ways of preserving food and dates back to the 7th century B.C. It is, however, due to the large catches of herring in the 19th century that marinades emerged on European markets. Even today the herring is the basic raw material for marinades, although they are also made from sprat, sardine, and the gadoids.

There are three basic kinds of marinades, i.e., cold, cooked, and fried marinades.

B. COLD MARINADES
1. Maturing

Fish in a solution of acetic acid and salt take a few days to change physical and sensory properties. The muscular tissue becomes soft and dull, and can easily be skinned and boned. The marinating bath usually contains 4 to 4.5% acetic acid and 7 to 8% salt, and, after marinating, 1 to 2.5% and 2 to 4%, respectively. Acetic acid causes the structural proteins to swell considerably and some collagen fractions in the connective tissue and muscle membranes to dissolve. At the same time, muscular proteins denature. When the sodium chloride concentration is small, some of the proteins dissolve; as the concentration grows, denaturating changes take place. These processes reduce the mass of the raw material by 15 to 20% on the average. The synergism of the acetic acid and salt makes the flesh of the fish become more firm and less prone to swelling.

The acidic conditions of the marinades, pH 4 to 4.5, make the tissue cathepsins much more active. This results in the degradation of some muscle proteins into peptides and amino acids. This gives the marinade the proper texture and flavor.[14,15]

2. Factors Affecting the Quality and Shelf Life of Cold Marinades

Some undesirable changes caused by cathepsins occur in the marinades in storage. The meat becomes less firm, the texture becomes greasy, the brine gets turbid following protein degradation, and the fat from the muscle is released. It has been observed that heterofermentative lactic acid bacteria can grow in marinades, while bacteria causing the hydrolysis of lipids do not. *Betabacterium buchneri* causes amino acids to degrade, the process leading to the formation of carbon dioxide and other decarboxylation products, such as γ-aminobutyric acid formed from glutamic acid. These products bind acetic acid, and the pH of the marinade rises, thus enabling mold, yeasts, and proteolytic bacteria, for example, *B. subtilis* to grow. The optimum temperature for this group of bacteria is between 30 and 37°C, but there are some Betabacteria which can already develop at 4°C.[15,16] The growth of the bacteria is slowed down with the salt concentration of at least 6.5%. The acetic acid used in marinating has a preserving effect due to the sensitivity of the microbes to high concentration of hydrogen ions and the undissociated acid particles. The preserving effect of the acid depends on its concentration. For longer storage, a semiproduct of high concentration of acid is prepared. Thus, the final acid content in the marinating bath should amount to 2.5%, which is an equivalent of 2.3% acid content in the fish tissue. The salt present in the marinating bath causes dehydration of the tissue resulting from osmotic processes and checks the hydrolysis of proteins caused by enzymes. A higher salt content, therefore, extends the shelf life of marinades. However, if the salt content in the tissue is higher than 4.5%, the product becomes too salty and will not be accepted by consumers. In addition, too high concentrations of acid and salt impair the flavor of the marinade.

The optimum temperature of the marinating process is between 10 and 12°C. With lower temperatures, the process is too slow; higher temperatures can make the muscular tissue too soft, which is caused by the activation of tissue and bacteria enzymes. The storing temperature of 0 to 8°C ensures high quality of the marinades for several weeks.

If salt and acetic acid are to penetrate well into the tissue, the marinade must be stirred properly while being produced; otherwise, a favorable breeding ground is created for anaerobic bacteria which may be responsible for the reddening of the tissue and the inappropriate quality of the product. During the entire manufacturing process as well as in storage, the fish tissue should be completely immersed in the bath. If the amount of brine is insufficient, the contact of the fish tissue with air can lead to the fish fat becoming rancid. This can be prevented if the brine amounts to 40% of the total mass of the product.

To extend the shelf life of cold marinades, substances reducing water activity such as glucose, saccharose, or xylose are used. Unfortunately, they are effective only in high concentrations; saccharose, for instance, needs a concentration of 15 to 20% to lower the activity of heterofermentative lactic acid bacteria.[15] For the sake of taste, a 12% saccharose content is considered to be the maximum level of sugar in the fish tissue of cold marinades.[17]

In some countries of western Europe, hydrogen peroxide is used in the production of marinades. This makes the tissue color lighter and by -SH group oxidation into sulfoxides checks the activity of cathepsins. Hydrogen added to the bath (50 to 100 mg/1 kg) of the solution takes a few days to degrade. Among the preservatives which are widely used in marinating are benzoic and sorbic acid sodium and potassium salts, as well as ethyl and propyl esters of the *p*-hydroxybenzoic acid. These are added in quantities equivalent to 0.1 to 0.2% benzoic or sorbic acids in the product. The application of these substances is difficult due to their low solubility in water.[16,17]

The use of hexamethylenetetramine is objected to for health considerations, as it makes the formation of formaldehyde possible. On the other hand, the use of this chemical combined with low temperature of storage reduces the risk of spoilage of cold marinades to the minimum.

3. Manufacturing Procedures and Products

The highest quality product is obtained from fresh fish. Marinades made from frozen or salted fish have a less tender texture. The technological process (Figure 1) begins with washing the fish in running water. Depending on the technical equipment of the plant, fish are cut, deheaded and gutted, or filetted mechanically or by hand. When marinades are

158 Seafood: Resources, Nutritional Composition, and Preservation

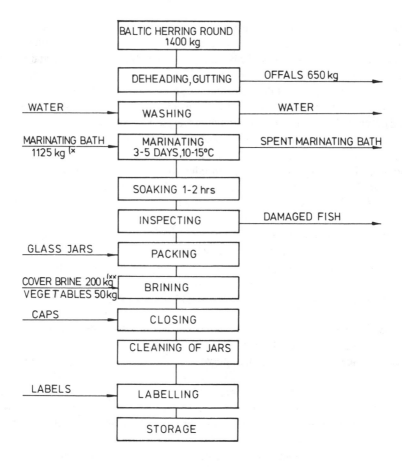

FIGURE 1. Flow sheet for producing 1000 kg of cold marinade from Baltic herring. For brine composition, see Tables 1 and 2.

made from salted fish, desalting is carried out in basins with running water. The time of this operation depends on the salt content in the tissue, the fish species and the force of the water stream. Desalting salted herrings, for instance, from the level of 20% to 3 to 4.5% salt content takes from 8 to 24 h.[16]

A second washing removes the remains of scales and blood residuals. The fish is allowed to drip dry and then placed in stoneware, acid-proof steel, or concrete basins, previously filled with a sodium chloride and acetic acid solution, i.e., the marinating bath. The fish-to-bath proportion should be at least as 1.5:1 and the temperature of maturing should be kept between 10 to 15°C. The fish has to be stirred so as to prevent it from clustering. The semiproduct can be regarded as fit for further processing when the muscular tissue can easily be boned, is of an even light-pink color, sweetishly sour taste, and has the desired flavor. The average time of marinating at 10 to 15°C is between 2 and 8 d, and depends on the fish species and the kind of initial processing. The matured product is then packaged together with the previously prepared cover brine. The most typical packaging of marinades is in twist-off glass jars or easily opened cans. The shelf life of cold marinades at 0 to 8°C is 14 d, with the 2 to 4% salt content and 1 to 2.5% acetic acid content in the tissue.

To avoid dependence on seasonal deliveries of the raw material, a semiproduct is prepared in Europe. It takes the form of heavily marinated fish. Deheaded and gutted fish or filets are put into barrels and covered with marinating bath containing 7% acetic acid and 15% salt. The fish-to-bath proportion should be as 2:1. The barrels, after closing, are stored for

2 or 3 d at about 15°C, during which they must be rolled a few times. They can then be left standing for 6 months at 0 to 5°C, or 3 months at 12°C. The final product is then made by packaging the fish together with a bath containing up to 2% acetic acid and 1% salt, so as to make their respective contents in the final product comply with the existing norms. The shelf life of marinades produced in this way is identical with those after standard processing.[18]

An example of a typical cold marinade is the butterfly herring filet in clear vinegar brine, with black pepper, mustard seeds, and slices of onion and carrot. This type of product is sold in Germany under the trade name of "Bismarck herring". In delicatessen products, clear brine could be replaced with mayonnaise or remoulade. Another kind of cold marinade is the collared herring filets — rolled filets with a seasoning of pickled onion and cucumber slices in the center. The German name of this product is "rollmops".

Cold marinades are also made from deheaded and gutted fish. On the German market this product is known as "delikatess herring", while in restaurants it is served as "home-style prepared".

C. COOKED MARINADES

These are preserves for which the fish, after initial treatment with salt and acetic acid, is cooked or blanched and then, in the process of packaging, covered with a gelatin solution containing salt, acetic acid, and seasonings. The purpose of the thermal processing is to make the material ready-to-eat. In the past, the fish, cut into pieces, was first treated with a solution of acetic acid and salt and then steamed. That was inefficient, as the material lost up to 40% in weight and the salt and acetic acid leaked out of the tissue. Today blanching is used, which reduces the losses to 25 to 30% and ensures a permanent control of the composition of the blanching bath. After a 10- to 15-min blanching in a solution containing 3% acetic acid and 6.5% salt, the fish tissue contains 0.4% of the acid and 1.5% salt. With a 1:1 fish-to-bath proportion, the pH of the tissue after blanching is as high as 6. When the pH is that high, microbes can breed, including *Clostridium botulinum* as well as bacteria which liquify gelatin: *Pseudomonas, micrococci, pneumonococci,* and *heterofermentative* lactic acid bacteria.[16,19] If the packaging is not airtight, the product with the pH of about 6 can develop a mold growth. Thus, the lowering of the pH to not more than 4.6 becomes indispensable. The necessary amounts of acetic acid and salt are supplied with the gelatin solution used as jelly cover brine.

Salt and vinegar penetrate into the tissue of cooked marinades through membranes damaged during the thermal processing, together with the water present in the gelatin solution. The respective concentrations of acid and salt become more or less equal a few days after the product has been made. The jelly brine covering the fish prevents lipids from oxidation, and the seasonings it contains add to the taste of the product.

The salt and acetic acid contents in the fish are of crucial importance for the shelf life of cooked marinades. On the average, the product contains 1 to 2% of the acid and 2 to 4% salt. The application of acetic acid gives the marinades a very distinct sour taste and a special smell. It also makes the pH higher than 4.6. This has to be reduced in view of the threat from *C. botulinum*. Today this is done with the help of citric acid. When 25% of the total of acetic acid is replaced by citric acid, the pH is reduced to 3 and the sourness of the product decreases. Saccharose added to the jelly brine at 8 to 15% reduces water activity, thus preventing the growth of some bacteria. To avoid mold growth, various preservatives are used, e.g., sorbic or benzoic acid salts.

The shelf life of cooked marinades largely depends on the technology and the preservatives used; in Germany, for instance, it is 6 months. In Poland, the shelf life of a product containing 1.5% acetic acid, 0.5% citric acid, 2 to 4% salt, 8% saccharose, and 0.1% of sodium benzoate is 28 d at 0 to 8°C.

160 *Seafood: Resources, Nutritional Composition, and Preservation*

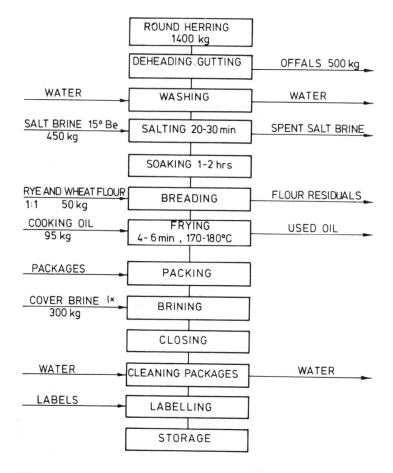

FIGURE 2. Flow sheet for producing 1000 kg of fried marinade from herring in acetic brine. 100 kg of brine contains: acetic acid 10% solution, 40 kg; salt, 3 kg; sugar, 0.5 kg; and seasonings, 0.15 kg in the spring-summer period.

Cooked marinades are produced from many fish species, e.g., herring, cod, mackerel, salmon, and dogfish.

D. FRIED MARINADES

These are salt- and acetic acid-preserved fish products which have been made fit for human consumption by frying (Figure 2). Like cooked marinades, they are products which do not need maturing. In the process of frying, the weight of the fish is reduced by 20 to 30% due to water losses. A herring before frying contains 68% water, 18% proteins, and 13% fat; the respective contents after frying amount to 53, 27, and 19%.[16] The flour-coated fish are fried in vegetable oil at 160 to 180°C. The effect of the frying is the formation of brown products of Maillard reaction on the surface, which give the marinades the characteristic look and taste. Cover brine is added and the fried fish is packed. When the product is stored, salt and acetic acid diffuse into the tissue. The initial acetic acid content in the brine of 2.5% is reduced to 1.3% when the diffusion process is over, i.e., after 2 or 3 d. With an initial content of 3.4%, a 1.8% acid content in the brine is obtained after the same period of time.[16] Another characteristic is an increase in the weight of the product of about 20%, the amount of water absorbed depending on the fat content.

Since the outer layers of the fish are virtually sterilized in the frying, the shelf life of fried marinades is longer than that of cold or cooked ones. At 0 to 8°C, they can be stored for as long as 1 year, the shelf life depending on salt and acid contents in the tissue. The microbiological spoilage of fried marinades, resulting in the brine becoming turbid, is caused by lactic acid bacteria, such as *Lactobacillus plantarum* and *L. casei*.[19] The commonly used preservatives such as sodium and potassium salts of sorbic and benzoic acids do not affect these bacteria at all, as opposed to the *p*-hydroxybenzoic acid esters. One of the main sources of infection in the production of fried marinades is the flour dust, which can contain spores or vegetative forms of bacteria. The growth of bacteria is prevented by packaging the product tightly and storing it at 0 to 8°C.

Fried marinades are packaged in twist-off glass jars or easily opened cans. In Poland, fried marinades must comply with the following standards: salt content 1.5 to 3.5%, acetic acid content 1 to 2%, the fish must amount to at least 80% of the net weight of the package, and the shelf life of such products is declared to be 2 weeks at 0 to 8°C.

TABLE 1
Composition of 100 kg of Marinating Bath

Type of material	Salt (kg)	10% Acetic acid solution (kg)
Fresh or frozen fish	6—8[a]	40—60[a]
Salted fish	2—3[a]	40—60[a]

[a] Concentration applied in the spring-summer period.

TABLE 2
Composition of 100 kg of Cover Brine

Component	Period Spring-summer (kg)	Period Autumn-winter (kg)
Acetic acid 10% solution	30	20
Salt	4	3
Sugar	2	2
Seasonings total	0.1	0.1

REFERENCES

1. **Levanidov, I. P.**, *Fish Salting (Elements of Theory and Practice)*, Vol. 63, Pacific Scientific Research Institute of Marine Fisheries and Oceanography, Vladivostok, 1967.
2. **Voskresensky, N. A.**, *Principles of Fish Salting, Smoking and Drying Technology*, Gidrometpishcheprom, Moscow, 1953, 3.
3. **Ruljov, N. N.**, *Primary Processing of the Atlantic Herring*, Kaliningrad Publishing, Kaliningrad, 1960, 3.
4. **Ruljov, N. N.**, *Atlantic Herring Salting on Board Ships*, Kaliningrad Publishing, Kaliningrad, 1964, 3.
5. **Shenderjuk, V. I.**, *Mildly Salted Fish Production*, Moscow, Pishch. Prom., 1976, 3.
6. **Minder, L. P.**, Influence of some factors of fish weight in salting, *Tr. VNIRO*, 23, 35, 1952.
7. **Tereshchenko, V. P.**, Study of peculiarities of completed salting of fresh and frozen Baltic herring, physical and chemical investigation methods of fish products and raw resources, *Tr. KTIRPIZ*, 52, 16, 1973.
8. **Covendon, D. K.**, Studies on salting and drying of fish with special preference to changes in nitrogenous constituents, *Indian Food Packer*, 29, 4, 1969.
9. **Ritzskes, T. M.**, Artificial ripening of maatyes-cured herring with the aid of proteolytic enzyme preparations, *Fish. Bull.*, 69(3), 647, 1971.
10. **Lujipen, A. F. and Lujipen, M. G.**, Fish products and production of delicatessen items, 1955, No. 5.
11. Fish technology, *Food Prod. Dev.*, 14(11), 16, 18, 1980.
12. Proposals of wholesale trade concerning the nematode problem, 11 Fisch. Mag., 1987, Nr. 11, 10.
13. Minced Fish Technology: A Review, FAO Fish. Tech. Paper No. 216, Food and Agriculture Organization, Rome, 1981, 72.
14. **Meyer, V.**, Problems of spoilage of canned fish products. VII. Investigations on amino acids formation in marinades from herrings, Veröff Inst. Meeresforsch. Bremerhaven, 8, 21.
15. **Kreuzer, R.**, Investigation on biological factors causing spoilage of fish products and its effects. Organisms and environment, *Arch. Fischereiwiss.*, 8, 104,
16. **Meyer, V.**, Marinades, in *Fish as Food*, Vol. 3, Borgstrom, G., Ed., Academic Press, New York, 1965, chap. 5.
17. **Bykowski, P., Kowalewski, W., and Wocial, M.**, Methods of extending the shelf life of cold marinades. Studia i Materiały, Morski Instytut Rybacki, Gdynia, 1981, 5(in Polish).
18. **Bykowski, P. and Pawlikowski, B.**, Mass transfer kinetics in marinating process. Studia i Materiły, Morski Instytut Rybacki, Gdynia, 1981, 27 (in Polish).
19. **Zaleski, S.**, *Marine Food Microbiology*, Wydawnictwo Morskie, Gdańsk, 1978, chap. 18 (in Polish).

Chapter 10

SMOKING

Kazimierz B. M. Miler and Zdzisław E. Sikorski

TABLE OF CONTENTS

I.	Introduction	164
II.	Wood Smoke	164
	A. Generation and Chemical Composition	164
	B. Physical Properties	166
	C. Contribution to Sensory Properties of Smoked Fish	167
	1. Color Formation	167
	2. Contribution to Flavor	167
	3. Impact on Texture	168
	D. Preserving Action	168
	1. Antioxidative Action	168
	2. Antimicrobial Action	169
III.	Methods and Equipment for Smoke Production	169
	A. The Smoldering Method	169
	B. Smoke Production by Friction	169
	C. The Hydropyrolytic Process	170
	D. Smoke Production in a Fluidized Bed	170
IV.	Production of Smoke Flavorings	170
	A. Smoke Condensates	171
	B. Smoke Extracts	171
	C. Smoke Distillates	171
	D. Synthetic Flavorings	171
	E. Miscellaneous Flavorings	172
V.	The Smoking Process	172
	A. Engineering Aspects	172
	B. Technological Aspects	173
	1. Methods of Fish Smoking	173
	2. Unit Operations	173
	a. Dressing and Cutting	173
	b. Salting	173
	c. Arranging the Fish in the Smokehouse	174
	d. Drying and Heat Processing	174
VI.	Smokehouse Equipment	175
	A. Smokehouses	175
	B. Control Equipment	176
VII.	The Quality and Shelf-Life of Smoked Fish	176
	A. Quality	176

B. Shelf-Life 177

References.. 178

I. INTRODUCTION

Smoke curing is a processing method, wherein — due to the action of smoke constituents — the presalted fish attains a unique smoky odor, taste, and color. Most often these changes in sensory properties go along with a partial dehydration of the fish tissues and alterations in their texture. Initially these processes served primarily for the preservation of surplus food. However, with the advent of more effective conservation methods, e.g., pasteurization and cold storage, this incipient function of smoke curing lost its importance. Instead, the unique sensory features of smoked products became more important.

The prevailing smoking techniques nowadays consist of hanging fish in a draft of smoke, which is generated by smoldering sawdust, wood shavings, or the like. Although modern, often automated, equipment is used for this purpose, the basic principles of said method essentially are the same, as were used by our prehistoric ancestors. Nevertheless, the everspreading use of smoke flavorings and flameless methods of smoke generation announce the advent of a major breakthrough in the technology of smoke curing.

II. WOOD SMOKE

A. GENERATION AND CHEMICAL COMPOSITION

In most countries, curing smoke is developed from wood, in particular, from that of deciduous trees. All hitherto known methods of smoke production are based on the thermal degradation of wooden matter. Hence, it is the chemical constitution of wood and the process parameters that determine the composition and properties of smoke.

Disregarding the tree species, the elemental composition of wood is almost constant. Around 95% of the dry matter of wood consist of cellulose (~45%), lignin (20 to 30%), and hemicellulose. The amount of lignin is higher in conifers than in deciduous trees, whereas the opposite is true with regard to hemicellulose.

Cellulose is a polymer of D-glucose (mainly in its pyranose form), and its structure is much alike in all tree species. Its thermal decomposition yields anhydroglucose, carbonylic compounds, and derivatives of furan. The proposed pathways of this process were comprehensively surveyed by Fagerson.[1]

Hemicellulose is a complex of polymerized hexoses, pentoses, and uronic acids. During pyrolysis, it undergoes processes which essentially are similar to those occurring in cellulose. However, the presence of numerous acetyl and carboxyl groups in its structure gives rise to considerable amounts of acetic acid and carbon dioxide. In deciduous trees, hemicellulose consists predominantly of O-acetyl-(4-O-glucuron)xylan (80 to 90%), whereas in conifers, the main components are glucomannan (60 to 70%) and arabin-(4-O-methylglucuron)xylan (15 to 30%).[2] This explains the higher yield of carboxylic acids in smoke produced from hardwood, as compared to their amount in smoke from softwood. Smoke obtained from firwood was found not to contain fatty acids with chains longer than C_5 (crotonic acid), while that from alderwood had acids with up to C_9-chains (pelargonic acid).[3]

Lignin is a polymer composed of derivatives of cinnamylic alcohols (p-coumaric, coniferyl, and sinapilic). In the cambial juices of deciduous trees (beech), these alcohols occur in the ratio of 1:10:9, whereas in conifers this ratio is about 2:13:1, respectively.[4] During pyrolysis, the derivatives of these alcohols may get oxidized to the respective p-hydroxycinnamylic acids, which are transformed into phenols via radical reactions, whose pathways were proposed by Fiddler et al.[5] and Tressl et al.[6] The thermal degradation of p-coumaric acid yields phenol (C_6H_5OH) and its alkylated derivatives, that of ferulic acid — guaiacol — and its homologues, while that of sinapilic acid yields syringol and its alkyl-substituted derivatives. Hence, smoke from deciduous trees contains considerable amounts of syringol, which is found in minute quantities only in smokes derived from conifers.[7,8] The tree species does not influence the qualitative composition of polynuclear aromatic hydrocarbons (PAH).[9] It may, however, have some impact on their quantitative pattern, although this is governed mainly by the process parameters, i.e., temperature and the access of oxygen.

Curing smoke consists of a vast number of organic compounds. According to a recent review,[10] the number of positively identified phenols amounts to 84 individuals, that of carboxylic acids is 35, alcohols — 12, esters — 10, lactones — 13, aldehydes — 21, ketones — 68, ethers — 5, furans — 9, aliphatic hydrocarbons — 22, aromatic hydrocarbons — 74, and nitrogen compounds — 8.

According to Rusz,[11] the thermal decomposition of 1 g of wood yields: ~2.5 mg phenols (as C_6H_5OH), ~30 mg carboxylic acids (as CH_3COOH), and ~90 mg carbonyl compounds (as CH_3COCH_3). Although these data may vary with changing process parameters, they nevertheless are a magnitude estimate.

The impact of processing parameters upon the thermal degradation of wood was explored by several authors, and advanced mathematical models were proposed.[12] The yield (Y) of volatile degradation products can be described by the following formula:[13]

$$Y[\%] = 100 \cdot [(k_1 - k_2)/k_1] \cdot [1 - \exp(-k_1 \cdot t)] \quad (1)$$

It depends exponentially on the retention time (t) of wood in the degradation zone, and in the same way follows the changes in temperature, because both rate constants (k_1 and k_2), do so by virtue of the known Arrhenius equation.

Although cellulose, hemicellulose, and lignin to a great extent are linked with each other by means of chemical bonds,[2,14] during thermal degradation wood behaves as if it were merely a mixture of these constituents.[15] With rising temperature, it first loses moisture and its low molecular components. At 170°C, their partial pressure may suffice to cause inflammation in the presence of an external source of fire (inflammation point), and at 270 to 290°C self-ignition may occur.[16] According to Kuriyama,[17] hemicellulose gets degraded within 180 to 300°C — pentosans at the lower, and hexosans at the upper limit of this interval. Cellulose is decomposed at 260 to 350°C, and lignin within 300 to 500°C, although it starts losing some amount of its methoxyl groups already at 260°C. An intense degradation of lignin takes place at temperatures above 400°C. An elevation of the temperature beyond 500°C results merely in splitting off some amounts of hydrogen from the charred wood. The pyrolysis of wood proceeds endothermally below 180°C, and becomes exothermic above this point.[16] After ignition, the glow zone of freely smoldering sawdust has a temperature approximately within 860 to 940°C.[18] When the sawdust bed is aerated, its temperature may achieve ~1300°C.[19]

With the exception of charcoal, all products of wood pyrolysis are volatile at the temperatures encountered in the degradation zone. Their volume exceeds by 500 times that of the material they are formed from. Effusing at high speed from the inner parts of the wood, they react with atmospheric oxygen, thus preventing its access to the degradation zone.

Temperature and oxygen concentration affect the yield of smoke constituents. The amount of phenols, carbonyl compounds, carboxylic acids, and polynuclear hydrocarbons was found to depend curvilinearly (bell-shaped curve) on the product of temperature and air flow rate in a static bed of smoldering sawdust.[3,7,9,20] In a fluidized bed, the yield (Y) of phenols follows the changes in temperature in a way described by the following formula:[10]

$$Y = (c/T) \cdot \exp(A_1 - B_1/T)/[1 + (c/T) \cdot \exp(A_2 - B_2/T)] \qquad (2)$$

Here c is a factor characteristic for the smoke generator, T[K] stands for the bed temperature, and the constants A and B are the parameters of the Arrhenius plot of the formation (subscript 1) and decay (subscript 2) reactions, respectively. These parameters were found to depend parabolically on oxygen concentration. The maximum yield of guaiacol or syringol and their para-substituted derivatives was found at temperatures within 400 to 600°C, while that of phenol (C_6H_5OH) and its para-alkylated homologues at temperatures some 300°C higher.[10]

B. PHYSICAL PROPERTIES

In general, smoke constituents have boiling points greatly exceeding the temperatures encountered in smokehouses. Hence, the bulk amount of these compounds is suspended in the gaseous phase of smoke in form of tiny liquid droplets. The dispersing phase consists predominantly of air with a small admixture of CO_2, CO, CH_4, C_2H_4, and vapors of the substances present in smoke particles. The dominating share of air causes the gaseous phase of smoke to have physical properties similar to those of air. The particulate (dispersed) phase of smoke contains approximately 90% of all smoke matter, and consists of liquid droplets, whose average radii range from 0.08 to 0.14 μm.[21]

Smoke particles scatter light, attenuating its intensity proportionally to the concentration of particulate matter in smoke, and inversely to their radii.[21,22] Brownian motions result in the coalescence of smoke particles (aging of smoke), and cause them to deposit on dry surfaces. Temperature gradients, e.g., in the vicinity of smoke-duct walls, evoke radiometer forces acting on the particles. These forces are the principal agent causing the deposition of smoke on dry surfaces.[21] In addition, the particles always are under the influence of gravitational forces, and if the smoke stream is diverted by an obstacle or is in the state of turbulence, they are subjected to centrifugal forces, which enhance their deposition, evoked by temperature gradients or Brownian motions.

Smoke particles always bear some electric charge, which can be considerably increased in the presence of a corona brush discharge. In that case, the deposition of particles is enormously increased due to the existence of an electrostatic field, or by self-dispersion of unipolar charged smoke clouds.[23]

Although smoke particles readily settle on dry surfaces, they do not contribute more than 5% of the total deposit of smoke compounds on conventionally smoked fish.[24] Smoke constituents are transferred to fish mainly by means of diffusion of their vapors, present in the dispersing phase. The diffusion rate of smoke compounds is approximately proportional to the concentration of their vapors, which, in turn, is related to their concentration in the smoke particles. As the mass concentration of particulate matter is proportional to the optical density of smoke,[22] so the diffusion rate of smoke components also depends on this density.

The volatility of smoke components increases with rising temperature, and depends on their latent heat of evaporation and boiling point. For this reason, both the concentration of smoke constituents in the dispersing phase and their quantitative pattern vary at differing temperatures. This explains why the total amount and composition of smoke compounds in the product depends on the temperature applied in the smoking process. In addition, the partition of smoke constituents between water and oil is an important physical factor that influences the perceptual quality of the smoky flavor, too. Partition ratios for smoke compounds in a water-fish oil system have to be determined.

C. CONTRIBUTION TO SENSORY PROPERTIES OF SMOKED FISH
1. Color Formation

The color of smoked sprats and sardines is characterized by the dominant wavelength 574 to 577 nm.[25,26] Data for other fish species may differ due to the variations in the pigmentation of their skin. The dominant wavelength and the brightness of color in sprats are independent of the time and temperature of smoking. However, the purity of color increases asymptotically with elapsing time of smoking. The value of the asymptote is related to the smoking temperature by means of the Arrhenius plot.[25,27] Successful experiments with developing color in fish smoked solely in the dispersing phase of smoke[24,28] indicate that this process is substantially a result of chemical reactions. These have been shown to be reactions of the Maillard type, wherein glycolic aldehyde and methylglyoxal are the smoke components, playing the dominating role. The possible pathways of said reactions were suggested by Ruiter.[29]

The yield of color development in smoked fish is susceptible to the wetness of their surface. A relative smoke humidity within 65 to 70%, corresponding to 12 to 15% moisture contents in the outer layers of the fish, is deemed to offer the best results.[29] This stands in agreement with the practical experience that neither too wet nor too dry fish readily develop color during smoking.

The glossy surface of smoked fish is a factor highly appealing to the consumer. Gloss is always developed in fat fish due to the presence of a thin, oily film on their surface. However, lean fish attain a glossy appearance only when a film of polymerized extractable proteins is formed on their surface. In order for this polymerization to take place, the moisture contents in the superficial layers of fish must not exceed 65%.[29]

2. Contribution to Flavor

The flavor of smoked foods results from the composite action of smoke constituents, heat and salt, as all these factors induce physical and chemical changes in the product. The role of smoke components consists primarily in developing the characteristic smoky odor and taste. They interact also with proteinaceous matter, inducing some changes in the texture of fish. This effect, however, is negligible, compared to that induced by heating, drying, or salting.[30]

From practical experience, it is well known that the odor of smoke-cured food is distinctly different from that of smoke itself. Therefore, the term "smoky" was proposed for denoting the odor of smoked food.[15] Due to the interaction of smoke compounds with proteins — reported elsewhere[30-32] — the smoky odor is a composite sensation, in part evoked by the products of these interactions. The dominating aromatizing agents, however, are the smoke components themselves.[33] The osmic activity of many smoke constituents is well known.[34]

There is common agreement nowadays that the phenolic constituents of smoke have the leading share in imparting the smoky flavor to foodstuffs. Other osmically active components play an auxiliary role, rounding up the overall aroma and introducing additional notes, thus giving rise to the multitude of varieties of the smoky flavor.[35] From among all smoke phenols, only those that distill off within 76 to 89°C at 5.33 hPa (4 mmHg) were found to bear the smoky odor.[36] According to Kulesza et al.,[37] a pleasant smoky flavor is associated with the presence of syringol, guaiacol, and their 4-alkylated derivatives. Fiddler et al.[38] and Lustre and Issenberg[39] are of the opinion that syringol, guaiacol, 4-methylguaiacol, and eugenol belong to the potential carriers of this flavor. Zir Olsen[40] points to syringol, *trans*-isoeugenol, 4-methylsyringol, and 4-allylsyringol as the dominant contributors to said flavor. Radecki et al.[41] found that neither syringol nor 4-methylsyringol, nor 4-ethylsyringol alone exhibit the smoky flavor. However, when mixed up in a ratio of 4:3:1, these substances develop a flavor very much resembling that of smoked foods. Based on the results of multiple regression analysis, Gudaszewski[42,43] found a significant correlation between the amount of syringol in the product and the frequency of describing the flavor of said product as smoky. Consequently, this author suggests using the amount of syringol in the product as the criterion of its smokiness.[43] Working with syringol and 4-methylsyringol fractions obtained by means of preparative scale GLC, Sznajdrowska[10] demonstrated the smoky odor to be a sensation evoked by the simultaneous action of both these compounds and their chromatographic associates (mainly *cis*-isoeugenol). The odor of a solution, containing ~55% of 4-methylsyringol (+ trans-isoeugenol) and ~45% of syringol (+ *cis*-isoeugenol), was indiscernable from that of a smoke flavoring, which itself was rated as "typically smoky" by 89 from among 100 members of the sensory panel.

Hence, in developing the smoky flavor, the leading role is probably played by substances, which when separated by GLC have retention volumes identical or very similar to those of syringol and 4-methylsyringol. However, the multitude of variations in the smoky flavor is probably due to the presence of other osmically active smoke constituents, e.g., carbonyls, furans, heterocyclic compounds, etc. Additional variations originate from the differing temperatures, applied during smoking, and the fat-to-moisture ratio in the smoked product.

3. Impact on Texture

Common experience supplies plenty of evidence for the tenderizing action of the smoke-curing process upon the fish tissue. In hot-smoked products, this results mainly from the heat denaturation of proteins, while in cold-smoked fish it is caused predominantly by the action of proteolytic enzymes. Smoke components also seem to affect the textural properties of smoked foods.[30,44] In some cases, they exhibit a tenderizing activity, while in others they make the tissues tougher.[44] As yet, no theoretical explanations were found for these phenomena, and there is a general lack of theories concerning the thermoviscoelastic properties of muscle tissues.

D. PRESERVING ACTION
1. Antioxidative Action

As has been shown by Kurko,[45] from among all smoke constituents, only those with an active phenolic function possess a marked antioxidative activity, which becomes more pronounced in compounds with a higher boiling point. Most active are the vicinal polyhydroxyphenols, e.g., pyrogallol and resorcinol. In monohydroxyphenols, the activity depends to some extent on the substituent, located at the "para" position with regard to the hydroxylic group. The highest activity is exhibited by 4-methylguaiacol, 4-vinylguaiacol, and 4-*trans*-propenylsyringol. Less active are guaiacol, syringol, 4-methylsyringol, and 4-vinylsyringol. Other monohydroxyphenols do not contribute significantly to the antioxidative activity of smoke compounds.[46]

The antioxidative activity (a_A) is proportional to the concentration of the antioxidant (c_A):

$$a_A = b \cdot c_A \tag{3}$$

The constant b represents the specific activity of the antioxidant. Its value depends on the nature (and composition) of the agent and also on temperature and on the kind of fat used as test substance. For example, the specific activity of a Polish smoke flavoring (BRDW), tested in fish oil at 40°C is $b_{40} = 2048$, while at 80°C it is only $b_{80} = 352$.[47] Hence the retarding effect of smoke constituents upon the autooxidation of fish oil is more pronounced at lower than at higher temperatures.

Excessive amounts of antioxidants are known to exert prooxidative action. Smoke flavorings, consisting mainly of phenols, exhibited these adverse effects in lard when their concentrations were raised beyond 3710 ppm (AOM test) or 14,467 ppm (filter paper test at room temperature).[48]

2. Antimicrobial Action

Smoked fish is known to have a slightly extended shelf life, as compared to that of raw fish. Although this effect is attributed mainly to the action of physical factors, i.e., heat (hot smoking) or reduced water activity (cold smoking), in part it also results from the antimicrobial action of smoke constituents.

According to Kurko,[36] from among all smoke components the highest antimicrobial activity is exhibited by the carboxylic acids and phenols. Carbonyl compounds and esters generally are less potent, and hydrocarbons exert no influence at all. There are, however, exceptions from this general rule, and so formaldehyde was found to be more active than phenol.[49]

Depending on their concentration, smoke compounds either diminish the growth rate of microorganisms, or reduce their count. In the latter case, the actual count (N) is reflected by the known Watson equation, i.e.,

$$N = N_o \cdot \exp(-k \cdot t \cdot c^n) \tag{4}$$

Here N_0 stands for the initial count, t denotes the exposure time, and c the concentration of the agent. The symbols k and n represent constants.

Bacteria are more susceptible to the action of smoke compounds than yeasts and molds, the latter being the most resistant. The antimicrobial action is more pronounced in Gram-positive bacteria than in Gram-negative ones, and viable cells are more readily affected than spores.

The mode of action of smoke compounds upon microorganisms is still obscure in details. Carboxylic acids lower the pH of the millieu and exert a specific action in their undissociated state. Phenols manifest their antimicrobial activity only then, when they are not dissociated, which makes their activity pH dependent. This indicates the existence of some synergistic effects in the antimicrobial action of smoke compounds. Experimental evidence for such effects has been supplied by Incze.[49] Smoke compounds also enhance the lethal action of elevated temperatures upon the microflora of smoked products.

III. METHODS AND EQUIPMENT FOR SMOKE PRODUCTION

A. THE SMOLDERING METHOD

The oldest and still most widely used method of smoke production consists of smoldering wooden logs, shavings, or sawdust. Due to the spontaneous and exothermal character of the combustion process, this method is both the simplest and least expensive one. The temperature of the glow zone is high enough to bring forth a complete degradation of all constituents of wood. As a consequence, the application of thus-obtained smokes yields a smoked product with a fully developed aroma. The only drawback of the smoldering method is the impossibility of controlling the temperature of the glow zone. As a result, the smoke is produced at temperatures favoring the pyrolytic synthesis of PAH and very often shows variations in the quantitative pattern of smoke constituents.

There exists a wide variety of generators used for the production of smoldering smoke. Although they vary in construction details and ease of operation, they all work on the same principle of wood combustion, which constitutes the basis for the open fireplace and hearth. As a rule, generators used nowadays have a grated firebed and are equipped with automated feeders for the wooden material (often sawdust). In some constructions, the wood is fed on a conveyer belt, which enters the combustion zone. In the most modern designs, the smoke generator is operated by means of a computer program, compatible with (or being a subroutine of) the program that executes the whole smoking process.[50]

B. SMOKE PRODUCTION BY FRICTION

The principle of this method also consists of subjecting the wooden material to thermal degradation. It differs, however, from the smoldering method in the mode of developing heat, which is obtained by friction of the wooden log against a rotating disk or drum. The temperature at the friction interface can be controlled by varying the pressure exerted on the log or by changing the speed of rotation of the rotor. Its value, however, usually does not exceed 380°C.[51] As a consequence, the thermal degradation of lignin is less advanced than in the smoldering method, and the oxidation of the volatile degradation products is accomplished to a lesser degree. For this reason, the sensory features of products, smoked with friction smoke, differ somewhat from those obtained with smoldering smoke.[52]

Friction smoke generators are more or less modified products of the construction described by Rasmussen.[53] They gained much interest from 1955 to 1975. Nowadays they have lost much of their popularity, most probably due to the relatively high exploitation costs (energy consumption) and their noisy work.

C. THE HYDROPYROLYTIC PROCESS

The hydropyrolytic method of smoke production is characterized by effecting the thermal degradation of sawdust by means of overheated steam. It was invented by Fessmann for the production of liquid smokes and is covered by numerous patents. In the original version of this method,[54] the sawdust is fed to the degradation chamber by means of a controllable worm feeder. The degradation chamber is constructed in the form of a tilted pipe with perforated sidewalls. Steam at a temperature not less than 180°C (250 to 390°C at best) is blown through these perforations into the sawdust, causing the bed temperature to rise to 200°C. As a consequence of the relatively low temperature of wood degradation, the resulting volatiles are rich in carboxylic acids and carbonyl compounds; however, they bear a relatively poor load of phenols. In another version,[55] the hydropyrolytic generator was fitted with an additional chamber, wherein the volatile degradation products are oxidized with oxygen-enriched air. In this installation, the temperature of the sawdust bed can be raised to a level ensuring self-ignition of the wooden material, which renders the process into a smoldering one.

D. SMOKE PRODUCTION IN A FLUIDIZED BED

The use of fluidized beds offers the opportunity to conduct processes under highly uniform conditions of temperature and mass concentration. For this reason, their use for developing smoke is advantageous over other methods of smoke production. In particular, they render the process controllable over a relatively wide range of temperatures and oxygen concentrations.

The first generator for the production of smoke in a fluidized sawdust bed was designed by Nicol.[56,57] Its main item, the fluidization chamber, is a truncated cone into which sawdust is fed countercurrently to the upwards-directed stream of hot air or any other gaseous medium. The feeding rate of sawdust and the temperature of the gaseous phase are fully controllable. With air used as the heating medium, the bed temperature must not exceed 400°C, otherwise self-ignition of the wooden material may occur. In a version of the fluidizer, modified by Balejko,[13] smoke is produced at bed temperatures ranging up to 860°C without self-ignition taking place, when the oxygen concentration is reduced to 6%. The quality of thus-obtained smoke is comparable to that of smoldering smoke.

IV. PRODUCTION OF SMOKE FLAVORINGS

In recent years, smoke flavorings have gained increasing interest. They are sold as liquid smokes, smoking powders, gels, solutions in oil, aqueous suspensions, etc. According to the methods used for their production, smoke flavorings may be classified into (1) smoke condensates, (2) smoke extracts, (3) smoke distillates, (4) synthetic flavorings, and (5) miscellaneous flavorings. A comprehensive survey of the production methods has been presented by Kurko.[58]

A. SMOKE CONDENSATES

Smoke flavorings of this kind are produced by physical condensation of curing smoke or the volatile products of dry distillation of wood. The thereby-obtained pyroligneous liquids are filtered and concentrated by evaporation of surplus water. The product is standardized by controlling the final concentration of phenols and/or carboxylic acids.

Usually smoke condensates are aqueous products, readily miscible with water. There are, however, also oily condensates, as, for example, the product obtained by the method patented by Taylor.[59] According to this procedure, smoldering smoke enters the condenser kept at a temperature preventing the condensation of water vapor. The higher boiling constituents of smoke get condensed, while other components are fed back to the smoke generator. This method yields an oily smoke condensate, which is sold as the smoke oil.

Smoke condensates have been subject to much criticism because they often impart undesired, cresolic flavor notes to the product.[36]

B. SMOKE EXTRACTS

These smoke flavorings are produced by way of a more or less selective extraction of smoke constituents either directly from the smoke aerosol, or from pyroligneous liquids or the pitchy fraction of smoke condensates. In some cases water is used as the solvent while in others, the extraction is performed by means of organic solvents.

A method, typical for the production of smoke extracts, has been patented by Hollenbeck.[60] According to this procedure, smoldering smoke is blown into an absorption tower, fitted with ceramic packings, e.g., Rashig rings. Here it countercurrently meets water that is recycled on top of the tower until the concentration of carboxylic acids, expressed as CH_3COOH, in the aqueous solution attains the level of 6 to 7.2%. The solution is then passed through a cellulose filter and constitutes the product, known as CharSol.

The pitchy fraction of smoke condensates also serves as a raw material for the production of smoke extracts. The pitch is first solubilized in an aqueous solution of NaOH or KOH, and then extracted with an organic solvent inmiscible with water. The aqueous phase is next partly neutralized to pH 10.5. Then the liberated phenols are extracted with another portion of said solvent. After distilling off the solvent, this extract yields the phenolic fraction of the smoke flavoring. This is mixed in an appropriate ratio with a second fraction that is obtained by removing the solvent from the first extract and distilling the residue under vacuum (13 hPa) until reaching 220°C. This procedure is used for the production of the smoke flavoring, known as Scanrøg.

C. SMOKE DISTILLATES

These products are obtained by distillation of pyroligneous liquids, as well as by subjecting the pitchy fractions of smoke condensates to a fractionating distillation. Distillates, based on pyroligneous liquids, usually are obtained by means of steam distillation at normal pressure. Those produced from wood pitch are distilled under vacuum at elevated temperatures. An example of these is the Polish smoke flavoring, known as BRDW.[61] To obtain it, the wood pitch first is liberated from undesired substances, distilling off under 26 to 40 hPa until the temperature rises to 90°C. The remainder is fractionated under vacuum (13 hPa) and the fraction collected at temperatures being within 100 to 180°C constitutes the smoke flavoring.

D. SYNTHETIC FLAVORINGS

The progress made during the recent decade in elucidating the chemical composition of wood smoke gave rise to attempts aiming in producing smoke flavorings, composed entirely of synthetic compounds. An example of such products is the Russian flavoring, known as VNIIMP-1. According to Kurko,[58] it is produced by mixing a 10% aqueous solution of acetic acid with appropriate amounts of formic and propionic acids, and furfural. This mixture is fortified with some amounts of butyric, valeric, and caproic acids, and also with 1,3-dihydroxyacetone, diacetyl, guaiacol, o-cresol, and other not specified compounds. The proportions of the components were not published.

E. MISCELLANEOUS FLAVORINGS

There is a group of flavorings not produced by any of the aforementioned methods. They are prepared either as powders, made from desiccated smoked meat or fish scraps or plant materials, or in the form of extracts produced from said materials by leaching them with organic solvents, taken from the GRAS list. A typical product is the "natural ham aroma" produced by a patented method,[62] whereby smoked meat or fish trimmings are extracted with ethanol, and the concentrated extract constitutes the flavoring. Powdered flavorings usually are produced by smoking yeasts and hydrolyzates of yeasts or other proteins of plant origin, which after desiccation are comminuted.[63]

V. THE SMOKING PROCESS

A. ENGINEERING ASPECTS

The smoking process incorporates phenomena of heat and mass transfer from the smoke to the product, and vice versa. The processes of mass transfer involve both the transportation of smoke compounds to the product, as well as the transposition of moisture from the product to the environment. The heat and mass transfer taking place within the body of the smoke is effected by convection, whereas that occurring inside the product is brought forth by diffusion.

The principles of heat diffusion (conductive heat transfer) in solids and the mathematical solutions of this problem were surveyed comprehensively by Carslaw and Jaeger.[64] Similarly, the in-depth mathematical treatment of diffusive mass transfer is given in the fundamental book of Crank.[65] From among the solutions, presented by said authors, many can be applied directly for solving problems of heat or mass transfer in fish in those cases, when the shape of the fish body can be simply described by means of the regular coordinate systems, e.g., rectangular, cylindrical, or spherical polar. Solutions for problems requiring the application of more sophisticated coordinate systems can be found by following the outlines presented by Moon and Spencer.[66] An example of this is the solution of heat conduction in whole sprats.[67]

In process engineering, the diffusion of heat or mass in solids of regular shape usually is traced by means of dimensionless parameters and their interrelations, i.e.,

$$\phi = f(Bi, Fo, m) \tag{5}$$

where ϕ represents the dimensionless temperature or mass concentration, Bi stands for the Biot's number, Fo denotes the Fourier's number, and m characterizes the position ratio. Knowing the values of Bi, Fo, and m, the actual temperature or mass concentration is found easily from the respective nomographs.

In hot smoking, the temperature in the kiln usually changes with elapsing time, and so does the concentration of smoke constituents in the dispersing phase of smoke. This, in turn, induces changes in the temperature and concentration of smoke components on the surface of the fish. These changes have to be taken into account in the boundary conditions when solving the respective diffusion problem. Solutions are then obtained either by using Laplace transforms or applying the Duhamel theorem. The use of said procedure for solving temperature conduction in hot-smoked mackerel has been published by Sznajdrowska.[68]

Due to its anatomical constitution, the fish body is an extremely heterogeneous and heterophasic system. Hence, it is anisotropic with regard to diffusive processes and the diffusion constants are time dependent. In addition, many important smoke components, e.g., phenols and aldehydes, react with constituents of the tissues, which induce alterations in the respective concentration gradients. As yet, these facts have not been taken into account in papers published in accessible literature. These phenomena may be responsible in part for the scattering of experimental data concerning heat conduction and mass transfer during smoking of fish.

The simultaneous diffusion of heat and moisture, taking place during drying, constitutes a specific problem that is dealt with in a separate chapter. The general solutions of this problem are comprehensively treated by Crank[65] and more detailed aspects are discussed elsewhere.[69-71]

B. TECHNOLOGICAL ASPECTS
1. Methods of Fish Smoking

There are two methods used: cold and hot smoking. In cold smoking, the proteins of raw fish turn edible as a result of their enzymatic ripening, while in hot smoking this is accomplished due to their thermal denaturation. In both methods, the applied unit operations are similar; however, different parameters of time and temperature are used. The temperature in the kilns does not exceed 30°C during cold smoking, while in hot smoking it is not lower than 60°C. Consequently, the products of these two smoking methods differ in their sensory properties and in their shelf life. In both methods, various techniques of dressing, salting, smoke development and its deposition, heating, cooling, and packaging are used, depending on the fish species and the demanded specifity of the product.

2. Unit Operations
a. Dressing and Cutting

Depending on the size and properties of the fish, as well as on the demanded features of the product, various techniques of splitting and cleaning are applied. Small fish, e.g., sprats, are always smoked whole, ungutted. This saves labor and prevents excessive dehydration of the product. Also many other, somewhat larger species often are smoked without splitting, if their skin is not too thick and their shape provides for proper smoke and heat penetration and an adequate drying rate. Examples are herrings as bloaters, red herrings, or hot-smoked bucklings. However, in seasons of heavy feeding the herrings should be gutted. Eels, because of their impervious skin, are eviscerated regardless of their size to enable the smoke and heat to penetrate through the belly cavity. Haddocks are gutted and split along the backbone to aid drying and smoking. For the same reason, large fish are filleted or cut into smaller portions.

b. Salting

Fish intended for hot smoking is salted to a content of ~2% NaCl, a level which satisfies the consumer demand for a proper salty taste of the product. The duration of salting, as well as the fish to salt ratio, or the concentration of the brine depends on the species and size of the fish and on its fat contents. The factors influencing the rate of salt penetration are discussed in a preceding chapter.

Salting brings about a slight decrease in the breaking strength of the connective tissues. This is probably due to the fact that salt lowers the rate of moisture losses during the subsequent stages of the hot-smoking process.

Salting of fish intended for cold smoking not only adds a salty note to their taste, but also contributes to the development of the desired cured flavor and texture of the product. According to various procedures, fish may be salted by mixing in some proportion with salt or by brining in salt solutions — most often about 80% saturated. If dyes are used in the process, they usually are added to the brine. Brown sugar and other flavorings or sodium nitrite, if approved by the supervising agencies, can also be incorporated in the brine used for special cures, e.g., for chubs or salmon. As raw materials for cold smoking also salted fish can be used. In this case, the excessive amount of salt must be leached out with water before the fish is put into the smokehouse.

The conditions existing in many fish processing premises do not guarantee the required hygienic standard which would exclude any risk of contaminating the product with pathogenic bacteria. The contamination can be spread over new raw material by repeatedly using the same brine for salting. Many species of bacteria found in fish can survive salt concentrations up to 20%, and so their count in the brine increases with its repeated use. Therefore, it is important to control the microbial contamination of the brine, if the latter is intended to be used several times.

c. Arranging the Fish in the Smokehouse

Depending on the size of the fish and the equipment of the smokehouse, different techniques are used to expose the raw material to the action of smoke, draft, and heat. Small fish frequently are smoked on wire mesh sheets or on conveying bands. Smoking on wire mesh sheets or even on mesh layers made of plant material is practiced in many artisan smoke ovens. In modern smokehouses, the fish are exposed to the smoke hanging on metal speats or on hooks. The speats are pierced either through the eyes or the gills and mouth. Some species, e.g., split herring, are tentered, i.e., hung in rows tail down on pairs of hooks, run into wooden bars. Others, e.g., deheaded gutted whiting, are tied in pairs by the tail and hung over wooden bars.

d. Drying and Heat Processing

Drying is aimed to reduce the moisture content in the raw material according to the demanded yield of the product. In hot-smoked fish, the yield, referred to the weight of the pretreated raw material, is 70 to 80%, and that of many cold-smoked commodities usually is 55 to 60%. Higher weight losses decrease the water activity, thus extending the shelf life of the product. However, at the same time, they diminish the juiciness of the smoked fish. The following semiempirical formula may be used to calculate the time (t) necessary for lowering the moisture content in the product to the desired level:[72]

$$t = \frac{1}{k} \cdot \ln[(w_o - w_e)/(w_t - w_e)] \tag{6}$$

where

$$k = 2.7 \cdot v^{0.2} \cdot c_f^{-0.3} \cdot \left[\left(\frac{T}{100}\right)^{3.0} + 1.3 \cdot \varphi\right] \cdot 10^{-3} \tag{7}$$

The symbols used in these formulas have the following meaning:
k, rate constant (1/h); w_o, initial moisture content (kg/kg dry matter); w_e, equilibrium moisture content (kg/kg dry matter); w_t, final moisture content (kg/kg dry matter); v, flow rate of smoke or air in the smokehouse (m/s); c_f, fat content in the fish (%); φ, relative humidity in the smokehouse (%); and T, temperature in the smokehouse (°C).

During hot smoking, the proteins present in fish tissues undergo thermal denaturation. Around 70 to 80% of the proteins is denatured already at 50°C, and this share rises up to 95% at 60°C. Thus, heating the fish to approximately 70°C in the center of its thickest part is sufficient to make it well-done and to gelatinize the collagen in the connective tissues.

The thermal treatment also brings about inactivation of most of the vegetative forms of the microflora. In order to eliminate the risks imposed by the presence of *Clostridium botulinum* toxins in hot-smoked fish, the Good Manufacturing Practice regulations in the U.S. require the fish to be heated at least for 30 min at a temperature of 82.2°C in the center of its thickest part and to have a brine concentration in the products of at least 3.5%. If the final product will have a brine concentration of at least 5%, then the process may be carried out at an internal temperature of 65.6°C with unchanged time of duration.

Fish threaded on speats tend to tear under their own weight, if the relative humidity and temperature in the kiln sufficiently weaken the connective tissue. The tearing of fish results from changes in the connective tissues, which take place due to the thermolysis of collagen at high air humidity. The gelatinized tissues, not yet strengthed by the tanning action of smoke components, lose their mechanical strength and break. At 100% relative humidity and a temperature of 60°C, Baltic herring tears from speats under its own weight in only 16 min. At lower humidities, the rate of losing moisture in fish is higher than that of the thermohydrolysis of collagen and the danger of tearing is reduced. Based on experimental data collected by Tilgner and Markowski,[73] the upper limits of the relative humidity, at which no tearing does occur, may be related to temperature as follows

$$RH = 374.17 - 79.25 \cdot \ln(T) \tag{8}$$

where RH is the relative humidity in the smokehouse (%) and T is the temperature in the smokehouse (°C). The above formula is valid for the temperature range 35 to 90°C at the 0.05 level of statistical significance.

VI. SMOKEHOUSE EQUIPMENT

A. SMOKEHOUSES

Fish can be successfully smoked in very simple devices, e.g., an inverted barrel fitted with supports for speats or wire mesh sheets, and outlets for the smoke. Such smoking ovens made of iron sheets, bricks, or other locally available materials are used in artisan technology. In old European canneries or smoking premises, there still are traditional chimney-type kilns in operation, in which heat and smoke are generated by burning logs and smoldering wooden chips and sawdust. In these smokehouses, the temperature, draft, and humidity of smoke or air are difficult to control, and to a large extent depend on weather conditions and the skill of the operator. In order to produce smoked fish of fairly uniform quality, the operator must rearrange the speats during smoking because of temperature, draft, and humidity differences in various parts of the kiln. Smoking in these smokehouses is a labor-consuming task — in particular when no mechanization is available, and takes a long time, as the heat and mass transfer processes are not carried out at optimum conditions.

Modern mechanical kilns are fitted with devices for mechanically forced air or smoke circulation, and for controlling the temperature and humidity inside the smokehouse. Most often smoke is supplied from an external generator, although in some constructions the smoke developer is located in the door of the smoking unit, e.g., in the Allround-System "Rondair".[74] Smoking kilns, originally developed at the Torry Research Station, have gained much popularity and are now available in various sizes and used both for cold and hot smoking. In large enterprises, smoking tunnels or towers are used often. In these units, the product is carried continuously on chain conveyers or trolleys, passing successively the drying, smoking, and heat-processing sections. In European countries, the Kvaerner-Brug tunnel has found a wide application. Modern smokehouses operate at programed operation times. In the most advanced designs, all operation steps are executed by means of a computer program.[50]

Electrostatic smoking units are not very widespread in the industry. Most existing installations are equipped with infrared radiators and are used for continuous smoking of small fish, e.g., sprats or herring. A different type is used for smoking oil, which is subsequently used in the canning of sprats.

There is an increasing tendency to use smoke flavorings instead of curing smoke. In this case, all operations, except the mode of applying the smoke constituents to fish, are the same as practiced in the conventional (draft) smoking process. Therefore, this kind of smoking is usually performed in conventional smokehouses. The smoke flavorings are applied to fish by means of diverse techniques. In the most simple design, the flavoring is added to the brine and the smoke constituents thus are absorbed together with salt by the fish tissues (immersion smoking). More frequently the smoke flavorings are vaporized or nebulized in the kiln. The effects of this method are much the same as those obtained by conventional (draft) smoking. A typical example of using the nebulization technique are smokehouses operating in the Penova system.[75] Smoke flavorings may be also deposited on fish electrostatically,[76] and the fish is subsequently dried and/or subjected to heat processing in any of the known kilns.

B. CONTROL EQUIPMENT

To operate a smokehouse reliably, measuring instruments and effective control equipment are indispensable. There exist a wide variety of devices for measuring and controlling the flow rate and temperature of the gaseous medium in the kiln and the temperature inside the smoked product. Similar instruments are used in all branches of the food industry and are familiar to food technologists. Equipment for controlling humidity of air also is widespread in food processing plants and easy to operate. However, when the humidity sensors are located in the smokehouse, they become contaminated with smoke compounds and, if proper maintenance is not provided, the indications and operation of the control instrument may be erratic. Therefore, it is of utmost importance to follow strictly the maintenance instructions of the supplier.

Particular problems are linked with the control of smoke density. All hithero known smoke generators operate on an all-or-none schedule and there is always a considerable time lag in changing their output. In addition, the most interesting parameter is the actual mass concentration of smoke compounds in the dispersing phase of smoke. As yet, no control instruments exist for the instantaneous measurement of this parameter. An indirect method consists of controlling the optical density of smoke, which at a constant temperature is linked with the concentration of smoke vapors in the gaseous phase.

The optical density (D) is defined as

$$D = \log(I_o/I_t) \qquad (9)$$

where I_0 is the intensity of the incident light beam and I_t is the intensity of the transmitted light beam.

Hence, it can be easily controlled by measuring the intensity of the light beam falling on a layer of smoke of known thickness and the intensity of the transmitted light beam. The measurements are performed by means of photoelectric instruments and the indications can be fed back to the smoke generator or bypassing devices. Needless to say, the maintenance instructions must be strictly followed in order to keep the sensor clean from any smoke deposits. Photoelectric smoke density meters are produced based on the construction principles developed at the Torry Research Station.[77,78]

VII. THE QUALITY AND SHELF LIFE OF SMOKED FISH

A. QUALITY

In smoked fish, the contents of proteins and lipids is higher than in the respective raw materials, as the loss of moisture exceeds that of lipids and soluble proteins. Also, brining of the fish prior to smoking causes negligible leaching of the proteins, generally below 1% of the total protein content of the tissues. The chemical changes in the functional groups of the amino acid residues due to smoke are limited in extent, and do not have any significant influence on the nutritional value of the proteins in the product. Also, extensive autooxidation of lipids does not take place in the presence of smoke compounds, many of which exhibit an antioxidative activity. Small losses of vitamins can result from dripping and oxidation and depend on the temperature. The effect of smoking and drying on the retention of nutrients in fish has been recently discussed elsewhere.[79]

Smoked foods contain up to ~0.5 g of smoke constituents in 100 g of tissue. Most published reports deal with compounds which impart the desirable sensory properties or extend the shelf life. The total content of phenols has been proposed as an objective index in the quality evaluation of smoked products. They are present in quantities varying from ~5 to ~60 mg/100 g of tissue. However, the smoky flavor is linked only with a narrow group of these components (see Section II.C.2) and no exact measurements are available as yet.

Fish smoked in smoldering smoke always contain detectable amounts of PAH. According to Steinig,[80] their quantity varies from 0.4 to 3.3 ng/kg, depending on the smoking conditions. In the skin, the amount of PAH varied within the range 0.77 to 61.00 ng/kg. The fish were more heavily contaminated when smoke was developed inside the smoking kiln than when supplying it from an external generator. Also, hot smoking resulted in a higher PAH content as compared to cold smoking. In the interest of the consumers, government agencies in many countries have imposed upper limits on the content of PAH in smoked foods. For example, in the West Germany and Austria the quantity of benz(a)pyrene in smoked products must not exceed 1 µg/kg, and in Finland the use of smoke flavorings containing said compounds in excess to 30 µg/kg is banned.[81] The contents of PAH and of N-nitroso compounds of carcinogenic activity in various smoked fish products have been recently discussed elsewhere.[82]

Smoked fish is characterized by the golden color of its surface and the smoky aroma of the meat. As the formation of the typical color is important for the quality, many producers use coloring agents to intensify this feature and make it more uniform. According to traditional requirements, the surface of hot-smoked fish should have a glossy appearance. Lack of gloss is caused by protein denaturation in the frozen raw material. Other sensory properties such as texture, juiciness, and saltiness, although not being characteristics of smoked foods only, also influence the overall quality of smoked fish. Objective indices for color, gloss, texture, succulence, flavor, and saltiness in hot-smoked herring and sprats were proposed by Tilgner and Baryłko-Pikielna.[83]

B. SHELF LIFE

Smoked fish are generally perishable commodities and should be kept under refrigeration. Their shelf life depends on many factors, mainly the species and initial quality of the raw material, the concentration of salt and the corresponding water activity in the meat, the temperature regime during smoking, the contents of smoke components, the type of packaging, the hygienic standard of the premises, and the temperature of storage. Lightly hot-smoked fish, stored at 4°C, generally have a shelf life of 2 weeks, while cold-smoked fish, more heavily salted and exposed to the action of smoke for at least 6 to 8 h, can be kept refrigerated in good quality for about 2 months. Species with a low moisture content, e.g., the eel, are more resistant to spoilage than others, while smoked chunks of fish with large exposed meat surfaces, with holes, and containing much moisture are more susceptible to putrefaction. Within the temperature range 6 to 12°C, the Q_{10} values for hot-smoked halibut, buckling, and eel are 2.81, 2.49, and 1.88, respectively. When the temperature range is extended to 6 to 20°C, these values change to 2.85, 2.59, and 1.75, respectively. An increase of the initial bacteria count by two orders of magnitude shortens the shelf life of halibut by 50% at least.

REFERENCES

1. **Fagerson, I. S.**, Thermal degradation of carbohydrates. A review, *J. Agric. Food Chem.*, 17, 747, 1969.
2. **Kin, Z.**, *Hemicelluloses: Chemistry and Application*, Państw. Wyd. Roln. i Leśne, Warsaw, 1980, chap. 1 to 3 (in Polish).
3. **Kłossowska, B. M.**, Influence of Thermal Degradation Conditions on the Contents of Low Molecular (Up to C_{10}) Monocarboxylic Acids in Wood Smoke, Ph.D. thesis, Instytut Przemysłu Mięsnego i Tłuszczowego, Warsaw, 1978, (in Polish).
4. **Freudenberg, K.**, Lignin. Its constitution and formation from *p*-hydroxycinnamyl alcohols, *Science*, 148, 595, 1965.
5. **Fiddler, W., Parker, W. E., Wasserman, A. E., and Doerr, R. C.**, Thermal decomposition of ferulic acid, *J. Agric. Food Chem.*, 15, 757, 1967.
6. **Tressl, R., Kossa, T., Renner, R., and Koppler, H.**, Gas chromatographic-mass spectrometric investigations on the formation of phenols and aromatic hydrocarbons, *Z. Lebensm. Unters. Forsch.*, 162, 123, 1976.
7. **Olkiewicz, M. J.**, Influence of Thermal Degradation Conditions on the Contents of Phenols in Wood Smoke, Ph.D. thesis. Instytut Przemysłu Mięsnego i Tłuszczowego, Warsaw, 1977 (in Polish).
8. **Toth, L.**, *Chemistry of Smoke Curing*, Deutsche Forschungsgemeinschaft, Verlag Chemie, Weinheim, 1982.
9. **Obiedziński, M. W.**, Influence of Thermal Degradation Conditions on the Contents of Benz(a)pyrene in Wood Smoke, Ph.D. thesis, Instytut Przemyslu Mięsnego i Tluszczowego, Warsaw, 1977.
10. **Sznajdrowska, W. B.**, Production of Wood Smoke in a Fluidized Bed under Conditions Yielding the Optimal Composition of the Phenolic Fraction. Optimization of Process Parameters, Ph.D. thesis, Academy of Agriculture, Szczecin, Poland, 1989 (in Polish).
11. **Rusz, J.**, Investigation of factors important for the production of wood smoke used in smoke curing of meat and of meat products, *Tehnol. Mesa,* Special Ed., 10, 1962.
12. **Kansa, E. J., Perlee, H. E., and Chaiken, R. F.**, Mathematical model of wood pyrolysis including internal forced convection, *Combust. Flame,* 29, 311, 1977.
13. **Balejko, J.**, Production of Wood Smoke in a Fluidized Bed under Conditions Yielding the Optimal Composition of the Phenolic Fraction. Construction of a Fluidized Bed Smoke Generator, Ph.D. thesis, Academy of Agriculture, Szczecin, Poland, 1987.
14. **Kin, Z.**, *Lignin: Chemistry and Application,* Wydawnictwo Nauk-Techn., Warsaw, 1971, chap. 1 (in Polish).
15. **Gilbert, J. and Knowles, M. E.**, The chemistry of smoked foods. A review, *J. Food Technol.,* 10, 245, 1975.
16. **Patzak, W.**, On the theory of wood combustion, *VDI Forsch.,* 552, 1972 (in German).
17. **Kuriyama, A.**, The thermal decomposition of woody substance, *Tehnol. Mesa,* Spec. Ed., 5, 1962.
18. **Miler, K. B. M.**, The production of wood smoke. Temperature of the combustion zone, *Tehnol. Mesa,* 7(3), 1, 1966.
19. **Borys, A., Jr., Kłossowska, B. M., Obiedziński, M. W., and Olkiewicz, M. J.**, Influence of combustion conditions on the composition of polynuclear hydrocarbons, and carbonylic, carboxylic and phenolic compounds in wood smoke, *Acta Aliment. Pol.,* 3, 335, 1977.
20. **Borys, A., Jr.**, Influence of Thermal Degradation Conditions on the Contents of Carbonylic Compounds in Wood smoke, Ph.D. thesis, Instytut Przemysłu Mięsnego i Tłuszczowego, Warsaw, 1977 (in Polish).
21. **Foster, W. W.**, Some of the Physical Factors Involved in the Deposition of Wood Smoke on Surfaces with Ultimate Reference to the Process of Smoke Curing. Ph.D. thesis, University of Aberdeen, Scotland, 1957.
22. **Foster, W. W.**, Attenuation of light by wood smoke, *Br. J. Appl. Phys.,* 10, 416, 1959.
23. **Foster, W. W.**, Deposition of unipolar charged aerosol particles by mutual repulsion, *Br. J. Appl. Phys.,* 10, 206, 1959.
24. **Simpson, T. H. and Foster, W. W.**, Mechanisms of smoke deposition, *Tehnol. Mesa,* Spec. Ed., 47, 1962.

25. **Dziel, A.**, Influence of Smoking Conditions upon the Colour of Smoked Baltic sprats, M.Sc., thesis, Academy of Agriculture, Szczecin, Poland, 1987 (in Polish).
26. **Senesi, E., Bertolo, G., Torregiani, D., Di Cesare, L., and Caserio, G.**, The utilization of Mediterranean sardines by means of smoking, in *Advances in Fish Science and Technology*, Connell, J. J., Ed., Fishing News Books, Farnham, England, 1980, 290.
27. **Mysik, B.**, Model Experiments on the Kinetics of Colour Development on the Surface of Smoked Products, M.Sc. thesis, Academy of Agriculture, Szczecin, Poland, 1985 (in Polish).
28. **Tilgner, D. J., Sikorski, Z., Urbanowicz, H., and Nowak, Z.**, Smoke curing with the dispersing phase of various curing smokes, *Tehnol. Mesa,* Spec. Ed., 62, 1962.
29. **Ruiter, A.**, Color of smoked foods, *Food Technol.,* 33, 54, 1979.
30. **Daun, H.**, Interaction of wood smoke components and foods, *Food Technol.,* 33, 66, 1979.
31. **Krylova, N. N., Bazarova, K. I., and Kuznetsova, V. V.**, Interaction of smoke components with meat constituents. Paper No. 38, VIIIth Eur. Congr. Meat Res. Inst., Moscow, 1962.
32. **Kozłowski, Z.**, Changes in the Amount of Smoke Phenols during Storage of Meat Tissues. Ph.D. thesis, Technical University Politechnika Gdańska, Gdańsk, 1965 (in Polish).
33. **Tilgner, D. J., Miler, K. B. M., Promiński, J., and Darnowska, G.**, The sensoric quality of phenolic and acid fractions in curing smoke, *Tehnol. Mesa,* Spec. Ed., 37, 1962.
34. **Kim, K., Kurata, T., and Fujimaki, M.**, Identification of flavour constituents in carbonyl, non-carbonyl, neutral and basic fractions of aqueous smoke condensates, *Agric. Biol. Chem.,* 38, 53, 1974.
35. **Potthast, K. and Eigner, G.**, Recent results on the composition of curing smoke. I. Preparation and analysis of aroma constituents from curing smoke, smoked meat products and smoke preparations manufactured by means of various technologies, *Fleischwirtschaft,* 68, 651, 1988 (in German).
36. **Kurko, V. I.**, *The Chemical and Physicochemical Foundations of the Smoking Process*, Wyd. Przem. Lekkiego i Spoz., Warsaw, 1963, chap. 1 and 2 (in Polish).
37. **Kulesza, J., Podlejski, J., Góra, J., Kolska, J., and Stołowska, J.**, A novel technology for the preparation of a smoke flavouring, *Acta Aliment. Pol.,* 3, 287, 1977.
38. **Fiddler, W., Wasserman, A. E., and Doerr, R. C.**, "Smoke" flavour fraction of a liquid smoke solution, *J. Agric. Food Chem.,* 18, 934, 1970.
39. **Lustre, A. O. and Issenberg, Ph.**, Phenolic components of smoked meat products, *J. Agric. Food Chem.,* 18, 1056, 1970.
40. **Zir Olsen, C.**, Smoke flavouring and its bacteriological and antioxidative effects, *Acta Aliment. Pol.,* 3, 313, 1977.
41. **Radecki, A., Bednarek, P., Bołtrukiewicz, J., Cacha, R., Rapicki, W., Grzybowski, J., Halkiewicz, J., and Lamparczyk, H.**, Analysis of a commercial smoke flavouring. I. Separation and identification of higher phenol fractions, *Bromatol. Chem. Toksykol.,* 8, 179, 1975 (in Polish).
42. **Gudaszewski, T.**, Influence of Heat Processing Upon the Amount of Selected Smoke Phenols and the Aroma in Meat Products — On the Example of Luncheon Meat, Ph.D. thesis, Academy of Economy, Wroclaw, 1984 (in Polish).
43. **Gudaszewski, T.**, The aroma of smoked meat products. I. Siringol as the index of smoke aroma, *Fleischwirtschaft,* 67, 1523, 1987 (in German).
44. **Sink, J. D.**, Application and effects of solid and liquid smoke technologies in the manufacturing of meat products, in *20th Anniversary Smoke Symp. Proc.,* Red Arrow Products, Mishicot, WI, 1981, 52.
45. **Kurko, V. I.**, The role and importance of individual smoke phenols in inhibiting the oxidative deterioration of smoked meats, paper at the XIIth Eur Meet Meat Research Workers, Sandefjord, 1966.
46. **Chomiak, D.**, Investigation of the Antioxidative Properties of Wood Smoke. Ph.D. thesis, Szkoła Główna Gospodarstwa Wiejskiego, Warsaw, 1977 (in Polish).
47. **Czyżewska, E.**, Antioxidative Activity of a Smoke Flavouring in Fish Oil, M.Sc. thesis, Academy of Agriculture, Szczecin, Poland, 1984 (in Polish).
48. **Chomiak, D. and Goryń, A.**, The inhibiting effect of smoke flavourings (SF) upon the autoxidation of lard, *Acta Aliment. Pol.,* 27, 223, 1977.
49. **Incze, K.**, The bacteriostatic action of a smoke solution and of smoke components, *Fleischwirtschaft,* 45, 1309, 1965 (in German).
50. **Maurer, H. and Söhne,** *MC-3 Computer — Operating Instructions,* Maurer H & Söhne, Insel Reichenau, 1985.
51. **Tilgner, D. J.**, Production and application of curing smoke, *Fleischwirtschaft,* 10, 751, 1958 (in German).
52. **Tilgner, D. J., Zimińska, H., and Wrońska-Wojciechowska, M.**, The chemical and sensorial characteristics of the steam volatile components in smouldering and friction smoke. *Tehnol. Mesa,* Spec. Ed., 35, 1962.
53. **Rasmussen, H. J.**, Fireless smokehouse smoker, *Food Eng.,* 28, 6, 65, 1956.
54. **Fessmann, G.**, Process and apparatus for preparing a smoking fluid and smoking foodstuffs therewith. U.S. Patent 3, 462, 282.

55. **Fessmann, G.,** A method of manufacturing a smoking agent, Patent Specification 1,262,925, London.
56. **Nicol, D. L.,** Improvements in and relating to the production of smoke, Patent Specification 781,591, London.
57. **Nicol, D. L.,** Production of smoke, Canadian Patent 591,846.
58. **Kurko, V. I.,** *Principles of Smokeless Smoke Curing,* Legkaja i Pishchevaja Promyshlennost, Moscow, 1984 (in Russian).
59. **Taylor, F. E.,** Method of producing smoke oil and product, U.S. Patent, 3,152,914.
60. **Hollenbeck, C. M.,** Aqueous smoke solution for use in foodstuffs, U.S. Patent 3,106,473.
61. **Kulesza, J., Podlejski, J., Góra, J., Kolska, J., Stolowska, J., Kozlowski, J., Miler K. B. M., Czajkowska, T., and Rutkowski, Z.,** Method of producing a smoke flavouring, Polish Patent 85985.
62. **Moller, H. G.,** Method of producing an aroma concentrate and the products obtained thereby, U.S. Patent 3,663,237.
63. **Tolin, S.,** Smoked hydrolyzed vegetable protein materials, U.S. Patent, 3,000,743.
64. **Carslaw, H. S. and Jaeger, J. C.,** *Conduction of Heat in Solids,* 2nd ed., Oxford University Press, London, 1959.
65. **Crank, J.,** *The Mathematics of Diffusion,* corrected reprint of the 1956 edition, Oxford University Press, London, 1957.
66. **Moon, P. and Spencer, D. E.,** *Field Theory for Engineers,* Van Nostrand Reinhold, Princeton, NJ, 1961.
67. **Chlaszczak, A. K.,** Diffusion of Heat in Non-Conventionally Shaped Solids, M.Sc. thesis, Academy of Agriculture, Szczecin, Poland, 1986 (in Polish).
68. **Sznajdrowska, W. B.,** Heat diffusion in the hot smoking process of fish, *Zesz. Nauk. Akad. Roln. Szczecin. Ser. Rybactwo Morskie i Technol. Zywn.,* No. 108, 129, 1984 (in Polish).
69. **Krischer, O.,** *The Scientific Foundations of Drying,* Springer Verlag, Berlin, 1956 (in German).
70. **Keey, R. B.,** *Drying Principles and Practice,* Pergamon Press, Oxford, 1972.
71. **Strumillo, Cz.,** *Principles of the Theory and Technique of Drying,* 2nd ed., Wyd. Naukowo-Techn., Warsaw, 1983 (in Polish).
72. **Nikitin, B. M.,** Investigation of Heat and Mass Transfer Processes in Hot Smoking of Small Fish, Thesis, Leningradskii Tekhnologicheskii Institut Kholodilnoi Promyshlennosti, Leningrad, 1965 (in Russian).
73. **Tilgner, D. J. and Markowski, B.,** Effect of thermal denaturation on the mechanical resistance and texture of animal tissue, *Prace Morskiego Instytutu Rybackiego,* Gdynia, No. 12/B, 127, 1964 (in Polish).
74. Allround-System "Rondair" — Function and Operating Instructions, Maurer, H. & Söhne, Insel Reichenau, 1983.
75. **IWEMA Food Machinery A/B.,** IWEMA Röksystem. System Penova, IWEMA Information.
76. **Brøste Industri A/S.,** Manufacturing of smoked bacon by electrostatic application, Scansmoke Information, No. 134.
77. **Jason, A. C.,** A recording smokemeter, *Food Manuf.,* 31, 3, 112, 1956.
78. **Brown, A. G. & Co,** Torry Brown Smoke Density Integrator, A. G. Brown & Co. Publication 11.
79. **Burt, J. R., Ed.,** *Fish Smoking and Drying, The Effect of Smoking and Drying on the Nutritional Properties of Fish,* Elsevier, Barking, England, 1988.
80. **Steinig, J.,** The contents of 3,4-benzpyrene in smoked fish in dependence of the smoking method, *Z. Lebens. Unters. Forsch.,* 162, 235, 1976 (in German).
81. **Walker, E. A.,** Some facts and legislation concerning polycyclic aromatic hydrocarbons in foods, *Pure Appl. Chem.,* 49, 1673, 1977.
82. **Sikorski, Z. E.,** Smoking of fish and carcinogens, in *Fish Smoking and Drying. The Effect of Smoking and Drying on the Nutritional Properties of Fish,* Burt, J. R., Ed., Elsevier, Barking, England, 1988, chap. 6.
83. **Tilgner, D. J. and Barylko-Pikielna, N.,** An attempt to establish indices of sensory quality (on the example of smoked fish), *Prace Morskiego Instytutu Rybackiego,* Gdynia, No. 11/B, 141, 1960 (in Polish).

Chapter 11

CANNING

Marian Naczk and Alekseevna Svetlana Artyukhova

TABLE OF CONTENTS

I. Introduction 182

II. Principles of Heat Sterilization 182
    A. Effect of Heat on Microorganisms 182
        1. Introduction 182
        2. Death of Microorganisms 182
        3. Factors Affecting the Destruction of Microorganisms 183
        4. Order of Destruction of Microorganisms 183
        5. Thermal Death Time and Thermal Resistance Curves 185
        6. Sterilization Value of Heat Process 186
    B. Process Calculations 186
        1. General Methods 186
        2. Mathematical Methods 188
            a. Introduction 188
            b. Heating and Cooling Curves 188
            c. Ball's Formula Method 189
            d. Modification of Ball's Formula Method 190
    C. Heat Processing Methods 190
        1. Steam Processing 190
        2. Processing in Water 191
        3. Flame Sterilization 191
        4. Aseptic Canning 191

III. Technological Aspects of Production of Canned Seafoods 191
    A. Introduction 191
    B. Unit Operations in the Canning of Seafoods 191
        1. Primary Processing 191
        2. Heat Treatment prior to Canning 193
        3. Packing and Sealing 193
        4. Heat Sterilization and Cooling 193
    C. Production of Canned Seafoods 194
        1. Mackerel 194
        2. Salmon 194
        3. Tuna 195
        4. Shrimp 195
        5. Clams 195

IV. Changes in Seafood Quality During Heat Sterilization 195

References 197

I. INTRODUCTION

The process of preserving food packaged in hermetically sealed containers was first described by Nicolas Apert[1] in 1810. He packed food in a wide-mouth glass bottle, then corked and heated it in boiling water. About half a century later, Luis Pasteur[2] provided a scientific explanation for Apert's work. He discovered the relationship between the presence of microorganisms and the spoilage of foods. The work of Madsen and Nyman[3] and Chick[4] laid the foundation for the science related to the death rate of spoilage-causing microorganisms. In 1920, Bigelow and co-workers[5] developed the first method for calculation of the minimum safe-heat sterilization process required for canned food products based on a scientific approach. In 1945, Otto Rahn[6] first applied the principle that microorganisms die according to a logarithmic order in the food preservation area. Recently, the use of advanced mathematical methods and computers led to the development of more rapid and accurate calculations of heat-processing parameters.

The primary objective of thermal processing is the destruction of microorganisms capable of causing public health hazard, as well as those capable of causing spoilage of the packaged products. Heat sterilization is based on lowering the probability of survival of vegetative forms of bacteria or bacterial spores of concern. Spore formers from the genera *Bacillus* (e.g., *B. coagulans* or *B. stearothermophilus*), *Desulfotomaculum* (genus containing very heat-resistant spores), and *Clostridia* are the microorganisms which normally cause spoilage due to underprocessing. The main public hazard of canned foods is *Clostridium botulinum*. The spores of *C. botulinum* are heat resistant and may survive when the heat treatment delivered to the product is insufficient. The health hazard is due to the ability of *C. botulinum* to grow under anaerobic conditions and to produce a toxin. The ingestion of this toxin is often fatal; therefore, it is the goal of the canning industry to have a zero-botulism outbreak. *C. botulinum* is not able to grow and produce toxin when the pH of the substrate is ≤4.7, so the botulism hazard will not exist if the pH is below 4.6. Therefore, a pH of 4.6 is generally considered to be the dividing line between low-acid and acid foods. Foods with pH >4.6 are considered to be low acid and foods with pH ≤4.6 are considered to be acid foods.[7,8]

The storage stability of canned foods is another important factor that has to be considered by the canning industry. The spores that cause spoilage of canned foods, resulting in economic losses, usually have greater heat resistance than those of *C. botulinum*. In order to achieve good storage stability, the product receives more severe heat treatment than that required for minimum safety.

The heat sterilization process also has other effects on the products, such as the destruction of nutrients, inactivation of enzymes, changes in texture, and other sensory properties.

II. PRINCIPLES OF HEAT STERILIZATION

A. EFFECT OF HEAT ON MICROORGANISMS
1. Introduction

Yeast has the least resistance to heat, followed by mold, and then bacteria. The vegetative forms of microorganisms are less resistant to heat than spores and are destroyed almost instantly at 100°C (373 K). Therefore, vegetative cells do not normally cause a problem in the sterilization of canned foods. Spores of *C. botulinum, C. sporogenes, C. bifermentans, C. butyricum, C. pasteurianum, C. perfringens, C. thermosaccharolyticum, D. nigrificans,* and *B. stearothermophilus* are very heat resistant and prolonged heating at high temperatures is necessary for their destruction. Therefore, they are of great concern when sterilizing canned foods.

2. Death of Microorganisms

The mechanism by which heat kills microorganisms is not yet fully understood. The

TABLE 1
Thermal Resistance of *Clostridium sporogenes* Spores in Different Canned Fish Products[11]

Packing medium	pH of product	$D_{121.1}$ (min)
Natural juice	5.8—6.8	0.60—0.70
Vegetable oil	5.8—7.0	0.70—0.75
Sauce	4.2—5.8	0.50—0.55

interruption of cellular function of the microorganism by heat may be due to the denaturation of critical proteins and nucleic acids in the cell. According to Rahn,[6] the death of bacteria has to be brought about by the reaction of a single type of molecule in the cell since the death of bacteria is a unimolecular or first-order bimolecular reaction.

The cell is truly dead if the molecule critical for the synthesis or reproduction of macromolecules such as DNA is inactivated. Such a cell cannot reproduce even though the cell may germinate, swell, and appear to be in the early stages of outgrowth.[9]

3. Factors Affecting the Destruction of Microorganisms

Thermal resistance of spores is affected by their inherent resistance and by environmental influences during the growth, formation, and the time of heating of the cells or spores.

Different strains of the same species grown in the same medium and under identical growth conditions may produce cells or spores having a wide range of resistance.

The spores have the maximum resistance to heat in the region of neutrality. Spores of *C. botulinum* show greatest thermal resistance at pH of 6.3 to 6.9, while *B. subtilis* spores show maximum resistance at pH of 6.8 to 7.6. The thermal resistance of most spores slightly decreases when pH is >7 and sharply falls off in the acid region.

Bacteria and spores are more resistant to dry heat than to wet heat. At 100 to 120°C (373 to 393 K), the maximum spore resistance occurs when the water activity ranges from 0.1 to 0.6.[10] However, a_w of canned fish products ranges from 0.86 to 0.99.

Fat and soluble proteins of fish may protect spores from the lethal effect of heat (Table 1). The protection by fat may be due to the localized absence of moisture. Salt in low concentrations (1 to 2%) also has a protective effect on the microorganisms. Addition of 2% NaCl to some foods may even double the resistance of certain spores. However, with increasing concentrations of salt, resistance of spores decreases rapidly.

4. Order of Destruction of Microorganisms

The death of bacteria exposed to wet heat is generally of logarithmic order. This means that microorganisms die in a geometric progression where in each successive time interval the same fraction of remaining viable cells die. The logarithmic model for the microbial destruction is described by the equation

$$U = D_T * (\log N_o - \log N_U) \tag{1}$$

where U is the equivalent heating time at the heating medium temperature, D_T the microbial decimal reduction time, N_0 the initial number of microorganisms, and N_U the number of microorganisms after heating.

The logarithmic order of bacterial destruction also means that theoretically the survivors can be reduced to less than one. However, some fraction will remain even after a long heating period. Thus, the number of survivors may become very small, such as one survivor in 10^3 units, one survivor in 10^{10} units, etc., but never reaching zero.

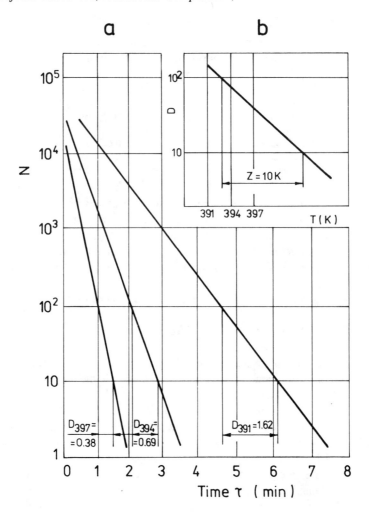

FIGURE 1. Survival curves (a) and thermal resistance curve (b) for *C. sporogenes* spores inoculated in canned sprats in oil.

The graph obtained by plotting the logarithm of the number of viable cells remaining in a suspension of bacteria or spores against the time of heating at a constant temperature is known as the survivor curve (Figure 1a).

The slope of the semilogarithmic survivor curve determines the decimal reduction time D_T. This is the time, in minutes, required to reduce the viable cells in suspension of bacteria to one tenth of their original number. The greater the D_T-value, the more resistant to heat are bacteria or spores. Since the death of bacteria is a unimolecular or first-order bimolecular reaction,[6] the D_T-value is related to the reaction rate constant k, as follows:

$$D_T = \frac{2.303}{k} \qquad (2)$$

The semilogarithmic model does not fit all experimental microbial thermal destruction data, but there is no other better model available at this time. Almost all shapes are possible for microbial wet-heat destruction curves. In about 40% of the heat destruction tests, the data form a straight line in a semilogarithmic system. In another 40% or so, the data form

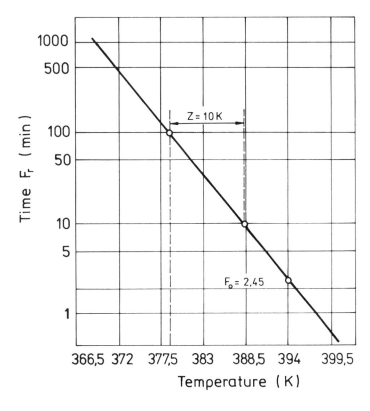

FIGURE 2. Thermal death time curve for *C. botulinum* spores.

a curve where the initial portion either shows a much lower (concave downward) or a much larger (concave upward) destruction rate. This is followed by a straight destruction line.[10]

5. Thermal Death Time and Thermal Resistance Curves

The thermal death time F is assumed to be between the longest heating time when the unit tests are positive for growth and the shortest heating time when the unit tests are negative, at a given temperature.

The value of F plotted on the logarithmic scale against the corresponding temperature on the linear scale provides a graph known as the thermal death time curve or TDT curve (Figure 2). The curve is described by an equation that was first introduced by Bigelow:[5]

$$\log F_T = (T_{ref} - T)/z + \log F_{ref} \qquad (3)$$

where F_T and F_{ref} are times required to destroy organisms at any lethal and reference temperatures, respectively; T is any lethal temperature; T_{ref} is the reference temperature; and z is the temperature coefficient of microbial destruction. Rearrangement of Equation 3 in an exponential form gives

$$L = F_{ref}/F_T = 10^{(T - T_{ref})/z} \qquad (4)$$

where L is the lethal rate defined as minutes at T_{ref} per minute at T.

Values of D_T plotted on the logarithmic scale against the corresponding temperature on the linear scale provide a graph called the phantom thermal death time curve or thermal resistance curve or thermal destruction curve (Figure 1b). This curve is described by the following equation:

$$\log D_2 - \log D_1 = (T_1 - T_2)/z \tag{5}$$

where D_1 and D_2 are D values corresponding to temperature T and T_2, respectively. For the same microbial spore crop and substrate, the semilogarithmic thermal death time curve and thermal resistance curve will be parallel.

The parameter z represents the number of degrees Fahrenheit, centigrade, or Kelvin necessary to cause the D_T-value to change by a factor of ten or required for the thermal resistance curve to traverse one logarithmic cycle.

The z-value is related to the temperature coefficient of reaction Q_{10} as follows:

$$z = 10/\log Q_{10} \tag{6}$$

The Q_{10}-value for many chemical and biological reactions is about 2. The Q_{10}-values for heat destruction of bacteria are much larger ranging from 2.2 to 4.6 for dry heat and from 8 to 20 for wet heat.

A z-value of 10°C (10 K or 18°F) is the general value used in calculating the lethal effect over the range of product temperatures during processing.

6. Sterilization Value of Heat Process

By substituting the sterilization value, F, for U into Equation 1, the following equation is obtained:

$$F = D_{ref} * (\log N_o - \log N_F) \tag{7}$$

where D_{ref} is the decimal reduction time for the microorganism of concern in the specific product at a specific reference temperature, N_o is the maximum initial microbial population of concern per container, N_F is the acceptable level of microbial survival per container, and F is the sterilization value or the equivalent time at a specific reference temperature.

This relationship is the basis for determination of the necessary sterilization value, F, for a container of product.[12] The sterilization value calculated for reference temperature of 121.1°C (394.1 K or 250°F) and z-value of 10°C (10 K or 18°F) is defined as F_0.

The initial contamination N_o of canned fish products ranges from 0.1 to 1 spore per gram and this depends on the sanitary and technological conditions of fish canneries.[13,14]

Pflug[15] introduced the term probability of nonsterile unit PNSU and suggested the use of PNSU as equivalent to N_F for calculating the sterilization value, F: for *C. botulinum* PNSU = 10^{-9}, for mesophilic spore-formers PNSU = 10^{-6}, and for thermophilic spore formers PNSU = 10^{-3} if product is stored below 30°C (303 K) or PNSU = 10^{-6} if the produce is stored at higher temperatures. In manufacturing operations, a PNSU of 10^{-6} means one nonsterile unit in 10^6 units. Pflug also proposed the use of $D_{121.1}$ = 0.2 min for calculating public health F_0-value, $D_{121.1}$ = 0.5 min for calculating F_0-value for preservation against spoilage by nonpathogenic mesophilic spores, and $D_{121.1}$ = 1.5 min for calculating F_0-values for perservation against spoilage by nonpathogenic thermophilic spores.

In designing heat-sterilization processes, the canning industry uses F_0 = 3.0 min for public health hazard and F_0 = 5 to 7 min for preservation against spoilage by mesophilic spores. For preservation against thermophilic spores, F_0 = 5 to 7 min is used if the canned products are stored below 30°C (303 K) or F_0 = 15 to 21 min is used if the products are stored at higher temperatures.[15]

B. PROCESS CALCULATIONS
1. General Methods

These methods provide the most accurate and straightforward estimation of the sterilization value, F, since the actual time-temperature data are used directly. The F value of

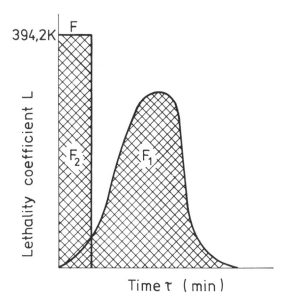

FIGURE 3. Lethality curve for canned food heat processing.

heat processing is obtained using graphic or numerical methods of integration to solve the following equation:

$$F = \int L * dt \qquad (8)$$

Bigelow et al.[5] first described the graphic method of calculation of sterilization value, F. They transformed the temperature into lethal rates and plotted the lethality curve (i.e., lethal rate vs. time). The area under the curve represents the sterilization value, F, at a reference temperature. The area can be measured by planimeter and converted to F-value using the unit area of the graph (Figure 3). Later, Ball[16] improved the method by introducing the hypothetical lethal rate equal to 1 min at a reference temperature of 121.1°C (394.1 K or 250°F) and proposed to calculate the lethal rate using this reference temperature.

Patashnik[17] described a numerical method for estimating the area beneath the lethality curve using the Trapezoidal Rule. The area is divided into equally spaced parallel cords with a time interval (Δt) between each cord. The sterilization value F is computed using the equation below (also see Table 2):

$$F_o = \Delta t \, \Sigma L_i \qquad (9)$$

where L_i is the lethal rate at temperature T_i.

The area under the lethality curve can also be calculated using Simpson's Rule of integration. However, differences in the results, using either method, are not great.

The general methods may also be used for designing sterilization processes. First, the sterilization values for several process times at a given temperature are determined. Then, the graph of delivered F_0-values vs. process time is prepared and the desired process time corresponding to the required F_0-value is selected. The use of this method in designing a process is very laborious compared to the mathematical method. However, the general method is the only available choice when the semilogarithmic heating curves are nonlinear.[9]

The general methods are very useful in process validation, in comparing the performance of the mathematical methods, and have become easier to use with the advent of computers.

TABLE 2
Calculation of Lethality, F_0, for Heat Sterilization Process for Tuna in Oil Packed in Can No. 3 (Fill Weight of 250 g) Using the Trapezoidal Rule

Time (min)	Temperature (°C)	Lethal rate L_1 (min. at 121.1° C/min at T)
0	47.0	0.0
5	53.0	0.0
10	61.0	0.0
15	75.0	0.0
20	86.0	0.0
25	97.0	0.004
30	103.0	0.015
35	107.5	0.044
40	110.0	0.077
45	112.0	0.123
50	114.0	0.194
55	116.0	0.308
60	117.5	0.435
65	118.5	0.548
70	106.5	0.035
75	92.0	0.0
80	74.0	0.0
85	45.0	0.0

Note: $\Delta t = 5.0$; $\Sigma L_i = 1.783$; $F_0 = \Delta t * \Sigma L_i = 5.0 * 1.783 = 8.9$ min.

Most data loggers of today contain small computers which can be programmed to calculate F_0-values using the general method. An example of a computer program usage is given by Pflug.[18]

2. Mathematical Methods
a. Introduction

These methods can be used efficiently in both design and evaluation of sterilization processes. They are also most helpful in calculating process time or sterilization value, F, when some processing conditions, such as retort temperature, initial temperature of the product, or container size, are changed. However, the semilog heating curve of the product should be a straight line. Ball's formula method[19,21] was the first mathematical model developed and is still the most widely used method. Since then, many modifications of this method have been presented.[20-22] In these methods, the time-temperature data are input as a temperature response parameter, f, and lag factor, j, which is obtained by appropriate analysis of heating and cooling curves.

b. Heating and Cooling Curves

The heating curve is obtained by plotting the logarithm of the differences between the temperature of the heating medium and the variable temperatures of the product. The sheet of graph paper is rotated 180° (Figure 4). The cooling curve is obtained by plotting the logarithm of differences between the variable temperatures of the product and the temperature of the cooling medium. The sheet of the graph paper is used in its normal position.

The beginning of the heating process should be adjusted to include lethal effect contributed by the come-up period of the retort. The retorts used for sterilization require a finite

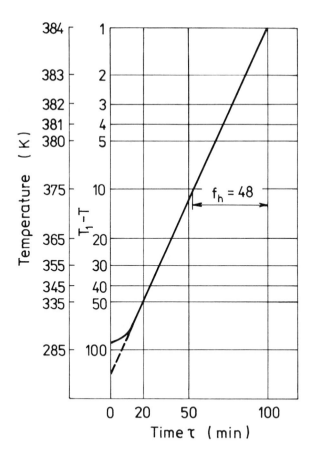

FIGURE 4. Semilogarithmic heating curve for canned Atlantic mackerel in natural juice packed into can No. 8 (fill weight of 350 g).

heating time to rise up to the operating temperature. The heating time measured from "steam on" to the time at which the process design temperature is reached is called come-up time, CUT. The CUT has an effect on the sterilization value, F. Ball[19] found that 42% of CUT is equivalent to the time at the heating medium temperature; therefore, the process time should be increased by 0.42 of CUT.

c. Ball's Formula Method

The equation of the straight-line semilogarithmic heating curve may be written as follows:[19]

$$B = f_h * [\log(j_h * (T_1 - T_0)) - \log g] \tag{10}$$

where B = Ball's time or process time that includes the 42% contribution of CUT; f_h = temperature reached by product at the slowest heating zone; $j_h = \dfrac{T_1 - T_a}{T_1 - T_o}$ heating lag factor; T_0 = initial product temperature; T_1 = retort temperature; and T_a = pseudo-initial temperature — an intercept at $B = 0$ of the extension of the line fitted linear portion of semilog heating curve.

Ball[19,20] tabulated f_h/U with respect to g, m + g, and z-values (where m + g is an equivalent of difference between heating and cooling medium temperatures). He found that variations in the z-value significantly affect the $f_h/U:g$ relationship, whereas the variations in m + g, normally found in heat processes, only have a minor effect on this relationship. When calculating the $f_h/U:g$ relationship, he assumed the cooling lag factor j_c to be 1.41, the temperature response parameter-cooling f_c to be equal to f_h, and the lag portion of semilog cooling curve to be a hyperbola. The $f_h/U:g$ relationship is independent of such process parameters as retort temperature, product initial temperature, container dimensions, cooling water temperature, and j_h.

The sterilization value of a process, F_0, is calculated using the equation below:

$$F_o = \frac{f_h}{(f_h/U) * F_i} \tag{11}$$

where f_i is the reciprocal of lethal rate at retort temperature.

In computing F_0, the log g-value must first be calculated from Equation 10. The corresponding f_h/U value may then be found from $f_h/U:g$ tables in the literature,[20,23] or could be calculated using polynomial algebraic equations developed by Steele et al.[24] and Vinter et al.[25] The polynomial equations are very useful tools in developing computerized methods of calculation using Ball's formula method. Tung and Garland[26] developed a number of computer programs providing rapid handling of heat penetration data for calculating lethality, data plotting, determination of thermal parameters f and j, and estimation of process time.

d. Modifications of Ball's Method

Ball and Olson[20] introduced a function which is defined as the ratio of the lethal value due to heating portion of the process, U_h, to the lethal value of the entire process, U. This function is useful in evaluating processes where the temperature response parameter of heating, f_h, and temperature response parameter of cooling, f_c, are different. The function ρ allows to calculate fractions of sterilization value, F, due to the heating and cooling separately.

Stumbo and Longley[27] and Stumbo[28] developed $f_h/U:g$ tables for process evaluation. This approach takes into account the variability in cooling lag factors, j_c.

Hayakawa[29] and Downes and Hayakawa[30] used circular functions to estimate the lethal effect of lag portion of semilog heating and cooling curves. For calculating lethality, the process is divided into four sections: heating lag portion, straight-line heating, cooling lag portion, and straight-line cooling. The lengths of these lag portions are estimated using an empirical relationship between f and j.

Hick[31] related the lethal effect of heating U_h with f_h and developed a table for calculating lethality of the heating portion of the process. Using the factor c (where $c = U_c/U_h$), he related the lethal effect of cooling, U_c, with f_c. The table of factor c, for calculating lethality of the cooling portion, was later provided by Pflug.[32] This method allows one to calculate directly the lethality of the heating and the cooling portion of the process.

An example of a computer program that combines Hick's heating[31] and Hayakawa's cooling models[29] is given by Kao et al.[33] This program is useful for hand-held calculators.

C. HEAT PROCESSING METHODS
1. Steam Processing

Saturated steam is commonly used for commercial sterilization of food packed in metal containers. During the heating period, steam condenses on the surface of the containers, resulting in large values of surface thermal conductance. This brings about a high rate of heat transfer from the heating medium through the container wall and into the outer layer of food. However, from this point, the penetration of heat into the coldest region of food is controlled by the thermal properties of the food itself.

Complete elimination of air is a very important factor in steam processing. This is brought about by a procedure known as venting. Vent design and the venting procedure depend on the type of retort used. It is only in the absence of air that the temperature and pressure of the steam are directly related.

2. Processing in Water

Water is commonly used as a heating medium for processing foods packed into glass containers. This protects the glass containers from thermal shock that may occur at the beginning of heating and cooling. This is due to the larger heat capacity of water. Therefore, heat added with steam or removed by cooled water brings about slow changes in the temperature. The glass containers are placed in retort and covered with cold water. Then compressed air is superimposed and water is heated to the desired temperature by steam. The air pressure is maintained in the retort throughout the heating and cooling phase of the process. Variations in water temperature throughout the retort can be quite large. Therefore, to ensure uniform temperature within the retort, circulation of water must be induced.

3. Flame Sterilization

Canned foods are heated through direct contact with gas flame at a temperature of about 1000°C (1273 K). Some forced convection is induced through the rotation of containers. The overall heat transfer coefficient is much lower than that for the conventional method of processing using saturated steam. Despite this, the flame sterilization process is up to five times faster than the conventional one. This is due to the very high temperature differences between the flame and the product. The Steriflamme is the most widely used flame sterilization system. In this, the containers are first preheated using live steam, passed through the flame, and then held at the process temperature for a short period. Finally, the containers are cooled with spraying water. The process may be used for sterilization of canned seafoods, such as shrimps and crab meat in brine.

4. Aseptic Canning

This is an ultra-high temperature processing method of great interest to the canning industry due to its potential for production of high-quality food products. In this system, liquid and semiliquid food is rapidly heated by steam injection or by using plate-type or tubular scrapped-surface heat exchangers. The food is then held in a holding tube for a short time (seconds) to obtain the desired sterilizing value, F_0. The temperature employed may be as high as 150°C (423 K). The product is then cooled in heat exchangers, and aseptically filled into containers. Containers are sterilized by superheated steam or hot air at about 260°C (533 K) prior to filling.

III. TECHNOLOGICAL ASPECTS OF PRODUCTION OF CANNED SEAFOODS

A. INTRODUCTION

The basic operations used in canning of marine products are shown in Figure 5. However, the order of unit operations used may differ from species to species, or from one type of canned product to another. For tuna, removal of skin, head, fins, dark meat, and bones follows steaming operations and for shellfish steaming usually precedes peeling or shucking. For canned fish in brine or in its natural juice, cooking in water or steaming is unnecessary. The basic principles of these operations are outlined below.

B. UNIT OPERATIONS IN THE CANNING OF SEAFOODS
1. Primary Processing

Detailed information concerning unit operations, such as bleeding, washing, heading,

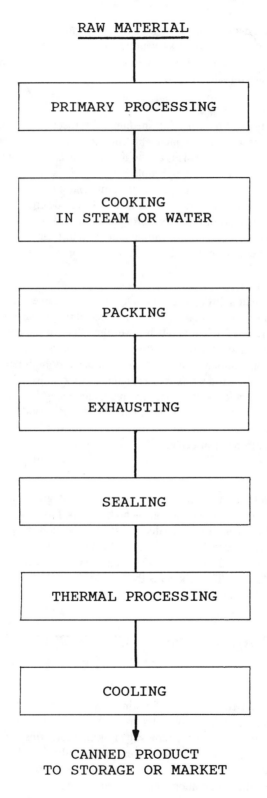

FIGURE 5. Flow diagram for canning of seafood products.

gutting, filleting, peeling, shucking, etc., used for the preparation of seafoods is provided in Chapter 5.

2. Heat Treatment prior to Canning

The objective of this operation is to decrease the content of moisture in fish to about 65%. This prevents dilution of sauce or oil by water released during heat sterilization. For shellfish, the heat treatment facilitates shucking and peeling of clams, shrimps, crabs, etc.

Seafoods may be immersed in boiling water or in brine (5 to 10% of salt) at 90°C (363 K) or exposed to live steam for up to 30 min. Among these, steaming is most commonly used. Fish is usually packed into containers and then steamed at 100°C (373 K) for 10 to 30 min. Losses in the fish weight range from 10 to 30% depending on the species, fat content, fish freshness, and heating parameters used.

For some canned fish products (e.g., those in tomato sauce), breaded fish may be fried in vegetable oil for several minutes at temperatures below 180°C (453 K). In some plants, fish may also be smoked for canned products in oil.

3. Packing and Sealing

Seafoods may be packed in metal or glass containers or retortable pouches. Among these, metal containers such as three- or two-piece cans, cylindrical or three-dimensional (usually squat) in shape, made from tin-plated steel or aluminum, are commonly used. However, glass jars are used for packaging fish marinades and some minced-type products.

Cans and jars are flushed with water under pressure or steamed before being filled. This eliminates microorganisms that otherwise would increase the initial bacterial load of the product. Seafoods are usually packed into containers by hand, while almost all canned tuna is filled mechanically. Cans, for products in sauce or oil, may then be steamed for 10 to 30 min. Following this, the packing medium such as water, brine, vegetable oil, tomato, mustard, or white sauce is added. The control weight of filled food is necessary. Overfilling may result in underprocessing of the food, in bulging of can ends, or even in splitting of seams. Therefore, a headspace of about 2.5 mm between the level of food and the inside surface of the lid is allowed.

Removal of air before sealing increases the stability of the canned product, due to minimizing oxidation of lipids and vitamins. Consequently, deterioration of food quality is retarded. This also prevents permanent distortion of can ends during heat processing. Removal of air may be accomplished by hot fill, injection of steam, or sealing containers using a vacuum-closing machine.

Cans are sealed as promptly as possible following the removal of air. Closing machines form a double seam that hermetically attaches lid to the body of the can and protects canned foods from spoilage by recontamination with microorganisms. The machines may operate at a speed of several hundred cans per minute. A visual inspection and tear-down examination of can seams should be done at regular intervals whenever a sealing machine is in use.

4. Heat Sterilization and Cooling

After closing, the containers are first washed by water, and then heated for a predetermined time at a given temperature in saturated steam or in water. Canned fish are examples of conduction-heating products and these are commonly processed in still or hydrostatic retorts. Still retort is a vertical or horizontal pressure cooker while hydrostatic retort is a continuous cooker in which the pressure in the sterilizing chamber is equilibrated by water pressure in the entrance and exit leg of retort.

Canned shellfish products are usually processed in still and agitating retorts. Clams, shrimp, and crabs in brine, water, and juice are examples of convection-heating products. Agitation by turning cans end-over-end or by spinning cans in an axial fashion induces a

TABLE 3
Heat Sterilization Conditions Recommended for Processing in Still Retorts for Some Marine Products in Brine Packed into 307 × 113 Cans[34]

Marine product	Minimum initial temperature (°C)	Retort temperature (°C)	Process time (min)
Tuna	−1	121.1	62.0
Salmon	2	121.1	61.0
Shrimp, gulf, large	7	121.1	16.0
Crabmeat, King[a]	5	121.1	40.0

[a] For cans without parchment liner.

forced convection within the cans. This significantly reduces process time, especially for processing canned shellfish in sauce.

Processing parameters depend on the type and size of the container, and type of canned seafoods. The National Food Processors Association in their latest revision of Bulletin 26-L recommended process times and temperatures for heat sterilization of some canned seafoods in still retorts.[34] An example of these conditions is given in Table 3. Processing conditions for processes in other sterilization systems and for other types of canned seafoods should be designed based on the results of appropriate heat penetration tests.

The containers are cooled immediately after steamoff by water to a product temperature of 40 to 45°C (313 to 318 K). Cooling rate should be at least 4° C/min in order to prevent overcooking of foods. This operation should be done under appropriate air pressure, especially for the larger can sizes to avoid seam straining. Severe seam straining may result even in leakage.

Canned seafoods are stored at a temperature of about 15°C (288 K) and a relative humidity of <75% for 1 to 2 months and then shipped. During this period, specific organoleptic properties are developed due to physicochemical changes in the product.

C. PRODUCTION OF CANNED SEAFOODS
1. Mackerel

The best quality canned products are obtained from fish rich in fat and over 25 cm long. The fish is dressed by splitting and removing the head, tail, fins, and viscera, by hand or by machine. The belly is then carefully washed, and the meat is cut crosswise into slices and soaked in brine at temperatures of about −3°C (270 K). The soaking time depends on the concentration of salt used. This operation removes any residual blood and prevents the formation of curd and turbid liquids during meat processing. After soaking, the meat is rinsed with fresh water and packed into containers. For mackerel in brine, the brine is added and the container is then vacuum-sealed. For mackerel in oil or sauce, the packed can is first cooked in live steam for 10 to 20 min, the liquids are drained, and the sauce or vegetable oil is added. The can is vacuum-sealed and processed, commonly, in still retorts.

2. Salmon

Different species of salmon, i.e., Chinook, Sockeye, Silver, Pink, and Chum, are first dressed using the so-called "iron chink" machine. This machine removes head, fins, and viscera from the fish. In some plants, salmon may be dressed by hand for egg recovery for caviar or bait. The fish is later conveyed to a sliming operation which removes remaining fins, bits of viscera, blood, etc. by machine or by hand. The fish is then washed, cut into can size lengths, slices, or chunks, and is filled into containers by hand or by machine. Salt, water, oil, or sauce is added, and the container is vacuum-sealed and processed.

3. Tuna

Different species of tuna namely Yellofin, Skipjack, Albacore, and Bluefin are first eviscerated, then washed in spraying water and cooked in live steam, until the final temperature of the backbone reaches 71°C (344 K). The average weight loss during cooking is 22 to 26%. The cooked fish is cooled to minimize flaking. The head, tail, fins, and skin are then removed and dark meat is scraped off. The meat is finally broken away from the bones in pieces or loins. The loins are filled into containers as solid or chunk pack. Smaller pieces and scrapings of meat are packed as flakes or broken into small uniform pieces and packed as a grated pack usually by machine. Salt and a packing medium such as brine, oil, water, broth, dressing, or sauce are added to the container which is sealed and processed.

4. Shrimp

Shrimp are deiced, thoroughly washed, and inspected for removal of broken, decomposed, and discolored individuals, as well as foreign debris. The heads and shells are then separated from the meat by a peeling machine. For the large shrimp, the sand vein is also removed. Following this, the meat is blanched in boiling brine. For the wet pack, the blanching time varies from $3/4$ to 3 min and for a dry pack from 8 to 10 min depending on the size of the shrimp. In some plants, precooked shrimps are first discharged into a cold water tank and then onto a drying belt. In other plants, the precooked shrimp are directly discharged from blancher to the drying belt. Next, the shrimp are graded and inspected once again. Shrimp, as whole, broken, or pieces, are packed into containers by machine or by hand. Next, brine, oil, or sauce is added, and containers are sealed and processed in still or agitating retorts. In the case of dry pack, shrimp are usually packed into containers lined with parchment paper and no liquid is added.

5. Clams

Clams are first washed to remove sand and mud, and then are usually precooked with steam. For preparation of clam juice, the first portion of condensed water which is collected after a brief steaming is discarded. The clams are then steamed again and the collected condensed water is used as juice. In some plants, however, washed clams are heated in boiling water for 4 to 5 min. Precooked clams are removed from shells by hand or by machine. The clam body is then slit on one side to remove the remaining sand and mud. The clams are washed again and the siphon, the side walls of the body, and the stomach are separated. The clams are packed into containers as whole, broken, chopped, chunk, cut, sliced, pieces, or minced meat and then water, brine, oil, broth, juice, or sauce is added. The containers are exhausted, sealed, and processed.

IV. CHANGES IN SEAFOOD QUALITY DURING HEAT STERILIZATION

The heat-sterilization process destroys not only viable microorganisms but also affects the desirable nutritive and organoleptic properties of food components such as proteins, sugars, fats, vitamins, as well as texture, flavor, color, etc. The goal of the canning industry is to produce canned foods which are microbiologically safe and have high nutritional value. Upon heat treatment, the content of many nutrients decreases exponentially, as does the number of viable microorganisms. However, the retention of nutrients is characterized by much higher D_T- and z-values than those of bacterial heat-resistant spores. The retention of nutrients can be estimated using Equation 7 where N_0 is replaced by C_0 defined as the initial content of nutrient, and N_F by C which gives the content of nutrient after heat processing.

Heat processing brings about denaturation of proteins which results in loss of solubility and enzymatic activity. Jack mackerel proteins begin to coagulate at 30°C (303 K) and

TABLE 4
Minimum Processing Time Required for Degradation of Proteins and Amino Acids (min)

Retort temperature (°C)	Hydrolysis of proteins	Loss of amino acids
110—112	90—120	80
115	80—100	80
120	60—85	60
125—130	60—80	60

coagulation of the last fraction of proteins ends at 80°C (353 K).[35] Hydrolysis of proteins may also occur after 90 min of heating at 110°C (383 K) and after 60 min of heating at 130°C (403 K). On the other hand, losses in amino acids can be observed after shorter periods of heating (Table 4). The extent of protein hydrolysis increases with increasing temperature and length of the heating period. Heating also results in an increase in the pH of meat by 0.3 to 0.6 units. The ability of proteins to bind calcium, magnesium, and phosphate ions also decreases significantly. An increase in the number of sulfhydryl, amino, hydroxy, and carboxyl groups due to changes in the configuration and unfolding of protein chains results. Prolonged heating of proteins at high temperatures may cause irreversible losses in sulfhydryl groups due to the formation and release of hydrogen sulfide.

Heat sterilization brings about slight changes in lipids due to their hydrolysis, oxidation, and polymerization. Products of lipid oxidation may react with nitrogenous substances in Maillard-type reactions, thus, reducing the biological value of canned foods.

Sugars are degraded by prolonged heating at high temperatures. Amino groups of proteins, peptides, and amino acids may react with sugars in browning-type (Maillard) reactions. The products of these reactions are complex mixtures of low- and high-molecular weight compounds[36] which may bring about changes in color and flavor of canned foods.

The extent of degradation of vitamins depends on the species and fat content of seafoods, and also on the sterilization parameters used. Vitamin B_1 is very labile to heat treatment (Figure 6). Losses of vitamin B_1, upon heating, ranges from 25 to 55%. Vitamin C added to canned fish with tomato sauce and vegetables is destroyed almost completely when heated. On the other hand, riboflavin and vitamins A, E, D, and PP are relatively heat stable in the absence of oxygen.

Heat alters the ability of meat to scatter and reflect light. While red meat changes its color to light-brown or brown, white meat becomes whitened. In addition, colored products may be formed as Maillard and carmelization reactions take place. Black deposits of ferrous sulfide may occur in the headspace of the can or even on the surface of shrimp, lobsters, crabs, and white meats from fish, as the result of reaction of hydrogen sulfide released during heating with iron ions.

Hydrogen sulfide is a major component of volatile substances released from meat and accumulated in the headspace of the container. Methane, ethane, propane, methyl sulfide, methanethiol, ammonia, and amines have also been identified. The content of ammonia may be used as a quality index for canned fish products.

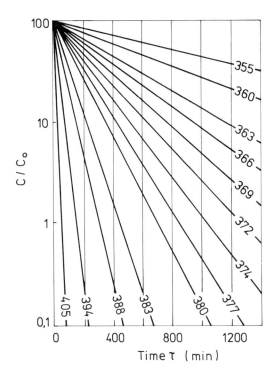

FIGURE 6. Retention curves for thiamine in meat heated at different temperatures (K).

REFERENCES

1. **Apert, N.**, L'Art de conserver pendant pulsieurs anees toutes les substances animales et ve vegetales, 1810, (Translated by K. G. Bitting, Chicago, 1920), in *Introduction to Thermal Processing of Foods*, Goldblith, S. A., Joslyn, M. A., and Nickerson, J. T. R., Eds., Avi Publishing Westport, CT, 1961.
2. **Goldblith, S. A.**, A condensed history of the science and technology of thermal processing, *Food Technol.*, 25, 1256, 1971.
3. **Madsen, T. and Nyman, M.**, Zur Theorie der Desinfektion, I, *Z. Hyg.*, 57, 388, 1907.
4. **Chick, H.**, An investigation of the laws of desinfection, *J. Hyg.*, 8, 92, 1908.
5. **Bigelow, W. D., Bohart, G. S., Richardson, A. C., and Ball, C. O.**, Heat penetration in processing canned foods, Bull No. 16-L, Res. Lab., National Canners Association, Washington, D.C., 1920.
6. **Rahn, O.**, Injury and death of bacteria by chemical agents, in *Biodynamica, Monogr. No. 3*, Luget, B. J., Ed., Biodynamica, Normandy, 1945, 9.
7. **Odlaug, T. E. and Pflug, I. J.**, *Clostridium botulinum* and acid foods, *J. Food Prot.*, 41, 566, 1978.
8. **Pflug, I. J., Odlaug, T. E., and Christensen, R.**, Computing a minimum public health sterilizing value for food with pH values from 4.6 to 6.0, *J. Food Prot.*, 48, 848, 1985.
9. **Pflug, I. J.**, *Textbook for an Introductory Course in the Microbiology and Engineering of Sterilization Processes*, 5th ed., Environmental Sterilization Laboratory, Minneapolis, 1982.
10. **Pflug, I. J. and Holcomb, R. G.**, Principles of thermal destruction of microorganisms, in *Desinfection, Sterilization, and Preservation*, Block, S. S. Eds., Lea & Febiger, Philadelphia, 1983, 751.
11. Instruction for the control of processing conditions in use and development of new heat sterilization processes for fish, invertebrates and seaweeds, Minrybkhoz, U.S.S.R., 1976, 68.
12. **Pflug, I. J.**, Calculating F_T-values for heat preservation of shelf stable, low-acid canned foods using straight-line semilogarithmic model, *J. Food Prot.*, 50, 608, 1987.

13. **Artyukhova, S. A.**, Study of the Microbial, Physico-Chemical and Thermo-Physical Criteria for the Development of Optimum Conditions for Heat Sterilization of Canned fish, Ph.D. thesis, Odessa, U.S.S.R., 1969, 175.
14. **Flaumenbaum, B. L., Tanchev, S. S., and Grishin, M. A.**, *Principles of Heat Sterilization for Foods*, Agropromizdat, 1986, 195.
15. **Pflug, I. J.**, Endpoint of preservation process, *J. Food Prot.*, 50, 347, 1987.
16. **Ball C. O.**, Mathematical solution of problems on thermal processing of canned food, University of California Publication Public Health, 1, 1928.
17. **Patashnik, M.**, A simplified procedure for thermal process evaluation, *Food Technol.*, 7, 1, 1953.
18. **Pflug, I. J.**, Heat sterilization, in *Proc. Int. Symp. Industrial Sterilization*, Phillips, G. B. and Miller, W. S., Eds., Duke University Press, Amsterdam, Netherlands, 1972, 117.
19. **Ball, C. O.**, Determining, by methods of calculation, the time necessary to process canned foods, Bull., 7-1, 37, National Research Council, Washington, D.C., 1923.
20. **Ball, C. O. and Olson, F. C.**, *Sterilization in Food Technology*, McGraw-Hill, New York, 1957.
21. **Hayakawa, I.**, A critical review of mathematical procedures for determining proper heat sterilization processes, *Food Technol.*, 32, 59, 1978.
22. **Merson, R. L., Singh, R. P., and Carroad, P. A.**, An evaluation of Ball's formula method of thermal process calculations, *Food Technol.*, 32, 66, 1978.
23. **Lopez, A.**, *A Complete Course in Canning*, 11th ed., The Canning Trade, Baltimore, 1981.
24. **Steele, R. J., Board, P. W., Best, D. J., and Willcox, M. E.**, Revision of the formula method tables for thermal process evaluation, *J. Food Sci.*, 44, 954, 1979.
25. **Vinters, J. E., Patel, R. H., and Halaby, G. A.**, Thermal process evaluation by programmable computer calculator, *Food Technol.*, 29, 42, 1975.
26. **Tung, M. A. and Garland, T. D.**, Computer calculation of thermal processes, *J. Food Sci.*, 43, 365, 1978.
27. **Stumbo, C. R. and Longley, R. E.**, New parameters for process calculations, *Food Technol.*, 20, 341, 1966.
28. **Stumbo, C. R.**, *Thermobacteriology in Food Processing*, 2nd ed., Academic Press, New York, 1973.
29. **Hayakawa, K. I.**, Experimental formulas for accurate estimation of transient temperature of food and their application to thermal process evaluation, *Food Technol.*, 24, 1407, 1970.
30. **Downes, T. W. and Hayakawa, K. I.**, A procedure for estimation of retention of components of thermally conductive processed foods, *Lebensm. Wiss. Technol.*, 10, 256, 1977.
31. **Hick, E. W.**, A revised table of P_h function of Ball and Olson, *Food Res.*, 23, 396, 1958.
32. **Pflug, I. J.**, Evaluating the lethality of heat process using a method employing Hick's table, *Food Technol.*, 33, 1153, 1968.
33. **Kao, J., Naveh, D., Kopelman, I. J., and Pflug, I. J.**, Thermal processes calculation for different z and j_c values using hand-held calculator, *J. Food Sci.*, 47, 193, 1981.
34. National Food Processor Association, Thermal processes for low-acid foods in metal containers, Bulletin 26-L, 12th ed., New York, 1982, 46.
35. **Markowski, B.**, Information on fish processing, *Zesz. Cent. Lab. Przem. Ryb.*, 15(7), 1, 1967.
36. **Safranova, T. M.**, Aminosugars of fish and invertebrates and their effect on product quality, *Pishch. Prom.*, 15, 1980.

Chapter 12

MINCED FISH TECHNOLOGY

Bonnie Sun Pan

TABLE OF CONTENTS

I. Formation of Functional Properties 200
    A. Formation of Gel Structure 200
    B. Enzymatic Disruption of Gel Structure 200
    C. Chemical Composition and Functional Properties 200
        1. Moisture 200
        2. Muscle Proteins 201
        3. Additives to Modify Functional Properties 202
            a. Macromolecular Extenders 202
            b. Cryoprotectants 204
            c. Fats and Oils 204

II. Raw Material 204
    A. Sources 204
    B. Quality Requirements 205
        1. Freshness 205
        2. Season of Catch 205
        3. Species 205

III. Processing 206
    A. Fish Mince (Surimi) and Processing 206
    B. Textural Quality of Minced Fish Products 206

References 208

I. FORMATION OF FUNCTIONAL PROPERTIES

A. FORMATION OF GEL STRUCTURE

Fish, shrimp, or cuttlefish being minced and formed into ball-shape products have been a type of traditional Chinese cuisine for a long history. However, they remained popular only in oriental diets and were manufactured on a kitchen-type processing scale until the success in developing the theory and technology for preparing frozen fish mince (surimi) by Japanese scientists, Nishiya, Takeda, Tamato and collaborators in 1961.[1] Today, minced fish products have evolved into continuous mass production of versatile products (Figure 1) and have gained favor in international markets.

The formation of myofibrillar protein network is responsible for the functional properties of surimi. It is this gel structure that brings about the elasticity and the textural strength of the products.

Since myofibrillar proteins are salt soluble, the grinding of fish with no salt added does not disrupt the myofibrillar structure, of which the M-lines and the Z-bands are still intact.[2] When fish meat is minced with salt, disintegration of the myofibrillar structure and formation of actomyosin network are observed.[2,3]

Setting of the mince at below-ambient temperature enhances the unfolding of protein helices and the interaction between the hydrophobic side chains resulting in a more uniform and thicker network as compared to those minced fish skip setting before heating.[2-5]

A firm gel network needs a balance between the protein-protein and protein-water interactions. The hydrophobic interaction and the disulfide linkages are the major forces that account for the integrity and strength of the gel network. A mechanism of oxidation-reduction and interchange of the sulfhydryl groups of myofibrillar protein with the sulfhydryl reagents was probably involved to reinforce the gel network.[6] Addition of cysteine or sodium bisulfite to the mince produced from frozen ground fish results in the recovery of reactive and total sulfhydryl groups and concomitantly improves the gel strength of the minced fish products.[7] Denaturation and interactions between the heavy chains reduce gel-forming capacity and lower the surimi quality.[8]

B. ENZYMATIC DISRUPTION OF GEL STRUCTURE

Fish mince being exposed to temperature ranged between 50 and 70°C either during setting or in slow heating causes reduction in gel strength of minced fish products.[9-11] This softening phenomenon is called "modori" in Japanese and has been attributed to the activity of muscle alkaline protease in minced fish products made from barracuda, carp, croakers, horse mackerel, and mullet.[12-18] Sardine also showed very high activity of this enzyme.[19]

Muscle alkaline protease found in fish bear similar properties, i.e., having optimal pH at 8.0 to 8.5, and optimal temperature between 50 and 65°C.[19] It is capable of hydrolyzing myofibrillar proteins.[20-23] In general, the occurrence of this enzyme in fish muscle is antagonistic to gel network formation. Setting of fish mince at temperatures below this range and accelerating the heating rate are key processing factors to avoid softening.

C. CHEMICAL COMPOSITION AND FUNCTIONAL PROPERTIES
1. Moisture

Since the myofibrillar protein network is responsible for the cohesiveness and textural strength of the minced fish product, an increase of moisture content dilutes the myofibrillar protein concentration. In general, gel strength is inversely proportional to moisture content in the range of 72 to 82%[3] as shown in Figure 2. The proportionality factor varies with species of fish.

The freeze-thaw stability of minced fish products is also moisture dependent. Increase in moisture content results in increases in expressible fluid.[24] In order to improve the freeze-

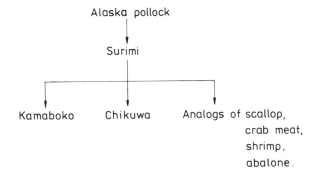

FIGURE 1. The Japanese model of surimi-related industries.

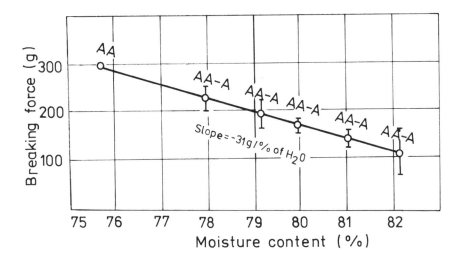

FIGURE 2. The effect of moisture content on the breaking force of minced squid products (From Pan, B. S., Lee, D. J., and Lin, L. P., *Advances in Fish Science and Technology*, Connell, J. J., Ed., Fishing News Books, Farnham, England, 1979, 232.)

thaw stability without reducing the moisture content of the frozen mince, it has become a common practice to add cryoprotectants.

2. Muscle Proteins

Sarcoplasmic proteins, the water-soluble fraction, interferes with the myofibrillar proteins from forming a cohesive and firm network by co-coagulation with the latter. Pelagic fish, of which the muscles are darker than bottom fish, have a higher content of heat-coagulable sarcoplasmic protein than the white fish. This is one of the reasons that minced fish is preferably made from white fish to ensure high elasticity.

Washing of mackerel or sardine increases the gel strength of the cooked products.[25,26] Proteolytic enzymes are among other enzymes present in abundance in the sarcoplasmic fraction. Myoglobin and hemoglobin are the part of the water-soluble proteins responsible for the color. Efficient washing reduces the content of the sarcoplasmic protein fraction and produces products of higher elasticity and whiter color.

Myofibrillar proteins, primarily the actomyosin, are salt soluble. During mincing with salt, actomyosin is solubilized to form gel, as proposed by Niwa and Miyake.[27] Myosins or myosin heavy chains are able to gel, the microstructure of which is very similar to that of

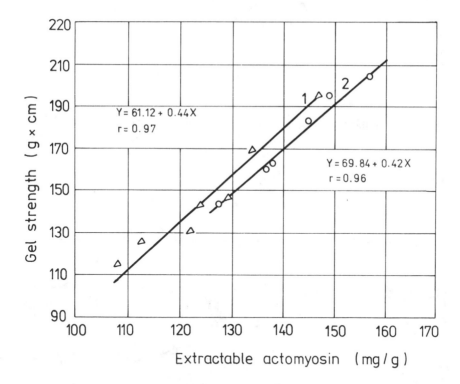

FIGURE 3. The effect of extractable actomyosin on the gel strength of the cooked products of the frozen ground (1) and the frozen mince (surimi) (2) of Falkland squid *Martialia hyagesi* after storage at −20°C for 3 months (From Lee, M. L. and Pan, B. S., Courtesy of Institute of Food Technologists).

actomyosin. However, actin alone does not form gel.[28] The weight ratio of actin to myosin changes the gel-forming ability of myosin. Increase in actin fraction decreases the rigidity of the gel.[29,30]

During frozen storage of round fish or fish mince, actomyosin undergoes denaturation as indicated by reductions in extractability and Ca-ATPase activity. The rate of freezing denaturation varies with species of fish. Usually cold-water fish are less susceptible to freezing denaturation than the warm-water fish.[31] The gel strength bears linear correlation with the actomyosin extractability (Figure 3) and Ca-ATPase activity (Figure 4) of minced fish products undergone freezing storage.[32] Prolonged chopping of fish meat may result in a temperature rise which accelerates protein-protein interaction leading to a decrease in gel-forming ability.[2,8] Warm-water fish tolerates higher temperature rise than the cold-water fish. Setting the mince at ambient temperature may also bring about protein-protein interaction for some species of fish.[8]

In summary of the effects of muscle proteins on gel structure and strength, it is undesirable to have much interactions between sarcoplasmic and myofibrillar proteins, nor to have much cross-linking among the myofibrillar protein itself. Either kind of interaction causes the gel-forming ability to decrease.

3. Additives to Modify Functional Properties

Food additives commonly used in minced fish products are described in the following sections.

a. Macromolecular Extenders

Starch is widely used at a level of 5 to 10% in minced fish products. During heating,

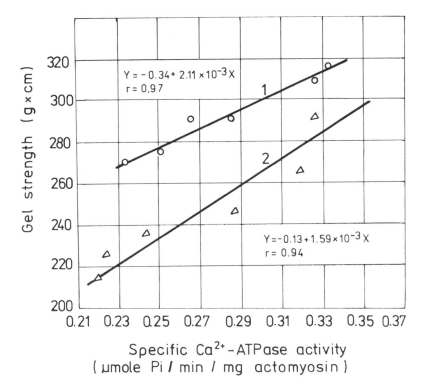

FIGURE 4. Effect of specific Ca^{2+}-ATPase activity on the gel strength of cooked products of the frozen mince (surimi) (1) and frozen ground Argentina squid *Illex argentinus* (2) after storage at $-20°C$ for 3 months (From Lee, M. L. and Pan, B. S., Courtesy of Institute of Food Technologists).

starch imbibes some water from the mince and becomes partially gelatinized and fills the pores of the protein network to reinforce it.[33] At the same time, starch acts as a humectant and improves the freeze-thaw stability of the minced fish products. However, pregelatinized starch having no granular structure induces mushy texture with no rigidity increase while addition of potato starch causes the rigidity of fish gel to increase dramatically.[34]

Starch from potato, corn, and cassava, and α-starch are commonly used. Modified starch with thermal stability is being tested to reduce the degradation of gel strength when the minced fish products are thermally processed.

Carbohydrate gums such as alginate, carboxymethylcellulose (CMC), and xanthan gums have been used in the development of surimi products. However, the xanthan gum particularly induces mushy texture by lowering the torsion rigidity and the strain at failure for the surimi product.[35] Carrageenan is used in gelling agent blend to improve freeze-thaw stability of surimi products.

Soy protein isolate (SPI) at 2% in boiled fish gel product and at 3 to 4% in fried and broiled products show no difference in gel strength from Alaska pollock products containing no SPI extender. Further additions of SPI in the minced Alaska pollock results in reduction of gel strength.[36] However, addition of up to 15% SPI to minced mackerel product still upgrades the gel strength of the products, probably due to the fact that gel strength of minced mackerel was lower than the minced Alaska pollock.[37]

Milk solids, egg white albumin, and gluten are other protein extenders being used in minced fish products. Their effects on textural modification vary with the species and freshness of fish and the type of minced products. Egg white also adds glossiness to the products.

b. Cryoprotectants

Freeze-thaw stability is another functional property, in addition to texture, of prime importance to the quality of surimi products. Syneresis and reduction in gel strength occur during frozen storage of some of this type of products. This concern led to the search for effective cryoprotectants.

Cryoprotectants applicable to minced fish products generally fall into five categories based on their chemical nature: (1) amino acids and peptides, (2) carboxylic acids, (3) mono- and disaccharides, (4) polyols, and (5) salts, mainly polyphosphates.

Many amino acids have cryoprotective effects. Among them, glutamate and aspartate are most effective.[38-42] They prevent the actomyosin from rapid decreases in solubility, viscosity, and ATPase activity. They also keep the actomyosin molecules from forming aggregates. Amino acids having relatively large hydrophobic side chains such as leucine and phenylalanine do not have cryoprotective effects.

Malonic, maleic, lactic, malic, tartaric, gluconic, and glycolic acids are among the carboxylic acids displaying most effective cryoprotective effects.[43]

Hexoses (glucose and fructose), and disaccharides (sucrose and lactose) are very effective. It has become a standard industrial practice to include sucrose in the surimi formulation to prevent freezing denaturation of fish muscle proteins. Reducing sugars may cause browning during processing and storage.

Polyols, especially glycerol, have long been used as biological cryoprotectants. Glycerol, ethylene glycol, and sorbitol, which have been considered as humectants in food processing, are effective cryoprotectants for surimi processing. Additions of 10% sorbitol and 1.5 to 3% glutamate to horse mackerel mince show synergistic effect on upgrading the gel strength of the end products.[44]

Salt, such as sodium chloride is a primary ingredient in fish mince. However, it is used to solubilize the actomyosin and to season the flavor. It does not serve as a cryoprotectant. Polyphosphates are widely used to improve water-holding capacity and to reduce thaw drip. Tripolyphosphates, pyrophosphates, and hexametaphosphates are more effective than orthophosphate. Mixtures of tripolyphosphate and pyrophosphate or of either phosphate or sugar are effective in improving water retention and gel strength.[45-47]

c. Fats and Oils

Other ingredients are added to fish mince depending on the type of products. Vegetable oil at 3 to 4% is often incorporated in molded products.[24] Incorporation of plastic fats improves freeze-thaw stability and prevents development of sponge-like texture. It also modifies the cooked gel to become less rubbery and minimizes the textural weakening effect of cooking especially when reaching temperature between 60 and 70°C.[48]

II. RAW MATERIAL

A. SOURCES

The gel-forming capacity of fish muscle proteins varies from species to species. For a given species, seasons of harvest and the conditions of postharvest handling influence the quality of the end products.

Traditionally, kamaboko, a kind of minced fish product with high elasticity, has mainly been made from lizard fish, croakers, and stroptoothed eel. Fish ham and sausage generally use tuna. Alaska pollock and Atka mackerel have only been used since 1960 because of their abundance in natural resources. The collaborative efforts of different expertise on preventing freezing denaturations of these fish by improving methods of harvesting, handling, processing, engineering, product developments, and marketing made underutilized fish the most valuable material to the surimi industry.

Fish being minced for use in further processed products are as follows:

Alaska pollock	Ocean perch
Atka mackerel	Pacific pollock
Atlantic and Pacific cod	Pike
Carp	Porgy
Cutlass fish	Rockfish
Cuttle fish	Saithe
Dory	Salmon
Eels	Sardine
Flounders	Sea perch
Grenadier	Sharks
Grouper	Sheepshead
Gunard	Shrimp
Haddock	Snapper
Hake	Tilapia
Halibut	Trevally
Herring	Trout
Hoki	Trumpeter
Horse mackerel	Tom cod
Lobster	Tuna
Mackerels	Warehou
Menhaden	Whiptail
Milkfish	Whitefish
Mullet	

Over 60 different species of fish have been used for surimi processing. However, Alaska pollock alone contributes to 40 to 50% shore-processed and 50 to 55% ship-processed surimi.[49] New fish material for kamaboko and the product properties are compiled and compared by Suzuki.[50]

Underutilized fish in sufficient quantity, i.e., squid, and shrimp by-catch, food grade-waste materials, and mechanically deboned fish, have been tested for development of new minced products.[51]

B. QUALITY REQUIREMENTS

Fish undergo seasonal and postharvest changes. The variation in raw materials can be very pronounced. Nevertheless, consistency in product quality is still required for good industrial production. Freshness of fish is the major factor to be controlled in minced fish processing.

1. Freshness

Freshness decreases with post-mortem time. As a result, gel strength of the product also decreases with the freshness of the raw material due to the decreases in extractable actomyosin and increases in pH of the post-mortem fish muscle (Figure 5).[33] The gel strength of the product is higher when it is made before the pH and NH_3 of raw material excels to logarithmic increase. Generally, good product quality is obtained when the fish is processed within 2 d provided that the fish is properly stored at chilling temperature.

2. Season of Catch

Fish caught during and after spawning are high in moisture and relatively low in lipid and protein as compared to those caught in feeding period. Consequently, minced fish made from the former fish catch has poorer quality than those from the latter.

3. Species

Different species of fish differ in chemical compositions of which the moisture and

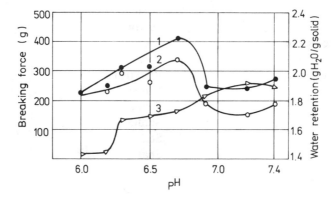

FIGURE 5. The effect of pH on the breaking force and water retention of minced squid product, buffered with phosphate. 1, Corrected breaking force, 2, breaking force, 3, water retention. (From Pan, B. S., Lee, D. J., and Lin, L. P., *Advances in Fish Science and Technology*, Connell, J. J., Ed., Fishing News Books, Farnham, England, 1979, 232.)

protein contents and the ratio of sarcoplasmic to myofibrillar protein are important to gel formation. They also differ in pattern and rate of post-mortem changes, of which the pH affects the actomyosin extractability and textural strength.

III. PROCESSING

A. FISH MINCE (SURIMI) AND PROCESSING

The fish are deheaded and gutted then put through a meat-bone separator. If a belt-drum-type meat separator is used, the drum perforations should not be too large to allow skin to pass through. The process scheme is as shown in Figure 6.

If pelagic fish or fatty fish are used, or high elasticity is required for the products, washing of meat is a necessary step, fish to washing water ratio is 5 to 7 w/v, or 5 to 10 w/v for batch process.[49,52]

Pelagic fish not only have higher content of sarcoplasmic proteins than the bottom fish, it also undergoes more rapid decrease in pH of post-mortem muscle. Both properties contribute to a poorer textural quality. Washing pelagic fish mince with water containing 0.5% sodium bicarbonate effectively increases the pH of mince and upgrades the textural quality as much as from grade D to grade AA for minced mackerel.[25,53]

Since mackerel and sardine are fatty fish, the fat contents can reach up to over 20%. A meat-fat separator has been introduced to remove the fat after the step of pH adjustment by washing with bicarbonate and has become essential for making pelagic fish surimi.[53]

The fish mince is either shaped into blocks and quickly frozen in a plate freezer or further processed into traditional products as steamed kamaboko, fried kamaboko, chickuwa, and other products.[50] Since 1960, frozen fish mince have been produced aboard ships or on shore in industrial scale and then transported to different processing plants of seafood analogue and traditional products, as shown in Figure 1. The thawing method becomes an additional factor affecting the quality of the minced fish products.

Good manufacturing practice is to be observed in minced fish processing plants to assure good quality of end products. A code of practice for minced fish may also be used as guidelines.[54] The energy input in the manufacture of these types of products are estimated being 5300 kcal/kg product.[55]

B. TEXTURAL QUALITY OF MINCED FISH PRODUCTS

The freshly prepared minced fish products are cooled overnight. Quality tests used in

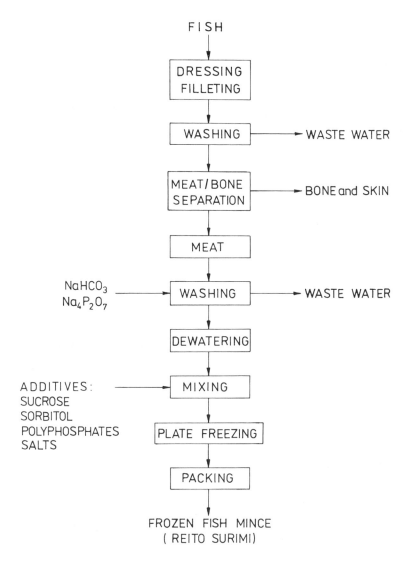

FIGURE 6. Flow chart of fish mince processing. NaHCO$_3$ is used to raise the pH of washing water when pelagic fish such as sardine or mackerel are processed.

the industry include instrumental measurements of textural determination of expressible water and folding test, which is the simplest but most widely used method for routine quality control.

A 3- to 5-mm thick piece is folded into halves and quarters.

- Grade AA: no cracks shown on folding into quarters
- Grade A: no cracks shown on folding into half
- Grade B: partly cracks shown on folding in half
- Grade C: cracks run through the folding edge
- Grade D: breaks into halves or fragments upon folding

Sophisticated instrumentation and evaluation methodologies are developed not only for industrial application but also for research and development of new products as well as for understanding the interrelation between the biochemical nature of fish proteins, chemical and physical treatments, and the textural quality of this fascinating type of seafood product.

REFERENCES

1. **Matsumoto, J. J.**, Technological solutions of fish processing in Southeast Asia, in *Recent Advances in Food Science and Technology,* Vol. 2, Tsen, C. C. and Lii, C. Y., Eds., Hua Shiang Yuan Publishing, Taipei, Republic of China, 1980, 179.
2. **Sato, S., Nakagawa, N., Tsuchiya, T., and Matsumoto, J. J.**, Electron microscopic study on the processes of preparation of kamaboko, *Bull. Jpn. Soc. Sci. Fish.,* 53, 649, 1987.
3. **Pan, B. S.**, Texture and chemical properties of minced fish products as affected by physical treatments, in *Role of Chemistry in the Quality of Processed Food,* Fennema, O. R., Chang, W. H., and Lii, C. Y., Food and Nutrition Press, Westport, CT, 1986, 225.
4. **Niwa, E. and Miyake, M.**, Physico-chemical behavior of fish meat protein. II. Reactivities of side groups of polypeptide chains during setting of fish meat paste, *Bull. Jpn. Soc. Sci. Fish.,* 37, 534, 1971.
5. **Niwa, E.**, Role of hydrophobic bonding in gelation of fish flesh paste, *Bull. Jpn. Soc. Sci. Fish.,* 41, 907, 1975.
6. **Itoh, Y., Yoshinaka, R., and Ikeda, S.**, Effects of inorganic reducing agents on the gel formation of fish meat by heating, *Bull. Jpn. Soc. Sci. Fish.,* 45, 455, 1979.
7. **Lan, C. C., Pan, B. S., and Jiang, S. T.**, Effect of reducing agents on protein denaturation of frozen minced lizard fish and textural properties of the cooked product, *J. Chin. Agric. Chem. Soc.,* 25, 159, 1987.
8. **Numakura, T., Seki, N., Kimura, I., Toyoda, K., Fujita, T., Takama, K., and Arai, K. I.**, Effect of quality of Surimi on cross-linking reaction of myosin heavy chain during setting, *Bull. Jpn. Soc. Sci. Fish.,* 53, 633, 1987.
9. **Tanikawa, E.**, *Marine Products in Japan,* Koseishi-Koseikaka, Tokyo, 1971, 365.
10. **Cheng, C. S., Hamann, D. D., and Webb, N. B.**, Effect of thermal processing on minced fish gel texture, *J. Food Sci.,* 44, 1080, 1979.
11. **Lee, C. M. and Toledo, R. T.**, Factors affecting textural characteristics of cooked comminuted fish muscle, *J. Food Sci.,* 41, 391, 1976.
12. **Makinodan, Y. and Ikeda, S.**, Studies on fish muscle protease. IV. Relation between Himodori of kamaboko and muscle proteinase, *Bull. Jpn. Soc. Sci. Fish.,* 37, 518, 1971.
13. **Ikeda, K., Kobashi, K., and Hase, J.**, Studies on muscle alkaline protease. V. Effect of carp muscular alkaline protease upon "modori" phenomenon in kamaboko production, *Bull. Jpn. Soc. Sci. Fish.,* 40, 1051, 1974.
14. **Ikeda, K., Kobashi, K., and Hase, J.**, Studies on muscle alkaline protease-VI purification of proteins which induce the "modori" phenomenon in kamaboko production and of cathepsin A from carp muscle, *Bull. Jpn. Soc. Sci. Fish.,* 40, 1051, 1974.
15. **Iwata, K., Kobashi, K., and Hase, J.**, Studies on muscle alkaline protease. VII. Effect of the muscular alkaline protease and protein fraction purified from white croaker and horse mackerel on the "himodori" phenomenon during kamaboko production, *Bull. Jpn. Soc. Sci. Fish.,* 45, 157, 1979.
16. **Deng, J. C.**, Effect of temperatures on fish alkaline protease, protein interaction and texture quality, *J. Food Sci.,* 46, 62, 1981.
17. **Lin, T. S., Su, H. K., and Lainer, T. C.**, Characterization of fish muscle proteases using radio-labelled protein substrates, *J. Food Sci.,* 45, 1036, 1980.
18. **Lainer, T. C., Lin, T. S., Hamman, D. D., and Thomas, F. B.**, Effect of alkaline protease in minced fish on texture of heat-processed gels, *J. Food Sci.,* 46, 1643, 1981.
19. **Makinodan, Y., Toyohara, H., and Ikeda, S.**, On the existence of acid, neutral, and alkaline proteases in fish muscle, *Bull. Jpn. Soc. Sci. Fish.,* 49, 109, 1983.
20. **Boye, S. M. and Lanier, T. C.**, Effect of heat-stable alkaline protease activity of Atlantic menhaden (*Brevoorti tyrannus*) on surimi gels, *J. Food Sci.,* 53, 1340, 1988.
21. **Yoon, I. H., Matches, J. R., and Rasco, B.**, Microbiological and chemical changes of surimi-based imitation crab during storage, *J. Food Sci.,* 53, 1343, 1988.
22. **Pan, B. S., Kuo, J. M., Luo, L. J., and Yang, H. M.**, Effect of endogenous proteinases on histamine and honeycomb formation in mackerel, *J. Food Biochem.,* 10, 305, 1986.
23. **Makinodan, Y., Toyohara, H., and Niwa, E.**, Implication of muscle alkaline proteinase in the texture degradation of fish meat gel, *J. Food Sci.,* 50, 1351, 1985.
24. **Lee, C. M.**, Surimi manufacturing and fabrication of surimi-based products, *Food Technol.,* 40, 115, 1986.
25. **Shiau, C. Y. and Pan, B. S.**, Effect of processing condition on properties of minced mackeral products, in *Recent Advances in Food Science and Technology,* Tsen, C. C. and Lii, C. Y., Eds., Hua Shiang Yuan Publishing, Taipei, Republic of China, 1981, 198.
26. **Noguchi, S. F.**, The effect of washing treatment of fish meat from pelagic species on the quality of surimi products, in *Recent Advances in Food Science and Technology,* Tsen, C. C. and Lii, C. Y., Eds., Hua Shiang Yuan Publishing, Taipei, Republic of China, 1981, 190.

27. **Niwa, E. and Miyake, M.**, Physico-chemical behavior of fish meat proteins. I. Behavior of polypeptide chains of proteins during setting of fish meat paste, *Bull. Jpn. Sco. Sci. Fish.*, 37, 877, 1971.
28. **Samejima, K., Hashimoto, Y., Yasui, T., and Fukazawa, T.**, Heat gelling properties of myosin, actin, actomyosin and myosin subunits in a saline model system, *J. Food Sci.*, 34, 242, 1969.
29. **Yasui, T., Ishioroshi, M., and Samejima, K.**, Heat-induced gelation of myosin in the presence of F-actin, *J. Food Biochem.*, 4, 61, 1980.
30. **Matsumoto, J. J., Chihara, S., Akahane, T., Tsuchiya, T., Noguchi, S., and Ookami, H.**, Application of differential scanning calorimetry to food technological studies of meats of fish and rabbit, in *Recent Advances in Food Science and Technology*, Tsen, C. C. and Lii, C. Y., Eds., Hua Shiang Yuan Publishing, Taipei, Republic of China, 1981, 218.
31. **Hashimoto, A., Kobayashi, A., and Arai, K. I.**, Thermostability of fish myofibrillar Ca-ATPase and adaptation to environmental temperature, *Bull. Jpn. Soc. Sci. Fish.*, 48, 671, 1982.
32. **Lee, M. L. and Pan, B. S.**, Comparison on the autolysis and freezing denaturation of Argentina and Falkland squid, submitted to Inst. of Food Technologists (USA), 1989.
33. **Pan, B. S., Lee, D. J., and Lin, L. P.**, Studies on a minced squid product; Effect of raw material and ingredients on the texture of the product, in *Advances in Fish Science and Technology*, Connell, J. J., Ed., Fishing News Books, Farnham, England, 1979, 232.
34. **Wu, M. C., Lanier, T. C., and Hamann, D. D.**, Thermal transitions of admixed starch/fish protein systems during heating, *J. Food Sci.*, 50, 21, 1985.
35. **Lanier, T. C.**, Functional properties of surimi, *Food Technol.*, 40, 107, 1986.
36. **Motohiro, T. and Numakura, T.**, Utilization of soy proteins in fish gel products. I. Optimum concentration of protein isolate in broiled-type products, *Bull. Faculty Fish. Hokkaido Univ.*, 29, 141, 1978.
37. **Pan, B. S., Shiau, C. Y., and Chen, S.**, Effect of extender on minced fish product, in *Recent Advances in Food Science and Technology*, Tsen, C. C. and Lii, C. C., Eds., Hua Shiang Yuan Publishing, Taipei, Republic of China, 1981, 85.
38. **Noguchi, S. and Matsumoto, J. J.**, Studies on the control of the denaturation of the fish muscle proteins during the frozen storage. I. Preventive effect of Na-glutamate, *Bull. Jpn. Soc. Sci. Fish.*, 36, 1078, 1970.
39. **Noguchi, S. and Matsumoto, J. J.**, Studies on the control of the denaturation of the fish muscle proteins during frozen storage. II. Preventive effect of amino acids and related compounds, *Bull. Jpn. Soc. Sci. Fish.*, 37, 1115, 1971.
40. **Noguchi, S. and Matsumoto, J. J.**, Studies on the control of denaturation of fish muscle proteins during frozen storage. III. Preventive effect of some amino acids, peptides, acetylamino acids and sulfur compounds, *Bull Jpn. Soc. Sci. Fish.*, 41, 243, 1975.
41. **Tsuchiya, T., Tsuchiya, Y., Nonomura, Y., and Matsumoto, J. J.**, Prevention of freeze denaturation of carp actomyosin by sodium glutamate, *J. Biochem.*, 77, 853, 1975.
42. **Ohnishi, M., Tsuchiya, T., and Matsumoto, J. J.**, Electron microscopic study of the cryoprotective effect of amino acids on freeze denaturation of carp actomyosin, *Bull. Jpn. Soc. Sci. Fish.*, 44, 755, 1978.
43. **Noguchi, S. and Matsumoto, J. J.**, Studies on the control of denaturation of fish muscle proteins during frozen storage. IV. Preventive effect of carboxylic acids, *Bull. Jpn. Soc. Sci. Fish.*, 41, 329, 1975.
44. **Noguchi, S., Oosawa, K., and Matsumoto, J. J.**, Studies on the control of denaturation of fish muscle proteins during frozen storage. VI. Preventive effect of carbohydrates, *Bull. Jpn. Soc. Sci. Fish.*, 42, 77, 1976.
45. **Noguchi, S., Shinoda, E., and Matsumoto, J. J.**, Studies on the control of denaturation of fish muscle proteins during frozen storage. V. Technological application of cryoprotective substances on the frozen minced fish meat, *Bull. Jpn. Soc. Sci. Fish.*, 41, 779, 1975.
46. **Okamura, K., Matuda, T., and Yokoyama, M.**, Effect of phosphate mixtures composed of pyrophosphate and tripolyphosphate upon the factor of water intake and the jelly strength of "Kamaboko", *Bull. Jpn. Soc. Sci. Fish.*, 24, 978, 1959.
47. **Matsumoto, J. J. and Noguchi, S.**, Control of the freezing-denaturation of fish muscle proteins by chemical substances, in *Proc. Int. Congr. Refrigeration*, Vol. 3, Washington, D.C., 1971, 237.
48. **Lee, C. M. and Abdollahi, A.**, Effect of hardness of plastic fat on structure and material properties of fish protein gels, *J. Food Sci.*, 46, 1755, 1981.
49. **Lee, C. M.**, Surimi process technology: mechanically deboned, washed and stabilized fish flesh is being increasingly used as a functional ingredient in fabricated seafood, *Food Technol.*, 11, 69, 1984.
50. **Suzuki, T.**, Kamaboko (fish cake), in *Fish and Krill Protein*, Applied Science Publishers, Barking, England, 1981, 89.
51. **Regenstein, J. M.**, The potential for minced fish, *Food Technol.*, 3, 101, 1986.
52. **Okada, M., Miyauchi, D., and Kudo, G.**, "Kamaboko" — the giant among Japanese processed fishery products, *Mar. Fish. Rev.*, 35, 1, 1973.
53. **Noguchi, S.**, Recent advances in utilizing and processing techniques in the Japanese fishery, Proc. 5th Int. Ocean Development Conference, Tokyo, Japan, Session, C2, 1978, 43.

54. **Limpus, L. G.**, FAO, Code of Practice for Minced Fish, FAO Fisheries Circular C700, Fish Production and Marketing Service Fishery Industries Division, Food and Agriculture Organization, Rome, 1977, 1.
55. **Watanabe, H.**, An estimation of energy input in the manufacture of fish meat paste product, *Bull. Jpn. Soc. Sci. Fish.*, 51, 1527, 1985.

Chapter 13

SANITATION IN MARINE FOOD INDUSTRY

Zenon M. Ganowiak

TABLE OF CONTENTS

I.	Objectives	212
II.	Sanitation Recommendations for Fishing Vessels	213
	A. Sanitary Design of Fishing Vessel and Facilities	213
	B. Equipment and Utensils Hygiene	213
	C. Handling the Catch on Board	213
	D. Unloading the Catch	214
III.	Hygienic Operation Requirements for Fresh Fish	214
	A. Hygienic Handling of Fish	214
	B. Hygiene of Raw Material Processing	214
IV.	Sanitation in Marine Food Manufacturing Plants	215
	A. Plant Construction and Sanitary Design	215
	B. Water Supply and Waste Disposal	216
	C. Equipment and Utensil Sanitation	217
	D. Personnel Hygiene and Food Handling Practices	217
V.	Fish and Shellfish Hygiene	218
	A. Health Hazards in Marine Fish Production	218
	B. Food-Borne Bacterial Diseases	219
	1. Marine Food Infections	219
	a. Salmonellosis	219
	b. Cholera	219
	c. *Vibrio parahaemolyticus*	219
	d. *Clostridium perfringens*	219
	2. Marine Food Intoxications	220
	a. Staphylococcal Food Poisoning	220
	b. Botulism	220
	3. Atypical Marine Food Infections	220
	C. Food-Borne Viral Diseases	220
	D. Food-Borne Parasitic Invasions	220
	1. Fish Parasites of Public Health Importance	221
	a. Anisakid Nematodes	221
	b. *Anisakis simplex*	221
	c. *Angiostrongylus cantonensis*	221
	d. *Capillaria philippinensis*	221
	e. *Diphyllobothrium latum*	221
	f. Trematodes	221
	2. Fish Parasites Not of Public Health Importance	222
	E. Biotoxins of Marine Fish and Shellfish	222
	1. Paralytic Shellfish Poisoning (PSP)	222

		2.	Ciguatera Poisoning..222
		3.	Tetraodon (Puffer Fish) Poisoning 223
		4.	Scombroid Fish Poisoning 223
	F.	\multicolumn{2}{l}{Special Marine Food Hygiene Problems in Developing Countries..223}
	G.	\multicolumn{2}{l}{Inspection Services ....224}
	H.	\multicolumn{2}{l}{FAO/WHO Standards and Codes of Practice for Fish and Marine Foods..224}

VI.	\multicolumn{3}{l}{Cleaning Facilities and Sanitizing Agents..224}
	A.	General Maintenance 224	
	B.	Cleaning in Marine Food Production 226	
	C.	Sanitizing Agents...227	
		1. Chlorine Compounds..227	
		2. Iodophors 228	
		3. Quaternary Ammonium Compounds 228	
		4. Steam or Hot Water 228	
	D.	Sanitary Control Program 229	

References..229

I. OBJECTIVES

Sanitation refers to all factors that relate to the contamination of marine foods, including the environment in which the marine organisms are caught, handling of the fresh raw product, and the cleanliness of the processing and storage facilities. The impact of sanitation depends upon the extent to which the people engaged in the fish industry will derive clear indications of how to improve the quality and public health safety of marine foods products. Sanitation measures adapted by the seafood industry are to be applied in accordance with the stage of the processing technology existing in each particular country. As processing becomes more complex, sanitation problems also increase in complexity, having always the following fundamental objectives:

1. To protect the public health from the risk of illness — whether it be from bacterial food poisoning, food-borne infections, or toxicity arising from either accumulation of toxic material from the environment or the use of naturally toxic marine organisms
2. To protect the wholesomeness of the product

Sanitation today is not merely the application of cleaning procedures; it is a constant and continuous task attached to the specific job of everyone from top management to any given employee within the plant. The modern meaning of sanitation encompasses practically every aspect of food production: preliminary aspect of sanitation on the vessel, plant layout, raw ingredients, processing techniques, processing equipment, packaging, storage conditions, cleaning procedures, microbiological testing, pollution control, sanitary inspection, personal habits, training, and attitudes, as well as management understanding and support.

The methods for achieving these objectives are usually the operations defined in codes of sanitary practices or good manufacturing practice/sanitation/GMP.[1]

II. SANITATION RECOMMENDATIONS FOR FISHING VESSELS

A. SANITARY DESIGN OF FISHING VESSEL AND FACILITIES

The fishing vessel should be designed for rapid and efficient handling of fish, ease of cleaning and disinfection, and should be of such material and construction as not to cause any damage or contamination to the catch. All surfaces with which the fish might come in contact should be of suitable corrosion-resistant material which is smooth and easily cleanable. Fish should be protected against exposure to high temperature and drying effects of sun and wind and handled so as not to cause contamination with bilge, water, sewage, smoke, fuel, oil, grease, or other objectionable substances.

If the vessel is engaged in processing of the fish, its design, layout, construction, and equipment should meet the requirements of shore establishments and the processing should be carried out under similar hygienic conditions.

It is most important to prevent water from carrying fish slime, blood, scales, and offal to parts of the vessel where effective cleaning is virtually impossible.

Proper drainage facilities are required to prevent a buildup of large quantities of melt water, blood, and slime. If drainage is inadequate, the bottom layers of the fish in the hold will be contaminated by the dirty liquid, especially during any periods of severe motion of the vessel.

There should be no sharp corners or projections in the hold or tank, as these will make cleaning difficult and may damage the fish. Contamination with fish slime, blood, scales, and guts will build up rapidly on surfaces in corners or around projections which are not smooth and impervious.

Only potable water or clean sea water should be used on fish and on surfaces with which fish might come in contact. If the fish is caught in polluted waters as occasionally happens, that water should not be used for washing fish or for preparation of refrigerated sea water or refrigerated brine or ice. Fish when alive are relatively resistant to a polluted environment but loses its natural defenses when it dies after being caught. All the plumbing and waste disposal lines servicing the vessel toilets, hand wash basins, or kitchen sinks should be large enough to carry peak loads, be watertight, and should not go through the fish holds where fish are being handled or stored.

B. EQUIPMENT AND UTENSILS HYGIENE

Fish handling, conveying, and storage equipment, used on board vessels, should be designed for rapid efficient handling of fish, be suitable for easy and thorough cleaning, and should be constructed so as not to cause contamination of the catch. In many areas wicker baskets are used for handling fish on deck. These are very difficult to clean properly, as slime, blood, scales, and small pieces of offal or parts of fish body become lodged within the framework. Containers with smooth, waterproof surfaces which are easy to clean and disinfect are recommended for handling fish on deck.

C. HANDLING THE CATCH ON BOARD

Before any fish come aboard, and between each haul, the gear, decks, boards, stanchions, and all other deck equipment which will come in contact with fish should be hosed down with clean seawater and brushed to remove all visible dirt, slime, and blood.

When fish are to be gutted, this should be done immediately after the fish are landed on deck. Where rapid gutting is not practicable whole fish should be washed and chilled as soon as it comes on deck. This helps to remove filth, particularly gut contents squeezed out of the fish in the net, and it helps to prevent excessive contamination during subsequent gutting and handling. Contamination of the catch by gutting offal can be prevented by dropping the guts into watertight containers. Fish should be thoroughly washed with clean seawater or potable water before being placed under refrigeration to remove all blood, slime, and pieces of gut. Harbor water which is always polluted in some way should never be used for washing fish.

D. UNLOADING THE CATCH

Unloading the fish from the vessel should be carried out in a careful hygienic manner and without delay. The use of hooks, shovels, forks, and other such implements for unloading the catch should be avoided in order that the fish suffer no damage. Tearing of the flesh reduces the value of the fish and accelerates spoilage. Care should be taken that fish are not damaged or contaminated during sorting, weighing, and transfer on shore in containers.

III. HYGIENIC OPERATION REQUIREMENTS FOR FRESH FISH

A. HYGIENIC HANDLING OF FISH

The fisherman should discard any fish that is diseased or is known to contain harmful substances, has undergone deterioration or any process of decomposition, or which has been contaminated with foreign matter to an extent which has made it unfit for human consumption. Poor handling of fresh fish on shore can ruin the best efforts of the fisherman. Fresh fish is often handled a number of times after it is landed, and the effects of bruising, contamination, or exposure to unduly high temperature will become apparent by the time the final product reaches the consumer.

B. HYGIENE OF RAW MATERIAL PROCESSING

Evisceration, filleting, and other operations in the handling of fish should be clean and hygienic. Precaution should be taken to protect the fish from contamination by rats, insects, birds, or chemical or microbiological contaminants during processing, handling, and storage.

Areas where fresh fish are received or stored should be so separated from areas in which final product preparation or packing is conducted as to prevent contamination of the finished product. Receiving and storage areas should be clean and readily capable of being maintained in a clean hygienic condition and should provide protection for the raw fish from deterioration and contamination.

All food contact surfaces should be smooth and free from pits, crevices, and loose scale, substances harmful to man. They should be unaffected by fish juices or other ingredients used and capable of withstanding repeated cleaning and disinfection. All work surfaces and containers, trays, tanks, or other equipment used for processing fish should be smooth, impervious, nontoxic material which is corrosion resistant and should be designed and constructed to prevent hygienic hazards and permit easy and thorough cleaning. In general the use of wood for this purpose is not recommended.

Fresh fish transport vehicles should be designed to allow adequate icing of fish to protect fish from warming up during transport and should be of such material and construction as to permit easy and thorough cleaning.

General sanitation in an establishment where fresh fish is processed for human consumption should be of the highest standard present in any food processing industry.

Fish, because of its highly perishable nature, requires strict adherence to specific hygienic requirements which should become a part of a daily operation routine of the plant.

All operation with fresh fish should be carried out in a manner and conditions suitable for the handling of food for human consumption.

IV. SANITATION IN MARINE FOOD MANUFACTURING PLANTS

A. PLANT CONSTRUCTION AND SANITARY DESIGN

The plant and surrounding area should be such as can be kept reasonably free from objectionable odors, smoke, dust, or other contamination. The buildings should be sufficient in size without crowding of equipment or personnel, well constructed, and kept in good repair. They should be of such design and construction as to protect against the entrance and harboring of insects, birds, or other vermin and to permit ready and adequate cleaning.

The location of a marine food processing establishment, its design, layout, construction, and equipment, should be planned in detail with considerable emphasis on the hygienic aspect, sanitary facilities, and quality control.

National or local sanitary authorities should always be consulted in regard to buildings codes, hygienic requirements of the operations, and sanitary disposal of sewage and plant waste. The food handling area should be completely separate from any part of the premises used as living quarters.

Buildings should preferably be constructed so that wet fish handling is carried out on the ground floor. This makes drainage easier and material handling can be assisted by simple conveyor systems, for example, to the cannery.

Floors should be hard surfaced, nonabsorbent, and adequately drained. They should be constructed of durable, waterproof, nontoxic, nonabsorbent material which is easy to clean and disinfect. They should be nonslippery and without crevices and should slope evenly and sufficiently for liquids to drain off to trapped outlets, fitted with a removable grill. If the floors are ribbed or grooved to facilitate traction, any grooving of this nature should always run towards the drainage channel. The junction between the floors and wells should be impervious to water and should be rounded for ease of cleaning. Concrete, if not properly finished, is porous and can be affected by oils, strong brines, weak ammonia, various detergents, and disinfectants. Concrete, if used, should be dense, of a good quality, and with a well-finished waterproof surface. Special treatments are available to prevent surface dust on concrete floors.

Damage to floors should be avoided by fitting trucks and trolleys with rubber wheels.

Walls should be smooth, waterproof, resistant to fracture, light colored, and readily cleanable. All sheeting joints should be sealed with a mastic or other compound resistant to hot water. Wall-to-wall and wall-to-floor junction should be rounded to facilitate cleaning. Pipes and cables should be sunk flush with the wall surface or neatly boxed in.

Windows should be filled with whole panes and those which open should be screened. The screens should be constructed so as to be easily removable for cleaning and should be made from suitable corrosion-resistant material. Insect-proof screens are required on all windows.

Doors through which fish or their products are moved should be sufficiently wide, well constructed of a suitable material, and should be of a self-closing type.

Both the doors and the frames of the doorways should have a smooth and readily cleanable surface.

Ceilings should be designed and constructed to prevent accumulation of dirt and condensation and should be easy to clean. In buildings where beams, trusses, pipes, or other elements are exposed, the fitting of a suspended ceiling just below is desirable to protect the fish products from falling debris, dust, or condensate.

The premises should be well ventilated to prevent excessive heat, condensation, and contamination with obnoxious odors, dust, vapor, or smoke. Special attention should be given to the venting of areas and equipment producing excessive heat, steam, obnoxious fumes, vapors, or contaminating aerosols. The air flow on the premises should be from the more hygienic areas to the less hygienic areas. Good ventilation is important to prevent condensation and growth of molds.

The light bulbs and fixtures suspended over the working areas where fish is handled should be of the safety type or otherwise protected to prevent food contamination in case of breakage. The by-products plant should be entirely separate from the plant for processing marine food for human consumption. Any processing of by-products not intended for human consumption should be conducted in separate buildings or in areas which are separated in such a way that there is no possibility for contamination of fish or seafood products.

B. WATER SUPPLY AND WASTE DISPOSAL

An ample supply of cold water should be available and an adequate supply of hot water of potable quality at a minimum temperature of 82°C should be available at all times during the plant operation. Standards of potability shall not be less than those contained in the International Standards for Drinking Water (World Health Organization, 1971). Ice should be made from water of potable quality and should be manufactured, handled, stored, and used so as to protect it from contamination.

All plumbing and waste disposal lines, including sewer systems, must be large enough to carry peak loads. All lines must be watertight and have adequate traps and vents. Disposal of waste should be effected in such a manner as not to permit contamination of potable water supplies. The plumbing and the manner of waste disposal should be approved by the official sanitary authority.

Adequate and convenient toilets should be provided and toilet areas should be equipped with self-closing doors. Toilet rooms should be well lit and ventilated and should not open directly into a food handling area. They should be kept in a sanitary condition at all times. There should be associated hand washing facilities within the toilet area and notices should be posted requiring personnel to wash hands after using the toilet.

The following formula could be used in assessing the adequacy of toilet facilities in relation to the number of employees:[2]

1—9 employees	1 toilet
10—24 employees	2 toilets
25—49 employees	3 toilets
50—100 employees	5 toilets
For every 30 employees over 100	1 toilet

Adequate and convenient facilities for employees to wash and dry their hands should be provided wherever the process demands. They should be in full view of the processing floor, and should be of type not requiring operation by hand or be fed by a continuous flow of potable water. Single-use towels are recommended, otherwise the method of drying hands should meet the requirements of the official agency having jurisdiction. The facilities should be kept in a hygienic condition at all the times. Machines and equipment should be so designed that they can be easily dismantled to facilitate thorough cleaning and disinfection. Containers used for handling fish should preferably be constructed of plastic or corrosion-resistant metal, and if of wood they should be treated to prevent the entry of moisture and coated with a durable, nontoxic paint or other surface coating that is smooth and readily washable. Wicker basket should not be used. Stationary equipment should be installed in such a manner as will permit easy access and thorough cleaning and disinfection. Fish-washing tanks should be designed to provide a constant change of water with good circulation, and to have provisions for drainage, and to be easily cleaned.

Equipment and utensils used for inedible or contaminated materials should be identified as such and should not be used for handling of fish and products intended for human consumption. Filleting boards and other surfaces on which fish are cut should be made of impervious materials which meet the physical requirements for cutting surfaces. Considerable microbial contamination of fillets and steaks is cuased by contact with the filleting and cutting boards. Wooden cutting surfaces are porous and quickly become water-logged. Being practically impossible to clean thoroughly, they are not recommended as suitable for this type of work.

Filleting and cutting boards should be frequently and thoroughly scrubbed and treated with disinfectant. Wherever practicable the boards should be continuously flushed with running potable water during use. The flushing water should contain 4 ppm of residual chlorine.[3]

It is recognized that the amount of microbial contamination on fillets and similar products is related to the amount of microbial contamination of the working surfaces. Clean surfaces become contaminated as soon as they are used, and consequently each fish that is filleted, after the first one, increases the surface contamination.

Filleting and cutting surfaces should therefore be cleaned during meal breaks and before resumption of production following other work stoppages. If they are not thoroughly scrubbed and disinfected, at least at the end of each working day, there may be a serious day-to-day carryover of microbial contamination. It has been proven that this contamination of both fillets and boards can be considerably reduced by continuous flushing with cold water. A further reduction in contamination has been observed when using chlorinated water for flushing.

Where it is desired and permissible to use dips, e.g., antioxidants or polyphosphates, the dangers of contamination must be fully appreciated. Microbial number will increase rapidly during use of these dips. This requires that the tanks be frequently and thoroughly cleaned and refilled with new solutions. The use of sprays instead of dips has been found to be a more efficient method for treatment of fillets or fish steaks. It eliminates an additional contamination with microorganisms, provides a continuously uniform solution strength, and lends itself to a better temperature control. No recirculations of the solution should be permitted, except if the solution is filtered, pasteurized, and cooled.

D. PERSONNEL HYGIENE AND FOOD HANDLING PRACTICES

All persons working in a marine food plant should maintain a high degree of personnel cleanliness while on duty and should take all necessary precautions to prevent the contamination of the fish, shellfish, or their products or ingredients with any foreign substance.

All employees should wear, appropriate to the nature of their work, clean, protective clothing including a head covering and footwear, all of which are either washable or disposable. The use of waterproof aprons where appropriate is recommended. Gloves used in the handling of fish should be maintained in a sound, clean, and sanitary condition and should be made of an impermeable material except where their usage would be incompatible with the work involved.

Hands should be washed thoroughly with soap or other cleansing agent and warm water before commencing work on every occasion after visiting a toilet before resuming work and whenever necessary. The wearing of gloves does not exempt the operator from having thoroughly washed hands.

Any behavior which can potentially contaminate the fish such as eating, smoking, chewing of tobacco or other materials, and spitting should be prohibited in any part of the fish handling areas.

No person who is known to be suffering from or who is a carrier of any communicable disease or has an infected wound or open lesion should be engaged in the preparation, handling, or transporting of fish or shellfish. Plant management should require that any

TABLE 1
Sources of Contamination, Infection, and Intoxication

Agents naturally present in aquatic habitats
    Ciguatera
    Paralytic shellfish poisoning
    Scombroid fish poisoning
    Vibrio parahaemolyticus gastroenteritis
    Vibrio cholerae non-01 gastroenteritis
    Vibrio vulnificus septicemia
    Botulism
Sewage pollution of aquatic habitats
    Typhoid fever
    Hepatitis non-B (A)
    Norwalk virus gastroenteritis
    Cholera
Workers, equipment, or environment of food processing or food service establishments
    Bacillus cereus gastroenteritis
    Clostridium perfringens enteritis
    Salmonellosis
    Shigellosis
    Staphylococcal food poisoning
    Streptococcus infections
Parasitic infections
    Diphyllobothriasis (human or animal feces)
    Anisakiasis (ingestion of infected fish)
    Some tropical diseases

Courtesy of F. L. Bryan, Elsevier, Amsterdam, 1987.

person afflicted with infected wounds, sores, or any illness, notably diarrhea, should immediately report to the management. The management should not allow any person known to be affected with a disease capable of being transmitted through food, or known to be a carrier of such a disease, or while afflicted with infected wounds, sores, or diarrhea to work in any area of a marine food factory in a capacity in which there is a likelihood of such a person contaminating fish or shellfish with pathogenic organisms.

Minor cuts and abrasions on the hands should be immediately treated and covered with a waterproof dressing of contrasting color and of a nature that it cannot be accidently detached; but if infection should occur subsequently, the worker should not be allowed to handle the fish. Adequate first aid facilities should be provided.

V. FISH AND SHELLFISH HYGIENE

A. HEALTH HAZARD IN MARINE FOOD PRODUCTION

The principal diseases transmitted to man by marine food are the bacterial infections. Bacterial infections constitute the largest proportion of fish- and shellfish-borne diseases. These infections are due either to direct contamination of the product by polluted water or to secondary contamination during landing, processing, storage, distribution, or preparation for consumption. Such contaminations are of particular importance when fish or shellfish are eaten raw or only lightly processed. According to Bryan[4] seafoods become contaminated, infectious, or toxigenic from one of four sources:

1. Agents naturally present in aquatic habitats
2. Sewage pollution of aquatic habitats
3. Workers, equipment, or other environment of food processing or foodservice establishments
4. Parasites (Table 1)

B. FOOD-BORNE BACTERIAL DISEASES

All food-borne diseases are classified as food infections or food intoxications. Although these classifications are somewhat arbitrary, food infections are those in which the bacteria present in the food at the time of eating grow in the host and cause disease. Food intoxications are those diseases in which bacteria grow in a food, producing a substance therein which is toxic in humans.

In the latter case, the bacteria grow in the food and in ordinary circumstances do not grow in the host; it is during the growth of the bacteria in the food that the poisonous substances or toxin are produced. The poisonous materials, in this case, are already present in the foods when they are eaten.

1. Marine Food Infections
a. Salmonellosis

There is a great risk of salmonella infection from fish and shellfish gathered in polluted water without adequate public health control and modern techniques of handling. Contaminations occur also through improper plant sanitation or more probably through improper personal sanitation of workers, who having had salmonellosis often become carriers of the organism for a period of time after the symptoms have gone. Such carriers excrete *Salmonella* bacteria in their faces. Carriers are a public health hazard because when they handle marine food during shucking, processing, or preparing transmit disease resulting from contaminated seafoods.

More than 1200 different serotypes of salmonella have been identified, and it is considered that all species are pathogenic to man.

b. Cholera

Although there is no evidence that contaminated fish cause cholera infection in man, epidemiological investigations have incriminated shellfish in outbreaks of the disease. Laboratory studies have indicated that *Vibrio* cholera persists in fish and shellfish at room temperature for 2 to 5 d and under refrigeration for 1 to 2 weeks.

c. Vibrio parahaemolyticus

It is recognized as a cause of fish-borne food poisoning and belongs to the marine pathogenic organisms almost exclusively associated with seafoods. *V. parahaemolyticus* is now believed to be responsible for over 50% of all cases of food-borne disease in Japan. The organisms have been isolated in marine waters, sediment, and fish and shellfish in various parts of the world; it is present in high numbers in warm water (so-called warm water bacterium). *V. parahaemolyticus* food poisoning seems to occur more often during warm weather, above 20°C, and to be closely associated with the consumption of raw, improperly cooked, or inadequately preserved seafood. The vibrio multiplies in marine foods more rapidly than do many other pathogenic organisms, but is usually reduced by freezing and heating. It rarely causes trouble in processed seafoods held at low temperatures. Good handling and processing will either eliminate the organism or prevent it from increasing to numbers which might be dangerous.

d. Clostridium perfringens

This organism reaches seafood from water, soil, mud, or through contact with surfaces of holds, containers, and equipment. *C. perfringens* has received more attention in recent years as a food-borne poisoning in which cooked fish dishes have been implicated. The control of *C. perfringens* poisoning would be relatively simple: the prompt application of temperatures below 4°C or above 54°C to foods after cooking which are not to be eaten immediately and the prompt application of temperatures below 4°C to foods left over from a meal.

2. Marine Food Intoxications

a. Staphylococcal Food Poisoning

A large number of foods have been incriminated in staphylococcal food poisoning outbreaks. Cooked seafoods belong to foods very often contaminated by workers, because the human is considered to be most important source of *Staphylococcus aureus* in food. Staphylococcal poisoning is a food intoxication in which the bacteria grow in the food and produce a very dangerous heat-stable toxin.

Of great importance in the prevention of outbreaks of Staphylococcal poisoning due to the ingestion of marine foods is the elimination of personnel from direct contact with foods when infections are present on their hands. This would include people with even small abrasions or wounds which are purulent or pussy.

b. Botulism

Clostridium botulinum type E spores are the most heat sensitive of the seven known types, and most outbreaks have been identified with raw or improperly processed seafoods such as fish or fish roe that has been fermented, smoked, or kept in vinegar. The organisms are of great public health importance because they can grow and produce toxins in fish without causing noticeable changes in its taste and odor. There are special types of *C. botulinum* spores that occur in small numbers on fish. However, these bacteria must grow and produce their special toxin before they are dangerous. They need the absence of both air and other competing bacteria to do this; therefore, most processing and holding procedures will stop their growth.

Only canned fish and some smoked fish offer any real hazard. Canning is designed to destroy *C. botulinum* and only gross error or mishandling should permit its growth. Inactivation of the toxin can be done by thorough heating of processed marine food just before serving.

3. Atypical Marine Food Infections

Fish and shellfish are implicated from time to time in outbreaks of food-borne illnesses due to microorganisms which are not typically fish bacteria, e.g., *Bacillus cereus*, Shigellosis, Streptococcal infections. In most cases this is not due to any special characteristic of the seafood but is caused by contamination and faulty handling in the restaurant or home.

Molluskan shellfish are an exception: they can and do accumulate undesirable bacteria from polluted water. Infectious hepatitis, salmonellosis, and dysentery have been caused in this way. Cholera and other enteric diseases have been disseminated by contaminated crabs as well as by bivalves.

C. FOOD-BORNE VIRAL DISEASES

Outbreaks of viral infections Non B-hepatitis (A) have occurred in Europe and parts of North America following the consumption of clams and oysters taken from seawater grossly contaminated with sewage; however, there is no evidence that viral hepatitis has been caused by shellfish taken from areas satisfying normal bacteriological standards. Norwalk and related viral gastroenteritis were also recently identified in Canada.[5,6] Raw clams were the usual vehicles. Contamination of clams were through human sewage from communities with no or inadequate sewage treatment facilities.

D. FOOD-BORNE PARASITIC INVASIONS

In areas where fish-borne helminths infecting man occur, the food habits of the people are the main factors in the incidence of helminthoses. Man becomes infected only if he ingests raw, insufficiently cooked or improperly processed fish.

The parasites of land animals are a major concern to health authorities but parasites of fish and shellfish are of minor importance because with few exceptions they cannot infect man. The only important problem is with *Anisakis* which can be picked up by eating raw or lightly cooked or pickled fish. Even moderate cooking will eliminate this hazard. The parasites are very sensitive to freezing.[7]

1. Fish Parasites of Public Health Importance
a. Anisakid nematodes

Within the family Anisakidae, species with the greatest potential for human infection are those that use fishes as either intermediate or paratenic hosts and warm-blooded vertebrates, usually marine mammals as final hosts. In the marine environment these include the species:[8] *Anisakis simplex, Pseudoterranova decipiens,* and *Phocascaris-Contracaecum* sp. These species use crustacean intermediate hosts and occur in fish as larvae that can infect the final host. *Hysterothylacium aduncum* has a similar life cycle except that fish host both larval and adult nematodes.

b. Anisakis simplex

A. simplex larvae occur in many marine fish. The most commonly reported source of infection in man is slightly salted raw herring. There is no obvious reaction in man when the first larvae migrate from the gut into the abdominal cavity, but the subsequent penetration of other larvae at the same site induces a severe allergic reaction as a result of the previous sensitization.

Anisakid larvae die at temperatures about 60°C. When raw or lightly marinated fish are prepared, it is best to freeze the fish first. Anisakid larvae are killed if held between -17 and $-20°C$ for 24 h, but are resistant to most curing and marinating and to a wide variety of chemicals, spices, and food additives.

As an effective prevention of invasion only deep-frozen fish should be used in recipes for various raw fish dishes.

c. Angiostrongylus cantonensis

It is a common nematode parasite of the lungs of rats in the Pacific Islands and Southeast Asia and causes eosinophilic meningitis in man. Although its usual intermediate host is a slug or land snail, the larvae pass through a paratenic host, e.g., freshwater prawn, land crab, and bonito, from which man is infected.

d. Capillaria philippinensis

C. philippinensis has been recognized as causing a syndrome in man called intestinal capillariasis, characterized by intractable diarrhea with malabsorption due to atrophic changes in the intestinal epithelium. The infection is believed to be caused by eating raw freshwater fish containing eggs of the nematode parasite. An unusual feature is that all stages of the parasite are found in the infected person; autoinfection is therefore possible.

e. Diphyllobothrium latum

The parasite has two types of intermediate host: copepods and fish. In man the plerocercoids develop into the adult tapeworms that generally cause debility and anemia. Plerocercoids of species other than *Diphyllobothrium* cannot mature into the adult tapeworm in man but migrate into skin or subcutaneaus tissues, causing the condition known as sparganosis. Methods that kill anisakid nematodes will also kill larval diphyllobothrid cestodes — therefore, both tapeworm and nematode infections are prevented by the same safety measures.

f. Trematodes

Over 40 species of trematodes belonging to 11 genera share the following epidemiological characteristics: their first intermediate hosts are mollusks, their second hosts are fish or crustaceans, and their final hosts are humans or animals eating raw fish. In man, many of these trematodes (fluke) parasitize the bile ducts, liver, and intestine. Others, such as Paragonimus, may invade the lungs or ectopic sites including the brain and heart.

The so-called salmon-poisoning fluke, is a trematode of fish-eating carnivores, known to infect people in the U.S.S.R. and U.S. Salmon are among the most commonly infected fishes and metacercariae remain viable through the marine phase of the salmon life cycle. Since metacercariae locate in virtually any fish tissue, ingestion of raw salmon flesh could lead to infection. The enzootic area as defined by the distribution of the snail host includes Washington, Oregon, and northern California.

2. Fish Parasites Not of Public Health Importance

One aspect of macroscopic parasites in marine fishes other than the human health concern is aesthetic. There are parasites that may affect the quality of marine fish flesh, but not the safety from a public health standpoint — they do not constitute a public health hazard.[9]

Myxosporidian protozoans may be common in some fish stocks, e.g., Pacific hake (*Merluccius productus* and blue whiting) and *Micromesistius poutassou*.

The parasites have characteristic spores and they often occur in marine fish tissue within cysts that are readily visible. *Myxosporidia* (genus *Kudoa*) are of major economic importance because they cause large, unsightly cysts that may render the fish flesh unmarketable.[10]

Another parasite group that occurs in the flesh of commercially important marine flesh is the Microspora. In fish, these protozoans usually occur within whitish, elongated cyst-like structures termed Xenomas that may be macroscopic.

E. BIOTOXINS OF MARINE FISH AND SHELLFISH

Only a small proportion of fish and shellfish species used for human consumption contain biotoxins of significance to man.

1. Paralytic Shellfish Poisoning (PSP)

The most common organisms associated with PSP are *Gonyaulax cantanella*, *G. tamarensis*, and *Gymnodinium brevis*. All are widely distributed, but PSP occurs only when relatively large numbers are present.

Edible filter-feeding mollusks, e.g., mussels, clams, and oysters, are the main source of the toxin for man. The buildup of the toxin in mollusks can occur in a few days, but its natural elimination may take several weeks. In small doses the toxin causes a tingling sensation of the mouth and lips; larger doses of toxin produced by certain marine dinoflagellates may cause severe neurotoxicity, collapse, paralysis, and death. There is no known antidote. There are 18 known naturally occurring PSP-toxins[11] (STX, saxitoxin; NEO, neosaxitoxin; and GTX, gonyautoxin). Usual cooking methods do not destroy paralytic shellfish-poisoning toxins.

In several areas where the population of toxic species of dinoflagellates develop annually, commercial shellfish species are routinely monitored for their toxic content.

Gathering them is prohibited when the concentration of the toxin exceeds the accepted level. Biological monitoring of the plankton is not a practicable way of assessing risk, since toxic plankton occurs only sporadically and shellfish remain toxic long after it has disappeared.

Other groups of invertebrates such as cephalopods (squid), abalone, crabs, and lobster may become toxic, but intoxication in man following their consumption is not connected with PSP — it is generally local and sporadic and does not require public health control measures.

2. Ciguatera Poisoning

It is a neurological disease acquired from contamination of seafoods by agents naturally present in aquatic habitats. The dinoflagellate *Gambierdiscus toxicus* is one source of ciguatoxin for the fish. Over 400 species of tropical fish, including snapper (Lutjanidae) and grouper (Serranidae) have been identified as sources of probably the most widespread form of intoxication from fish. The precise cause is unknown; food fish may suddenly become toxic and remain so for years. The toxin is heat stable. Symptoms of the poisoning include mild paralysis and gastrointestinal disturbances; in extreme cases, death occurs. Due to the lack of knowledge about the toxin and to its sporadic production, public health measures are not generally applicable.

3. Tetraodon (Puffer Fish) Poisoning

Puffer fish, mainly of the genus *Fugu* from the tropical regions of the Pacific, Atlantic, and Indian Oceans, are used as food after removal of the gonads and liver, which contain toxin in amounts varying according to the season. The toxin, which is heat stable, causes serious disease with a high mortality rate. Control is possible through public health measures to ensure that toxic organs are removed before the fish are used for food.

4. Scombroid Fish Poisoning

Scombroid fish poisoning is caused by ingestion of poorly cooled fish that have naturally high concentration of free histidine in their flesh. Tuna, bonito, mackerel, herring, sardines, and related fish species have been reported to become toxic following bacterial decomposition of histidine into histamine.

The toxin is heat stable and a variety of symptoms can be encountered including gastrointestinal (nausea, vomiting, diarrhea, abdominal cramps), cutaneous (rash, urticaria, edema), hemodynamic (hypotension), and neurological (flushing, itching, burning, tingling headache) symptoms.[12] Since histamine poisoning is an intoxication, the symptoms usually appear within minutes after eating the fish. A scombroid poisoning can occur when fish cooled too slowly after capture are eaten either fresh, frozen, or canned. Spreekens[13] noted that some psychrophilic bacteria are responsible for histamine production in mackerel exposed to temperature abuse due to delayed cooling on board and or during processing. She stated that also minor quantities of histamine in raw, basic material containing free histidine may be indicative of questionable safe quality.

F. SPECIAL MARINE FOOD HYGIENE PROBLEMS IN DEVELOPING COUNTRIES

Developing countries often have a climate that makes the handling and preservation of fish and shellfish difficult. Frequently there is a dearth of trained personnel and of resources, e.g., transport, electricity, water, salt, and ice. More important, there may be a lack of awareness of health hazards of modern sanitary practices. Many infections, occasionally of epidemic character, have arisen from inadequate handling or have been associated with fish and shellfish taken from polluted areas.

Other incidents have resulted from the practice common in some countries of consuming raw, partially cooked, slightly salted, or not efficiently smoked fish.

In many developing countries the production and consumption of molluskan shellfish are considerably high but the cleansing techniques such as relaying and purification are little known. Polluted shellfish may be made safe for human consumption by heat treatment, e.g., boiling, steaming, and canning.

Where mollusks are to be marketed in the raw state, removal of fecal organisms can be achieved either by relaying the shellfish on the seabed in areas where the seawater is unpolluted or by holding the shellfish in basins or tanks under conditions allowing the polluting bacteria or viruses to be removed naturally — a process known as purification or depuration.

In practice, most purification plants are situated in polluted areas, and the seawater used for purification is treated with chlorine, ozone, or UV light to remove fecal contamination. Such plants should be installed and operated under public health control.

A proposal to improve fish and shellfish hygiene must take into account the local economic and social background and the dietary habits of the consumers. Minimum sanitary requirements and education in this field of the public and of all personnel in the marine food industry are of prime importance.

Perhaps the most important single measure for improving fish and shellfish hygiene is the introduction or extension of refrigeration facilities or the use of ice, especially on board fishing vessels.

G. INSPECTION SERVICES

Many countries still do not have a specific program of sanitary inspection for fish and shellfish. Such programs aim at assuring to the consumer a safe, wholesome, and acceptable product. They are important in gaining the consumer's confidence, particularly in international trade, and they can help to prevent or lessen the effects of outbreaks of fish and shellfish-borne disease (Table 2).

A fish inspection program is most likely to succeed if it is developed as a cooperative effort between the government and the fishing industry authorities.

H. FAO/WHO STANDARDS AND CODES OF PRACTICE FOR FISH AND MARINE FOODS

The Joint Food and Agriculture Organization and World Health Organization (FAO/WHO) Food Standards Programme operates chiefly through the Codex Alimentarius Commission and its Executive Committee. The purpose of the commission, which is an intergovernmental body, is to protect consumers against health hazards in food and against fraud, to ensure fair practices in the food trade, and to facilitate international trade in foods.

One of the commission commodity committees is the Codex Committee on Fish and Fishery Products which has elaborated on the Standards and Codes of Practice to encourage good manufacturing practice (GMP) for a wide range of marine food products. As of 1988, 13 Final Codex Standards and 12 Recommended International Codes of Hygienic and Technological Practice have been established.

VI. CLEANING FACILITIES AND SANITIZING AGENTS

A. GENERAL MAINTENANCE

The cleaning operation shall be conducted in such a manner as to minimize the danger of contamination of marine food and food-contact surfaces. Detergents, sanitizers, disinfectants, and other supplies employed in cleaning and sanitizing procedures shall be free of significant microbiological contamination and shall be safe and effective for their intended uses. Clean and hygienic conditions are important for three reasons:

1. To prevent the risk of food poisoning
2. To assure the public that food is free from spoilage and prepared in clean surroundings by properly trained and supervised people
3. To ensure food is palatable and nutritious as well as safe

The producer can maintain bacterial hygiene only by cleaning the plant and equipment. There are several cleaning schedules open to use:

- End-of-production cleandown (EPC), which constitutes thorough cleaning and sanitizing of all plant equipment in the processing area

TABLE 2
Factors that Contribute to Seafood-Borne Diseases which Relate to Critical Control Points and Monitoring Procedure

Factors	Temperature	Time	Volume	pH	a_w	Hand washing	Handling procedures	Personal hygiene	Illnesses of worker	Surface cleanliness	Chlorine level	Construction, repair	Source	Sewage disposal	Ingredients, salt, NO_2	Dry storage practices
Eating toxic fish	x	x											x			
Eating raw fish	x	x											x	x		
Heat-process failure	x	x	x	o	o											
Handling after heating																
Gross contamination raw-cooked						x	x			x					o	
Bare hand contact						x	x	x								
Equipment surfaces							x	x	x	x	x					
Cooling water											x					
Sharp, rough surfaces												x				
Improper cooling	o															
Room/outside	x	x														
Large masses	o	o	x													
Improper cleaning	x	x		o						x	o					
Improper fermentation				x												
Inadequate acidification				x												
Improper drying	o	x			x											
Improper use/storage of chemicals							o								x	
Lapse of one or more days between preparation and ingestion	x	x														x

Note: x, essential operation to monitor and o, possible operation to monitor.

Courtesy of F.L. Bryan, Elsevier, Amsterdam, 1987.

TABLE 3
Types of Dirt Encountered in the Food Industry, Recommended Techniques, and the Degree of Cleanliness Achieved

Type of dirt	Technique	Cleanliness achieved
Fat	Remove with water 50°C and mechanical action, high pressure, steam jet, manual; emulsify with added cleaning agent	Sensorily clean
Protein		
Not dried on	Remove with water, manually or mechanically	Sensorily clean
Dried on	Soften — remove with mechanical force, high pressure, steam jet, manually	Adhesive layer often left behind
Dried on and burnt in	Soften — remove with mechanical force, high pressure, steam jet, manually	Crusts, coatings and adhesive layer often left behind

Courtesy of Schmidt, U., *Fleischwirtschaft*, 1983.

- Preproduction hygiene (PPH) involves inspection of the result of the EPC and may involve some sanitizing procedures prior to start of work
- Production hygiene, which embraces any cleandown procedures carried out during the work period and ranges from removal of debris, guts, etc., to periodic cleaning and sanitizing of equipment

The enlightened producer carries out all three cleaning schedules; although providing the EPC is effective, the PPH stage will usually not be necessary.

B. CLEANING IN MARINE FOOD PRODUCTION

Cleaning means the removal of objectionable matter from the surface. The plant is physically clean when all dirt, slime, blood, gurry, oil, and grease are removed from a solid surface. During cleaning procedures there will be a reduction in the bacterial numbers contaminating the surface; efficient cleaning means minimum one decimal reduction of the initial bacterial population.

Cleanliness is a visible attribute, so that inefficient cleaning is easily apparent during an inspection. Cleaning is made more effective by the use of a detergent which functions by facilitating the removal of dirt from a soiled surface. However, it is the cleaning technique and not the cleaning agent (detergent) that determines success in cleaning food processing plants. Treating with brushes and scrubbers is the most reliable method of cleaning dirty surfaces. Dirt is best removed with hot water (40 to 60°C) either mechanically or by using water pressure (30 to 60 bar). Dirt that will not be touched by mechanical cleaning methods can be removed in this way (Table 3).

The detergent as a cleaning agent is only one factor among many and should be neither overestimated nor underestimated. The detergents are necessary not so much to improve removal of dirt but to emulsify the fat which would otherwise be redeposited on the surface once the temperature of the water fell to below the melting point of the fat.

Modern synthetic detergents are produced from petroleum-derived, unsaturated hydrocarbons and sulfuric acid. Unlike soap, which are salts of fatty acids, they are efficient in hard or soft water and form no scum. A neutral detergent is suitable for most purposes, but care is needed to select one with the right formulation for the job in hand.

For equipment cleaning, hot freshly prepared solution should be used containing an accurately measured quantity of detergent. A good detergent has wetting ability, dissolves and emulsifies food debris, prevents scale formation, is easily rinsed, but at the same time does not promote adhesive surface.

TABLE 4
Relative Comparative Properties of Selected Chemical Sanitizing Agents

	Relative effectiveness		
	Chlorine	iodine	Quaternary ammonium
Gram + bacteria	Second in effectiveness	Most effective	Third in effectiveness
Gram − bacteria	Most effective	Second in effectiveness	Poor
Spores	Most effective	Second in effectiveness	Least effective
Thermoduric organisms	Second in effectiveness	Least effective	Most effective
Bacteriophage	Most effective	Second in effectiveness	Not effective
Affected by hard water	Second	Least	Most
Corrosiveness	Most corrosive	Slightly corrosive	Noncorrosive
Cause of off-flavors	+ (10 ppm)	+ + (7 ppm)	± (15 ppm)
Affected by organic matter	Most	Second	Least

Courtesy of Guthrie, R., Van Nostrand Reinhold, 1972.

The detergents fell into three main categories: alkaline, neutral, and acid. For the removal of fish slime, blood, scales, and dried and hardened fish residues from aluminum or stainless steel equipment, alkaline detergents are most often recommended. When used according to the instructions of the manufacturer, these detergents are noncorrosive to most metals and do not constitute a hazard to operatives using them.

After cleaning thorough drying is essential. Wet surfaces stimulate bacterial growth, dry surfaces discourage it.

C. SANITIZING AGENTS

A sanitizer is defined as an agent that reduces the number of bacterial contaminants to safe levels as may be judged by public health requirements. To be effective a detergent-sanitizer must possess excellent cleaning power because the sanitizing agents cannot kill organisms protected by layers of soil.

The sanitizer (disinfectant) effectiveness should result in multiplicated decimal (99.999%) reduction in the number of bacteria remaining on a surface which has been cleaned. The success of disinfection depends first on the efficiency of the cleaning that has preceded it, on the material and the nature of its surface, on the efficiency of the sanitizer, and on the technique applied. Sanitation is an invisible attribute and although a surface may appear clean it may harbor large numbers of bacteria and for this reason many types of chemical sanitizers are used.[14]

Sanitizing agents (compounds) approved for use in food processing plants fall into the following categories: chlorine compounds, iodophores, quaternary ammonium compounds, and steam or hot water (Table 4).

1. Chlorine Compounds

These are probably the most commonly used sanitizers in the marine food industry.

The use of chlorine prevents or greatly reduces the accumulation of microbial slimes on equipment that is continuously or frequently washed with chlorinated water. It also prevents the development of off-odors from fermentation decay. The use of chlorine permits longer time for technology operation by reducing the time for cleanup. The total bacterial counts of finished products are reduced when raw products are washed in chlorinated water. Chlorine compounds are useful in preventing spoilage and increasing shelf life of food.

Hypochlorite dissolved in water to give a chlorine level of 200 to 300 μg/g is a cheap and effective way of sanitizing plant and equipment which has been thoroughly cleaned. However, it is inactivated by organic material, and since it is mildly corrosive it must be thoroughly rinsed away after a contact of 15 to 20 min.

As a sanitizing agent the following suggested concentration of chlorine solutions in fish processing plants are advised:

Use	Available chlorine ($\mu g/g$)
Wash water	2—10
Rinse water on hands	50—100
Clean smooth surface (wash basin, urinals, glassware)	50—300
Clean smooth wood, metal or synthetic surfaces (new boxes, new table tops, conveyor belts, machines)	300—500
Rough surfaces (worn tables, old boxes, concrete floors, and walls)	1000—5000

Chlorination systems should not be relied upon to solve all sanitation problems. The indiscriminate use of chlorine cannot compensate for unsanitary conditions in a processing plant.

2. Iodophores

Iodophors are complexed iodine sanitizers. In complexing these sanitizers iodine is dissolved in synthetic detergents. This reduces the toxicity which causes skin irritation, staining, and odor found in other types of iodine solutions. The amber color of the solution is an index of germicidal power. The solution works effectively as a sanitizer as long as the color lasts. Iodophors are particularly suitable for hand dips and for partially porous surfaces:

Use	Available iodine ($\mu g/g$)
Hand dip	8—12
Smooth surfaces	8—35
Rough surfaces	125—200
Equipment and utensils	12—20

3. Quaternary Ammonium Compounds

These compounds come in many forms and in a wide variety of commercial products. They are less versatile than chlorine, but are better wetting agents and since they do not evaporate they provide a residual germicidal action. They are particularly effective in controlling mold growth on walls and ceilings of coolers. The major disadvantage of the compounds is that they leave a residual film. This residue must be removed from food processing surfaces before they are used.

There are many forms of these compounds. The label should be consulted for the recommended solution strength. Several generally suggested concentrates of quaternary ammonium compounds are

Use	Strength ($\mu g/g$)
Cooler walls and ceilings	500—800
Hand dips	50
Equipment	200

4. Steam or Hot Water

During cleaning with steam jet equipment and high-pressure hot water up to a temperature of 140°C and with or without a cleaning agent is sprayed onto the dirty surfaces under a pressure of 20 to 70 bar, using 350 to 1200 l of water per hour. Cleaning will only be efficient if temperature, pressure, application time, and amount of water used are so adjusted that the energy applied to the surface is sufficient to release and rinse off the dirt. The best cleaning effect on fatty dirt is achieved when the water is heated to 120°C and hits the dirt in the form of moist steam, achieved by mixing in cold water and in a fan-shaped jet. At temperatures below 100°C the distance between nozzle and surface should be between 5 and 20 cm if the surface is to be optically clean, but where the temperatures are above 100°C it is possible to have distances of 40 to 70 cm and to use less water and complete the work more quickly.[15]

To dissolve the fat that is always present with protein all that is needed is a temperature above the melting point of the fat, as with all other kinds of proteinaceous dirt, and a certain mechanical factor, whether applied manually or via water pressure.

D. SANITARY CONTROL PROGRAM

It is desirable that each fish processing plant in its own interest designates a single individual whose duties are preferably divorced from production to be held responsible for the cleanliness of the establishment. Such a person or his staff should be a permanent part of the organization or employed by the organization and should be well trained in the use of special cleaning tools, methods of dismantling equipment for cleaning, and in the significance of contamination and the hazards involved. A permanent cleaning and disinfection schedule should be drawn up to ensure that all parts of the establishment are cleaned appropriately and that critical areas, equipment, and material are designated for cleaning and or disinfection daily or more frequently if required.

More recently greater concern has been evidenced with the application of the hazard analysis critical control point (HACCP) system.[16] In this system cleaning and sanitation belongs to crucial factors which can provide a high degree of insurance for prevention and control of seafood-transmitted infections and intoxication. The components of the HACCP system are

- To determine hazards and assess severity and risks
- To identify critical control points
- To establish control measures and criteria
- To monitor critical control points
- To take action whenever the results of monitoring indicate that the process is out of control

REFERENCES

1. Current Good Manufacturing Practice (CGMP) Regulations, Code of Federal Regulation, Title 21, Parts 100 to 169, U.S. Government Printing Office, Washington, D.C., 1985.
2. **Doyle, J. P.**, Fish Plant Sanitation and Cleaning Procedures, University of Alaska, Sea Grant GH-83-6.6B, 1983.
3. **Cheng, J. W., Cook, D. W., and Kirk, J. R.**, Use of chlorine compounds in the food industry, *Food Technol.*, 39, 107, 1985.
4. **Bryan, F. L.**, Seafood-transmitted infections and intoxications in recent years, in *Seafood Quality Determination*, Kramer, D. E. and Liston, J., Eds., Elsevier, Amsterdam, 1987, 319.
5. **Morse, D. L. and Guzewich, J. J.**, Widespread outbreaks of clam and oyster associated gastroenteritis: role of Norwalk virus, *N. Engl. J. Med.*, 314, 678, 1986.
6. **Guzewich, J. J. and Morse, D. L.**, Sources of shellfish in outbreaks of probable viral gastroenteritis, *J. Food Prot.*, 49, 389, 1986.
7. **Myers, B. J.**, Anisakine nematodes in fresh commercial fish from waters along the Washington, Oregon and California coasts, *J. Food Prot.*, 42, 380, 1979.
8. **Olson, R. E.**, Marine fish parasites of public health importance, in *Seafood Quality Determination*, Kramer, D. E. and Liston, J., Eds., Elsevier, Amsterdam, 1987, 339.

9. **Kabata, Z. and Whitaker, D. J.,** Two species of Kudoa (*Myxosporea: Multivalvulida*) parasitic in the flesh of *Merluccius productus* in the Canadian Pacific, *Can. J. Zool.,* 59, 2085, 1981.
10. **Ganowiak, Z. M.,** Biological, histochemical and biochemical investigation on rats fed fish meat infested with parasitic protozoa (*Kudoa* sp.), *Acta Vet.,* 35, 245, 1985.
11. **Sullivan, J. J. and Wekell, M. M.,** The application of high performance liquid chromatography in a paralytic shellfish poisoning monitoring program, in *Seafood Quality Determination,* Kramer, D. E. and Liston, J., Eds., Elsevier, Amsterdam, 1987, 357.
12. **Taylor, S. L. and Summer, S. S.,** Determination of histamine, putrescine and cadaverine, in *Seafood Quality Determination,* Kramer, D. E. and Liston, J., Eds., Elsevier, Amsterdam, 1987, 235.
13. **Van Spreekens, K. J. A.,** Histamine production by the psychrophilic flora, in *Seafood Quality Determination,* Kramer, D. E. and Liston, J., Eds., Elsevier, Amsterdam, 1987, 309.
14. **Guthrie, R. E.,** *Food Sanitation,* Avi Publishing, Westport, CT, 1972, 158.
15. **Schmidt, U.,** Cleaning and disinfection of slaughterhouses and meat processing factories, *Fleischwirtschaft,* 63, 1188, 1983.
16. World Health Organization International Commission on Microbiological Specifications for Foods, Report on the WHO/ICMSF Meeting on Hazards Analysis: Critical Control Point System in Food Hygiene, VPH-82-37, World Health Organization, Geneva, 1982.

INDEX

A

Abalone, 21, 23
  chemical composition, 33
  collagen sugars, 40
  myofibrillar proteins, 38
  toxins, 222
Abductin, 40
Accelerated freeze drying (AFD), 130
Acceptability, 2
Acetic acid, marinades, 159, see also Marinades
Achromobacter, 66
Acinetobacter, 66, 67, 103, 105
Actinin, postharvest changes, 64
Actomyosin
  minced-type product, gel formation, 201—202
  protein composition, 38
  rigor mortis and, 61
Additives, minced-type products, 202—204, 207
Aeromonas, 66
Aeromonas hydrophila, 66
AFD, see Accelerated freeze drying
Aflatoxins, 136
Age, see Maturity; Reproduction
Agrowaste as drying fuel, 127—129
Air-blast freezers, 120
Alaska pollock, see also Pollock
  freezing, 117
  minced-type products, 201, 203—205
Albacore, 36, 47
Alcaligenes, 66
Alcohols
  fish protein concentrate preparation, 140, 141
  flavor and, 46—47
  lipid oxidation products, 117
  odor and, 69
Aldehydes
  flavor and, 46—47
  freezing and, 114
  lipid oxidation products, 117
  odor and, 69
Algae, 13—14, 42
Alginate, 121, 203
Alimentary tract, see Digestive tract
Alteromonas, 66, 67, 103, 104
Amines, see also Nitrogenous compounds; Histamine; Polyamines
  canning and, 196
  diamines, 71—72, 139
  dried fish quality, 139
Amino acids, 34—35
  abductin, 40
  dried fish quality, 139
  flavor and, 44—45
  minced-type product cryoprotectants, 204
  postharvest changes, 63—64
    bacterial activity and, 67
    freshness assessment, 71—72
    odor and, 69

salted products, ripening, 151, 152
Ammonia, 70, 102, 196
Ammonium bases, flavor and, 45—46, see also Quaternary ammonium compounds
Anchovy, 19
  chemical composition, 33
  protein quality, 36
  resource limitations, 27
  storage life, 97
Angiostrongylus cantonensis, 221
Anisakids, 218, 221
Anserine, 45
Antarctic krill, see Krill
Antarctic species, see Arctic/Anarctic species
Antibiotics, 101
Antioxidants, 139, 168
Aquaculture, 2, 6, 42
Arachidonic acid, 42, 43
Arctic/Antarctic species
  fluoride in, 52
  lipid composition, 42
  microflora, species of, 66
  protein composition, 36—37
Arginine, octopine and, 45
Aroma, see Odor; Sensory qualities
Arrhenius equation, 133
Arthrobacter, 66
Aseptic canning, 190
Aspergillus flavus, 136
Atka mackerel, 204, 205, see also Mackerel
ATP
  flavor and, 45
  postharvest changes, 56—57, 59
  rigor mortis and, 61
ATPase, 37, 202
Autolysis, 66—67, 98, 134
Autooxidation, 114, 117, see also Lipid oxidation

B

Bacillus species, 182
Bacillus cereus, 218
Bacillus stearothermophilus, 182
Bacillus subtilis, 105, 183
Bacteria, see Microorganisms
Bacterial diseases, 218—220
Balenine, 45
Ball's formula method, 189—190
Bass, 27
Beetles, 136, 137
Belly burst, 64
Benthic habitat, 9, 10
Benthic species, 11, 12, 65
Benzoic acid
  marinades, 157, 159, 161
  radiation vs., 107
  salted product, 154
Betabacterium buchneri, 157
BET isotherm, 131

Bicarbonate, 206
Biochemical changes, see Lipids; Postharvest changes; Proteins
Biology, 17—18
Bismarck herring, 159
Bisulfites, 102, 200
Black marlin, 37
Blanching, 159
Bleach, sanitizing with, 227—228
Bleaching, product, 101
Bleeding
  dried fish quality, 138
  shelf life of frozen product and, 120
Blood
  general biology, 18
  on-board processing, 95
Blowfly, 136
Bluefin, chilling, 98
Boats, see Fishing vessels
Body temperature, see Temperature, body
Bone/boning, 17
  cutting, 90
  filleting, see Filleting
  fish protein concentrate preparation, 140
  fluoride in, 52
  for marinades, 158
  minced-type products, 207
  mineral content and, 49
Bonito, 137
  families of commercial importance, 20
  parasites, 221
  postharvest changes, 64
  resource limitations, 27
  scombroid fish poisoning, 223
Bothidae, 20
Bottom deposits, 9, 10
Botulinus toxin, 66, 218, 220
  ionizing radiation effects, 105, 106
  modified atmospheres and, 103
  preservatives and, 102
Brain destruction, rigor mortis and, 62
Bream, 19, 97
Brine freezing, 120
Brining
  chilling in brine, 99—101
  composition of cover brine, 162
  dried product, insect spoilage and, 136
  before drying, 126, 127
  marinades, fried, 160
Buoyancy, lipids and, 41
Butterfly herring, 159
B vitamins, 47, 48, 196, 197, see also Vitamins

C

Cadaverine, 71—72, 139
Calcium, 49, 151
Calcium-ATPase, 38, 202
Callinectes sapidus, 33, see also Crab
Campylobacter, 67
Candida, 66
Canning
  botulism and, 220
  changes during heat sterilization, 195—197
  collagen and, 39
  families of commercial importance, 19, 20
  heat sterilization, principles of, 182—191
    microorganisms, 182—186
    process calculations, 186—190
    processing methods, 190—191
  production flow diagram, 192
  technology, 191—195
    production, 194—195
    unit operations, 191—194
Capelin, 64, 83
Capillaria philippinensis, 221
Carangidae, 19
Carbohydrates
  collagen sugars, 40
  gross chemical composition, 31—32
  minced-type product, 203, 204
  postharvest changes, 56—60
  sarcoplasmic enzymes, 37
Carbon dioxide
  marine habitat, 12
  smoke, 166
Carbon dioxide-enriched atmosphere storage, 103—104
Carbon monoxide, smoke, 166
Carboxylic acids
  marinades, see Marinades
  minced-type product cryoprotectants, 204
  postharvest changes, 59
  smoke, 170
  smoke flavorings, 171
Carboxymethylcellulose, 203
Carcinogens, smoked product, 165, 169, 177
Carnosine, 45
Carotenoids, postharvest changes, 68
Carp
  aquaculture, 2
  collagen sugars, 40
  connectin, 38—39
  minced-type products, 205
Carrageenan, 203
Castor oil fish, 41
Catfish, 2, 136
Cathepsins, 37, 38, 64
Caviar, 155
Cephalopods, see Octopus; Squid
Certification, 2
Cestodes, 221
Chemical changes
  drying and, 133—134
  freezing and, 112—114
  salting and, 149—151
  shelf life of frozen product and, 120
Chemical composition, 31—33
  minced-type products, 200—202
  smoke, 164—166

Chemical evaluation, 3, 138—139
Chemical methods, fish protein concentrate preparation, 141
Chikuwa, 201
Chilled sea water, 98—100
Chilling
  bacterial growth and, 67
  effects of, 94
  on-board, 94—100
    handling and processing, 94—95
    in ice, 95—98
    at subzero temperatures, 98—101
  rigor mortis and, 62
  shelf-life extension, 101—107
    modified atmospheres, 102—104
    preservatives, 101—102
    radiation, ionizing, 105—107
Chilling time, salted product, 154
Chioniectes, 16
Chlorine, 49
Chlorine-based sanitizing agents, 225, 227—228
Chlorpyriphos-methyl, 137
Cholera, 218, 219
Cholesterol, 65
Chromoproteins, 32, 36, 37
Chrosophrys auratus, 66
Chub, 174
Ciguatera poisoning, 218, 223
Clams
  canning, 195
  chemical composition, 33
  mineral content, 49
  protein quality, 36
  resource limitations, 27
  species of commercial importance, 14
  toxins, 222
  vitamin content, 48
Classification, gross chemical composition and, 32—33
Clostridium, 66, 182
Clostridium botulinum
  botulism, 220
  canning and, 182, 183, 186
  ionizing radiation and, 105, 106
  modified atmospheres and, 103
  preservatives and, 102
Clostridium perfringens, 218—220
Clupea harengus, 33, 51
Clupeidae, 19, 36, 48
Coastal vessels, 22—24
Cod, 17, 19
  chemical composition, 33
  collagen, amino acid composition, 40
  freezing
    ice crystal formation, 112
    lipid changes, 116—118
  lipid composition, 41
  marinades, cooked, 160
  minced-type products, 205
  mineral content, 50, 51
  modified-atmosphere storage and, 104
  muscle structure, 31
  postharvest changes
    enzymatic protein degradation, 64
    microbial population counts, 65
    microbial spoilage, 67
    rigor mortis, 62
  protein quality, 36
  quaternary amines, 45
  resource limitations, 27
  salting, 148, 152
  storage life, 97
  vitamin content, 47, 48
Coelacanths, 41
Cold marinades, 156—159
Cold smoking
  shelf life, 177
  texture and, 168
  unit operations, 173—175
Collagen
  muscle structure, 31
  protein composition, 39—40
  smoking and, 174, 175
Cololabis saira, 37
Color
  canning and, 196
  dried fish quality, 138, 139
  freezing and, lipid oxidation products, 117, 118
  marinades, fried, 160
  modified atmospheres and, 103, 104
  postharvest changes, 64, 68—70
  preservatives and, 102
  smoking and, 167
Condensates, smoke, 171
Conger, 27
Connectin, 38—39
Connective tissue, 69, see also Collagen
Consistency, see Texture
Constant rate drying, 130
Containers
  canning, see Canning
  marinades, fried, 161
  on-board processing, 96, 153
  salted products, 148, 153—155
Control process, smokehouse, 175, 176
Control program, sanitation, 229
Conveyer washers, 79
Cooked marinades, 159—160
Cooking, see also Canning; Heat processing
  collagen and, 39
  before drying, 126, 127
  shelf life of frozen product and, 120
Cooling, see Chilling; specific processes
Cooling curve, 188—189
Crab
  chemical composition, 33
  collagen sugars, 40
  dipeptides, 45
  flavor compounds, 45
  fluoride in, 52

homarine content, 46
minced-type product, 201
mineral content, 49
parasites, 221
postharvest changes, color changes, 68—69
resource limitations, 27
species of commercial importance, 16
toxins, 222
Crangon crongon, 15
Crassostrea gigas, 51
Crayfish, 48—51
Creatine, 45
Croaker, 20
   chemical composition, 33
   minced-type products, 204
   protein quality, 36
Cross-cut deheading, 80, 85
Crude protein, 34
Crustaceans, see also Crab; Lobster; Prawn; Shrimp
   flavor compounds, 45
   food chain, 11
   freezing, preparation for, 119
   lipids, 41
   nutritional composition, see Nutrition, composition of major groups of organisms
   postharvest changes, color, 68
   protein quality, 36
   resource limitations, 26, 27
   sarcoplasmic enzymes, 37
   species exploited, 15—17
   sulfur-containing compounds, 46
Cryogenic freezers, 120
Cryoprotectors, 114—115, 202—204
Culture techniques
   algae, 12—13
   fish farming, 2, 6, 42
Curing
   drying and, 126—128
   parasites and, 221
   smoking process, 174
Cutlass fish, 205
Cutters, 25
Cutting, see also Preprocessing
   for marinades, 157—158
   smoking process, 173—174
Cuttlefish, 14, 27, 205
Cyclic alcohols, 47
Cyclooxygenase, 43
Cysteine, 46, 69, 200

D

Daily intake, 6
Dark muscle
   connectin, 38—39
   gross chemical composition, 32
   lipid distribution, 44
   postharvest changes, 64, 69
   protein composition, 36, 37
Decatrienals, 117
Deheading

for marinades, 157—158
   operations, 80—88
   preparation for freezing, 119
Dehydration, frozen foods, 121
Deicing, conveyer washers and, 79
Demand, 6
Denaturation
   canned product quality changes, 195—196
   freezing and, 114, 116
   minced-type product, 201—202, 204
Depth, ocean, 9, 10
Dermestes maculatus, 136, 137
Desalting for marinades, 158
Desulfotomaculum, 182
Detergents, 226—227
Developing countries
   dried product storage, 136, 137
   hygiene problems, 223—224
Dewatering, minced-type products, 207
Diamines, 71—72, 139
Dichlorodifluoromethane, 120
Diet, fish
   digestive system and, 17—18
   families of commercial importance, 19, 20
   lipid composition and, 42, 44
   protein composition and, 34
   vitamin content and, 47
Diet, human
   food-borne diseases, 219—222
   health effects of fatty acids, 42—44
   nutrient composition, see Nutrition, composition of major groups of organisms
Diffusion rate, smoke particles, 166
Digestive tract
   biology, 17—18
   normal microflora, 66
   postharvest changes, 64—67
   processing, see Gutting
Dimethyl disulfide, 46
Dimethyl trisulfide, 46
Dimethyltrithiolanes, 46
Dipeptides, flavor and, 45
Diphyllobothriasis, 218, 221
Disease, fish, resource limitations, 26
Disinfectants, 227—229
Distillates, smoke, 171
Dogfish, 47, 60, 160
Dorado, 36
Dory, 205
Draft smoking, 176
Drag nets, 22
Dressing, smoking process, 173—174
Dried fish products, 137—139
Drift nets, 22, 26
Drum, 20
Drum scalers, 80—81, 84
Drum washers, 79, 83, 84
Drying
   dried fish products, 137
   families of commercial importance, 19, 20
   food-borne diseases and, 225

methods, 126—130
  agrowaste as fuel, 128—129
  curing and, 126—128
  factors in, 126
  mechanical, 129
  solar, 127, 128
  sun drying, 126, 127
principles of, 130—131
production of protein concentrates and preparations, 139—142
quality of fish, 137—139
rates, 130—131
smoking process, 174—175
sorption isotherms, 131—133
spoilage control, 134—137
taurine content and, 45

E

EDTA, 101
Eel, 17, 45, 204, 205
Egg albumin, 203
Eicosanoids, 42, 43
Elasmobranchs, quaternary amines, 45
Elastin, 40
Electrical drying, 127
Electrical scalers, 80
Electric charge, smoke particles, 166
Electric fishing unit, 21
Electronic freshness testers, 72
Electrostatic smoking units, 176
End-of-production cleandown (EPC), 224
Endoperoxides, 43
Engineering, smoking, 172—173
Engraulidae, 19
Enterobacter aerogenes, 67
Enterobacteria, irradiation and, 107
Enzymes, see also Proteases
  drying and, 134—135
  fish protein concentrate preparation, 141
  freezing and, 113, 116
  lipid oxidation, 43, 44, 64—65
  minced-type product, 200
  modified-atmosphere storage and, 103—104
  postharvest changes, 56—58, 64—65
  protein composition, 37
  salted products, ripening, 151, 152
  smoking and, 168
EPC, see End-of-production cleandown
Equilibrium moisture content curve, 131
Equipment
  food-borne diseases and, 225
  freezing, 119—120
  preprocessing, 79, 82, 84
  sanitation, see Sanitation
  smokehouse, 175—176
Escherichia coli, 67, 102
Ethane, 166, 196
Ethylene glycol, 204
Euphausia superba, 17
Evisceration, see Gutting

Exoskeleton
  color changes, 68—69, see also Color
  fluoride in, 52
Extenders, minced-type products, 202—204
Extracts, smoke, 171

F

F-actin, 38
Factory ships, 6—7, 25
Falling rate drying, 130—131
FAO standards, hygiene, 224
Fashion cut deheading, 82, 85
Fastac insecticide, 136
Fat-soluble vitamins, see Vitamins, fat soluble
Fatty acids
  composition, 41—44
  dried fish quality, 139
  frozen fish, 117
  lipid oxidation products, 117
  postharvest changes, 65
Fermentation
  dried fish products, 137
  before drying, 126, 127
  process, 153, 154
Filleting
  machine, 82
  operations, 84—87, 90
  preparation for freezing, 119
  sanitation, 214
  shelf life of frozen product and, 120
Fillets, 79
  freezing, equipment for, 120
  marinades, 157—158, 160
  rigor mortis and, 62—63
  salting, production methods, 153—155
Fins, 17
Fish
  biological characteristics, 17—18
  species exploited, 18—21
Fish farming, 2, 4, 42
Fishing gear
  developments in, 6—7
  types of, 21—22
Fishing lines, 21—22
Fishing vessels
  developments in, 6—7
  sanitation, 213—214
  types of, 22—25
Fish minces, see Minced-type products
Fish protein concentrate, 139—142
Fish traps, 22, 23
Flame sterilization, 190
Flavobacterium, 66, 67
Flavor, see also Sensory quality
  biological molecules affecting, 44—46
  canning and, 196
  dried fish quality, 138
  ionizing radiation effects, 105—106
  postharvest changes, 69—70
  salted products, 151, 152

salting and, 148
smoking and, 167—168
Flavorings
  marinades, 153, 154
  smoke, 170—172, 176
  smoking process, 174
Flounder
  chemical composition, 33
  freezing, lipid changes, 116
  minced-type products, 205
  mineral content, 50, 51
  preservative use, 101—102
  protein quality, 36
  quaternary amines, 45
  storage life, 97
Fluidized-bed blast freezers, 120
Fluidized-bed smoke production, 170
Fluke, northern, 20
Flukes (parasites), 221
Fly spoilage, 136, 137
Food-borne diseases
  bacterial, 219—220
  contributing factors, 225
  parasitic, 220—222
  toxins, 222—223
  viral, 220
Food chain, 12—13
Formaldehyde, 120, 157
Free fatty acids, see Fatty acids
Free radicals, see also Hydroperoxides; Lipid oxidation
  lipid oxidation, 43, 44
  temperature and, 133—134
Freeze drying, 127, 130
Freezer burn, 121
Freezers, types of, 119—120
Freeze-thaw process, minced-type product, 200—201, 203
Freezing
  commercial process, 119—122
  denaturation, minced-type product materials, 204
  deterioration in product, 114—119
  minced-type product, 200, 202, 206, 207
  parasites and, 221
  partial, 100
  postharvest changes, protein hydration, 68
  preserving action of, 112—114
  rate, 112, 119
  salted product, 154, 156
Freon, 120
Freshness, see also Quality
  chilling, see Chilling
  minced-type product raw materials, 205
  rigor mortis and, 60
Freshwater species
  crustaceans, 15
  lipid composition, 42
  quaternary amines, 45
Friction, smoke production by, 169—170
Fried marinades, 160—161
Fuel, drying, 127

Fugu, 223
Fungi, see Yeasts and molds

G

G-actin, 38
Gadidae, 19, 48, 50
Gadus morhua
  chemical composition, 33
  mineral content, 51
  protein quality, 36
Gambiordiscus toxicus, 223
Gaping, 62—63
Gas atmospheres, modified atmosphere storage, 102—104
Gases, 12, 166, 196, see also Ammonia
Gastroenteritis, 218—221
Gear, fishing, see Fishing gear
Gel
  frozen fish, 121
  marinades, cooked, 159
  minced-type products, 200, 201, 203, 204
  postharvest changes, protein hydration, 68
Gill cut for deheading, 82, 85
Gill nets, 26
Gills
  anatomy, 18
  microbial population counts, 65
  mineral content, 51
Glazing, frozen fish, 121
Glucose oxidase and glucose, 101—102
Glutamate, 204
Glutamic acid, 138
Gluten, 203
Glycerol cryoprotectants, 204
Glyceryl esters, 41
Glycine, 45
Glycogen, 56, 57
Goby, 36
Gonyaulax, 222
Grading
  freshness assessment, 69—70
  gross chemical composition and, 32—33
  operations, 78, 81, 82
  shrimp, 16
Gray weakfish, 20
Grenadier, 148, 152, 205
Grouper, 19, 205
Guanidine compounds, 45
Gum additives, 203
Gunard, 205
Gutting, 79
  bacterial growth and, 66
  dried fish quality, 138
  for marinades, 157—158, 160
  modified-atmosphere storage and, 104
  on-board processing, 95
  operations, 80—88
  preparation for freezing, 119
  sanitation, 214
  shelf life of frozen product and, 120

for smoking, 173
Gymnodinium brevis, 222

H

HACCP, see Hazard analysis critical control point system
Haddock, 19
  freezing, 112, 122
  minced-type products, 205
  postharvest changes, microbial spoilage, 67
  protein quality, 36
  resource limitations, 27
  storage life, 97
  vitamin content, 47
Hake
  minced-type products, 205
  postharvest changes, rigor mortis, 61
  protein quality, 36
  protozoan infection, 222
  resource limitations, 27
  storage life, 97
Halibut, 20
  chemical composition, 33
  fishing methods, 25
  freezing, 112
  minced-type products, 205
  mineral content, 50
  resource limitations, 26
  smoked, shelf-life, 177
  storage life, 97
  vitamin content, 47, 48
Haliotis kamschatkana, 33, see also Abalone
Halophilic bacteria, 135
Ham products, 204
Hazard analysis critical control point (HACCP) system, 229
Health, 2, see also Sanitation
  fatty acids and, 42—44
  nutrition, see Nutrition, composition of major groups of organisms
  smoked products and, 128, 177
Heat, insect larvae removal, 137
Heat conduction, hot smoking, 172, 173
Heating curve, 188—189
Heat processing, see also Cooking
  food-borne diseases and, 225
  smoking, 174—175
  sterilization, see Canning
Heat transfer, smoking, 172
Hepatitis, 218
Herring, 17
  chemical composition, 33
  deheading, 80
  filleting machine, 89
  fishing methods, 25
  freezing, lipid changes, 116, 118
  grading, 78
  marinades, 159, 160
  minced-type products, 205
  mineral content, 51
  postharvest changes, 64, 65
  preparation for freezing, 119
  protein quality, 36
  resource limitations, 26, 27
  salting, 150, 152
  scombroid fish poisoning, 223
  smoking, 173, 175, 176
  storage life, 97
  vitamin content, 47, 48
Hexamethylenetetraamine, 157
Hexanal, 46
High quality life, 121, 122
Hipoglossus stenolepis, 33, see also Halibut
Histamine
  dried fish quality, 139
  postharvest changes, 64, 67, 71—72
  scombroid fish poisoning, 223
Histidine, 45, 223
Hoki, 205
Homarine, 46
Homarus, 17, see also Lobster
Horizontal axis drum washers, 79, 84
Horse mackerel, 148, 150, 152, 205
Hot smoking, 168, 172, 173, 177
House fly, 136
Hydrogen peroxide, marinades, cold, 157
Hydrogen sulfide, 12, 46, 196
Hydrolysis, see also Autolysis; Lipolysis
  lipids, interactions of, 118—119
  minced-type product, 200
  salted products, ripening, 151, 152
Hydroperoxides, 43, see also Free radicals; Lipid oxidation
  frozen fish, 117
  lipid oxidation, 117
  postharvest changes, 72
Hydropyrolytic smoke production, 170
p-Hydroxybenzoate, 157, 161
Hyperbaric storage, 102
Hypobaric packaging, 104
Hypochlorite, sanitizing with, 227—228

I

Ice crystal formation, 112
Icing
  bacterial growth and, 67
  on-board, 95—97
  rigor mortis and, 62
  sanitation, 224
  storage life and, 96—98
  subzero processes, 98—100
  types of ice, 95, 96
Ilex, 14, 15, see also Squid
Ilex argentinus, 39
Immersion smoking, 176
Infection, meat texture and, 69, see also Microorganisms; Food-borne diseases
Infrared radiators, 176
Inosine, 70—71
Inosine monophosphate, 137, 138

Inosinic acid, 134
Insecticides, 136, 137
Insect spoilage, dried fish, 126, 134, 138, 139
Inspection, 2, 224, 225
Intelectron fish tester, 72
International cooperation, 3, 6
Interscience cooperation, 3
Invertebrates, see also Crustaceans; Mollusks; Shellfish; specific common names
  food chain, 11
  lipids, 41
  nutritional composition, see Nutrition, composition of major groups of organisms
  species exploited, 14—17
Iodophors, 228
Ionizing radiation, 105—107
Irradiation, 105—107

J

Japanese meagre, 20
Jasus, 17
Joy fish, 141

K

Kamaboko, 201, 204, 206
Ketones, 46—47, 117
Kilns, smoking, 175
Krill, 17, 20
  ATPase, 38
  fish protein concentrate preparation, 141
  fluoride in, 52
  freezing, lipolysis, 117
  microflora, species of, 66
  postharvest changes, 65, 68—69
  resource limitations, 26
  sarcoplasmic enzymes, 37
  sulfur-containing compounds, 46
K-sorbate, 102, 104, 157, 161
Kudoa, 222
Kvaerner-Brug tunnel, 175
K-value, 70—71

L

Lactic acid, postharvest changes, 59
Lactic acid bacteria, marinades, 155—156, 159—161
Lactobacillus, 103, 104
Lactobacillus plantarum, 161
Latimera chalumnae, 41
Lethality curve, 187—188
Leukotrienes, 43
Ligaments, protein composition, 40
Light
  marine habitat, 9
  photooxidation, 117
  seasonal cycles, 10, 11
Lines, fishing, 21—22
Ling, 36
Lipase, 65

Lipid oxidation, 42—44
  canning and, 196
  drying and, 133—135
  fish protein concentrate preparation, 140
  frozen fish, 114, 117—120
  postharvest changes, 65, 72
Lipids
  in canning, 183, 196
  composition, 41—44
  drying and, 131, 133—135
  equipment cleaning, 226, 229
  frozen fish, 116—120
  gross chemical composition, 31—33
  marinades, 155—156, 160
  minced-type products, 204, 206
  postharvest changes, 57, 64—65, 68, 69, 72
  salting and, 150—152
  smoked product, 166, 167, 175—176
Lipolysis
  canning and, 196
  frozen fish, interactions of, 118—119
  in frozen stored fish, 116—117
Lipoproteins, protein composition, 36, 37
Lipoxygenase, 43, 44, 116
Liquid nitrogen, 120
Liver
  lipid distribution, 44
  postharvest changes, 64
  vitamin content, 47
Lizard fish, 204
Lobster
  chemical composition, 33
  collagen, amino acid composition, 40
  freezing, preparation for, 119
  minced-type products, 205
  postharvest changes, 60, 64, 68—69
  species of commercial importance, 16—17
  sulfur-containing compounds, 46
  toxins, 222
  vitamin content, 48
Loligo, see Squid
Loligo pealei, 36
Loligo vulgaris, 14
Long liners, 24—25
Lutianidae, 19
Lysozyme, 37

M

Mackerel, 17, 19
  canned product quality changes, 195—196
  canning, 195
  chemical composition, 33
  chromoproteins, 37
  connectin, 39
  deheading, 80
  families of commercial importance, 20
  filleting machine, 89
  fishing methods, 25
  flavor compounds, 45
  freezing, lipid changes, 116—118

grading, 78
marinades, cooked, 160
minced-type products, 204—206
postharvest changes, 61, 64
protein quality, 36
resource limitations, 27
salting, 148, 150
scombroid fish poisoning, 223
Macrobranchium rosenbergii, 15
Macroelements, 49
Magnesium, 49, 151
Mahimahi, 67
Maillard reaction, 160, 196
Makaira mazara, 37
Mammals, marine, see Marine mammals
Manufacture, see also Operations; Production
    fish protein concentrates, 140—142
    marinades, cold, 156—157
    sanitation, 215—218
Marinades
    canning, 193
    cold, 156—159
    composition of bath, 162
    cooked, 159—160
    fried, 160—161
    parasites and, 221
Marine habitat, 9—13
Marine mammals
    food chain, 11
    lipids, 41, 42, 44
    parasites, 221
Marlin, 39
Martialia hyagesi, 202
Maturity, 44, 47, see also Reproduction
Meagre, 36
Meat quality, see Quality
Meat separation, 87, 89, 91, 207
Mechanical drying, 127, 129
Melanins, 68—69
Menhaden, 19, 205
Merluccius productus, 222
Metabisulfites, 102, 200
Metabolic products, bacterial, 67
Metabolism, see also Enzymes; Lipids; Proteins
    general biology, 18
    lipid composition and, 44
    postharvest changes, see Postharvest changes
Methane, 166, 196
Methanethiol, 46
Methionine, 46, 69
Methyl bromide, 137
Methyl mercury, 50
Micrococci, 66, 105, 159
Micrococcus, 66
Micrococcus radiodurans, 105
Microelements, 49—52
Microorganisms
    canning, heat effects, 182—186
    carbon-dioxide-enriched atmosphere and, 103—104
    drying and, 126, 134, 138, 139
    food-borne diseases, 219—223

    freezing and, 112
    marinades, 156, 159, 161
    postharvest changes, 57, 65—67, see also Postharvest changes
    preservatives and, 101—102
    processing and, see Processing; specific methods
    radiation effects, 105
    salted product, freezing and, 154
    sanitation, see Sanitation
    smoked products, 169, 174, 175
    washing, 78—79
Micropogon undulatus, 36
Microspora, 222
Milkfish, 205
Minced-type products
    canning, 193
    chemical composition, 200—201
    freezing, 119, 120
    functional properties, 202—204
    gel structure, 200
    processing, 206—207
    raw material, 204—206
Minerals
    composition, 49—52
        gross chemical composition, 31—32
        macroelements, 49
        microelements, 49—52
    dried fish quality, 139
Modified atmosphere storage, 102—104, 154—155
Modori, 200
Moisture content, see Water
Molds, see Yeasts and molds
Mollusks
    fishing gear, 21
    flavor compounds, 45
    food chain, 11
    freezing, preparation for, 119
    homarine content, 46
    lipids, 41
    mineral content, 49
    nutritional composition, see Nutrition, composition of major groups of organisms
    postharvest changes, microbial population counts, 65
    protein quality, 36
    resource limitations, 26
    sanitation problems in developing countries, 223
    sarcoplasmic enzymes, 37
    species exploited, 14—15
    toxins, 222
Moraxella, 66, 67, 103, 105
Moridae, 41
Morwong, 102
Mugil cephalus, 51
Mullet
    chemical composition, 33
    lipids, 41
    minced-type products, 205
    mineral content, 51
    protein quality, 36
    resource limitations, 27

storage life, 97
Musca domestica, 136
Muscle
  amino acid composition, 35
  fluoride in, 52
  freezing and, 112, 114
  homarine content, 46
  mineral content, 49, 51, 69, see also Postharvest changes
  salted products, ripening, 151
  smoking and, 168
  structure, 30—31
  vitamin content, 47
Mussels
  mineral content, 49, 51
  resource limitations, 27
  species of commercial importance, 14
  toxins, 222
Myofibrillar proteins
  composition, 37—39
  minced-type product, 200
    gel structure, 202
    raw material quality, 206
    salting and, 201—202
  postharvest changes, 61, 64, 69
Myofibrils, muscle structure, 31
Myosin, see Actomyosin
Myxosporidian protozoans, 222

N

Needlefish, 47
Nematodes, 221
Nephrops norvegicus, 60
Nets, 22—24
Nitrites, 101, 174, 225
Nitrogen, liquid, 120
Nitrogenous compounds
  canning and, 196
  flavor and, 44—46
  postharvest changes, 63—64
    bacterial activity and, 67
    freshness assessment, 70—71
    odor and, 69
  sarcoplasmic enzymes, 37
N-Nitroso compounds, 177
Nobbing, 79, 83, 88
Nonadienal, 46
Nonenal, 46
Northern fluke, 20
Norwalk virus, 218
Notohaliotis discus, 38
Notothenia, 52
Nototheniidae, 20
Nucleotides
  flavor and, 45
  freshness assessment, 70—71
  postharvest changes, 56—58
Nutrition, 2, 7
  canning and, 195—196
  drying and, 135, 139

fish protein concentrates, 140—141
Nutrition, composition of major groups of organisms
  flavor compounds, 44—46
  gross chemical composition, 31—33
  lipids, 41—44
    composition, 41
    distribution, 44
    fatty acid composition, 41—42
    fatty acid effects on human health, 42—44
  minerals, 49—52
  muscle of marine organism, 30—31
  proteins, 34—40
    myofibrillar, 37—39
    sarcoplamic, 35—37
    stromal, 39—40
    total, 34—35
  vitamins, 47—49
  water, 33—34

O

"Ocean" (product), 153, 154
Octenal, 46
Octopine, 45
Octopus
  collagen sugars, 40
  mineral content, 49
  octopine, 45
  resource limitations, 27
  species of commercial importance, 14
Octopus vulgaris, 14
Odor, see also Sensory quality
  dried fish, 138
  postharvest changes, 69—70
  salted products, 151, 152
  sulfur-containing compounds and, 46
Oils, see also Lipids
  minced-type product additives, 204
  salted products, 148
  smoke partitioning, 166
Ommastrephes bartrami, 14
On-board processing
  chilling, 95—101
  developments in, 7
  gutting and deheading unit for, 82, 97
  ionizing radiation, 106
  minced-type product raw materials, 206, 207
  salting, 152—153
  sanitation, 213—214
Oncorhynchus gorguscha, 33
Operations, see also Manufacture; Production
  canning, 191—194
  hygiene, 214
  minced-type products, flow chart, 207
  sanitation, 214
Orange roughy, 41
Ostreidae, 33, see also Oysters
Oxidation
  frozen foods, 120, 121
  lipid composition and, 44
  lipids, see Lipid oxidation

postharvest changes, 65
  color changes, 68—69
    enzymatic protein degradation, 64
    freshness assessment, 72
  salted products, ripening, 152
  smoking and, 168
  vitamin content and, 47
Oxygen
  general biology, 18
  marine habitat, 12
  smoke constituents and, 165—166
Oysters
  alcohols, unsaturated, 46—47
  chemical composition, 33
  food poisoning, 66
  freezing, 119, 120
  homarine content, 46
  mineral content, 49—51
  resource limitations, 27
  species of commercial importance, 14
  toxins, 222
  vitamin content, 48

P

Pacific rosefish, 20
Packaging, 2
  canning, see Canning
  dried product, insect spoilage and, 137
  frozen product, 121
  marinades, 158—161
  modified-atmosphere storage and, 104
  salted product, 148, 153, 155
Packing, in canning, 190
Pandalus borealis, 15
Pandalus jordani, 67
Panulirus, 17, see also Lobster
Paralithodes, 16
Paralytic shellfish poisoning, 218, 222
Paramyosin, 38
Parasites
  food-borne diseases, 220—222
  meat texture and, 69
  salted product, 154
  sources of contamination, 218
Pathogens, 66, see also Food-borne diseases
Peaneus blebejus, 102
Pecten, 40
Pecten alba, 51
Pectinidae, 33, see also Scallops
Penaeus monodon, 45
Peptide hydrolases, 151—153
Perch
  families of commercial importance, 20
  minced-type products, 205
  protein quality, 36
Perciformes, 36
Personnel
  health hazards, 218—219
  hygiene and food handling practices, 217—218
pH

dried fish products, 137, 138
food-borne diseases and, 225
frozen fish, 114
heat sterilization and, 183
marinades, 156, 159, 160
minced-type product, 200, 206
modified-atmosphere storage and, 104
postharvest changes, 57, 59—60, 64, 68
preservative use and, 101—102
protein composition and, 34
salted products, ripening, 152
sarcoplasmic enzymes and, 37
sorbate activity and, 102
Phosphates
  as minced-type product cryoprotectant, 204
  mineral content, 49
  postharvest changes, 56—58
Phosphine, 137
Phospholipids, 41
  drying and, 134
  freezing and, 116
  hydrolysis products, 117—118
  lipolysis and oxidation interactions, 118, 119
  postharvest changes, 64—65
Photooxidation, 117
Physical basis, salting, 149—151
Physical measurements, freshness testers, 72
Physical properties, smoke, 166—167
Phytoplankton, light and, 11
Pickled fish, storage, 155—156
Pickling, before drying, 126, 127
Pigment, see also Color
  lipid oxidation and, 118
  lipid-protein interactions and, in frozen fish, 119
  postharvest color changes, 68—69
Pike, 205
Pilchard, 19, 36, 47
Pindang, 137
Pirimphos-methyl, 137
Plankton, see also Krill
  food chain, 11—13
  resource limitations, 26
Plankton feeders
  digestive system, 17—18
  families of commercial importance, 19, 20
  fluoride in, 52
Plants, marine, 13—14
Platichthys flessus, 51
Platopecten magellanicus, 51
Pleuronectidae, 20, 36, 48, 50
Pneumonococci, 159
Pollock, 19
  actomyosin, 38
  minced-type product, 201, 203—205
  quaternary amines, 45
  vitamin content, 47
Pollution, 2
  gross chemical composition and, 32
  health hazards, 218
  microbial population counts and, 65
  sanitation, fishing vessel, 214

Polyamines
  dried fish quality, 139
  postharvest changes, 64, 71—72
Polyenoic acids, 41—43
Polynuclear aromatic hydrocarbons, 165, 169, 177
Polyols, 204
Polypaecilium pisce, 136
Polyphosphates, 204, 207
Polysaccharides, sarcoplasmic enzymes, 37
Polyunsaturated fatty acids, 41—44, see also Fatty acids
Porgy, 205
Postharvest changes
  carbohydrate degradation, 59
  catching, effects of, 56
  freshness assesment, 69—72
  lipids, 64—65
  meat, functional properties, 67—69
  microbial, 65—67
  minced-type products, 205—206
  nitrogenous compounds, 63—64
  pH changes, 59—60
  phosphate degradation, 56—58
  rigor mortis, 60—63
  sensory properties, 68—69
  sequence of, 56, 57
Post-mortem changes
  collagen and, 40
  minced-type product raw material quality, 206
Potassium content, 49
Potassium sorbate, see K-sorbate
PPH, see Preproduction hygiene
Practical storage life, 121, 122
Prawn
  flavor compounds, 45
  fluoride in, 52
  mineral content, 49
  parasites, 221
  preservatives, 102
  resource limitations, 27
  species of commercial importance, 15
  sulfur-containing compounds, 46
  vitamin content, 48
Predators
  digestive system, 17—18
  families of commercial importance, 19, 20
  food chain, 11
  lipid composition, 42
Preprocessing
  in canning, 191, 193
  chilling, see Chilling
  for marinades, 157—158
  marinades, fried, 160
  minced-type product raw materials, 206, 207
  operations, 78—91
    deheading and gutting, 80—88
    filleting, 84—87, 90
    grading, 78, 81, 82
    meat separation, 87, 89, 91
    scaling, 79—80, 84
    skinning, 86—87, 90, 91
    washing, 78, 79, 83, 84
  production line in, 92
  purpose of, 78
  sanitation, 213—214
  smoking process, 173—174
Preproduction hygiene (PPH), 226
Preservation, 2, see also specific methods
  mineral content and, 49
  preprocessing methods, see Preprocessing
  smoking, 168—169
Preservatives, 101—102
  marinades, 157, 159, 161
  modified-atmosphere storage with, 104
  vs. radiation, 107
  salted product, 154
Preserves, storage, 155—156
Process calculations, canning, 186—190
Process engineering, smoking, 172—173
Processing, see also specific processing methods
  chilling, see Chilling
  collagen and, 39
  food poisoning and, 66
  minced-type product, 202, 206—207
  on-board, 7
  preliminary, see Preprocessing
  protein composition and, 34
  regulation of, 7—8
  sanitation, 215—218, see also Sanitation
  vitamin content and, 47
  water and, 34
Production, see also Manufacture; Operations; Preprocessing
  canning
    methods of heat processing, 190—191
    products, 194—195
    unit operations, 191—194
  salted products, 152—155
  smoked product, see Smoking
Production line, processing, 92
Propylthioacetate, 46
Prostacyclin, 43
Prostaglandins, 43
Proteases
  fish protein concentrate preparation, 140, 141
  minced-type product, 200
  postharvest changes, 64, 69
  salting process, 151, 153
  sarcoplasmic enzymes, 37
  smoking and, 168
Protein concentrates, production of, 139—142
Proteins
  canned product, 183, 195—196
  composition of major groups of marine organisms, 34—40
  dried fish quality, 139
  equipment cleaning, 226, 229
  frozen fish shelf life, 114—116, 120
  gross chemical composition, 31—33
  marinades, 156, 160
  minced-type products, 201—202, 205—206
  postharvest changes, 60—64, 68

salted products, ripening, 151, 152
smoked product, 167, 168, 175—176
Proteolysis, see Proteases
Proteus, 67
Protozoans, 69, 222
Pseudomonas, 66, 67
   ionizing radiation effects, 105
   marinades, cooked, 159
   modified-atmosphere storage and, 103
   preservatives and, 102
Pseudomonas morgani, 67
Psychrobacter, 66, 67
PUFAs, 41—44, see also Fatty acids
Pufferfish, 45, 223
Purse seine, 22
Putrescine, 71—72, 139
Pyrethroid insecticides, 136
Pyrophosphates, 204

Q

Quality, 2
   canning and, changes during, 195—197
   collagen and, 39—40
   families of commercial importance, 19—21
   fish protein concentrates, 140—141
   frozen stored fish, deterioration of, 114
   inspection services, 224, 225
   marinades, 156—157, 161
   minced-type product, 205—207
   modified-atmosphere storage and, 104
   palatibility, 3
   postharvest changes, 65—67, see also Postharvest changes
      freshness assessment, 69—72
      rigor mortis, effects of, 62—63
      sensory properties, 68—69
   regulation of, 7—8
   salted products, differences in, 152
   smoked product, 176
Quality control, see Standards
Quaternary ammonium bases
   flavor and, 45—46
   sanitizing agents, 228
   TMA, see Trimethylamine/Trimethylamine oxide

R

Radurization, 105—107
Rancidity
   drying and, 134—135
   frozen fish, 117, 118
   lipid oxidation and, 117
   postharvest changes, 65, 72
   sun drying and, 126
Raw material, see also Preprocessing
   minced-type product, 204—206
   sanitation, 214
Rays, 45
Redfish, 27, 66
Red muscle, see Dark muscle
Red snapper, 66
Refrigerated sea water, 99—100
Refrigeration, 2
   bacterial growth and, 67
   dried product, insect spoilage and, 137
   postharvest changes, 57—58, 62, 67
   sanitation, 214, 224
Reproduction
   lipid composition and, 44
   meat texture and, 69
   minced-type product raw material quality, 205
   protein composition and, 34
   resource limitations and, 26
   temperature and, 11—12
   vitamin content and, 47
Reproductive organs, mineral content, 51
Resource limitations, 26, 27
Resources, 6
   availability and limitations of, 26, 27
   fishing boats, 22—25
   fishing gear, 21—22
   marine habitat, 9—13
      benthic, 9, 10
      depth, 9, 10
      food chain, 12—13
      gases, dissolved, 12
      light, 9
      salinity, 12
      temperature, 11—12
   organisms exploited for food, 13—21
      crustaceans, 13—17
      fish, biological characteristics, 17—28
      fish, families of commercial importance, 19—21
      mollusks, 14—15
      plants, 13—14
Rhincodon typus, 21
Rhodotorula, 66
Rigor mortis, 60—63
   bacterial growth and, 66
   minced-type product raw material quality, 205—206
   on-board processing, 95
   postharvest changes, 57
Ripening, salted fish, 151—152
Rockfish, 19, 36, 205
Rock lobster, 61, see also Lobster
Rollmops, 159
Rondair smoking kilns, 175
Rosefish, Pacific, 20
Ruvettus presiosus, 41

S

Sablefish, 33
Saithe, 205
Salinity, 12, 45
Salmon, 17
   aquaculture, 2
   canning, 195
   caviar, 155

chemical composition, 33
dipeptides, 45
families of commercial importance, 20
marinades, cooked, 160
minced-type products, 205
parasites, 222
protein quality, 36
resource limitations, 27
salting, 152
smoking process, 174
texture of meat, spawning and, 69
vitamin content, 47
Salmonella, 105, 218, 219
Salmonella typhimurium, 102
Salmonidae, 20, 36, 155
Salt, see also Brining; Salting
   canning and, bacterial protection by, 183
   dried product, insect spoilage and, 137
   drying and, 131, 133
   food-borne diseases and, 225
   marinades, 159, 161
   minced-type products, 201—202, 204, 207
   mineral content and, 49
Salt-free, fat-free dry basis (SFFFDB), 131, 132
Salting, see also Brining
   brine composition, 162
   dried product, 126, 127, 136
   marinades, 158, 160
   preservation technique, 148—156
      cans, 153—155
      caviar, 155
      evolution of, 148—149
      physical and chemical bases, 149—151
      production technology, 152—153
      ripening, 151—152
      storage of product, 155—156
   smoked product, 173—174, 177
Salting-in rates, 150—151
Sand dab, 20
Sanitation, 7—8
   cleaning facilities, 226—227
   control program, 229
   dried product, insect spoilage and, 136
   fish and shellfish, 218—224
      in developing countries, 223—224
      food-borne diseases, 219—222
      health hazards in production, 218—219
      inspection services, 224, 225
      standards, 224
      toxins, 222—223
   fishing vessels, 213—214
   manufacturing plants, 215—218
   operation requirements for fresh fish, 214
   sanitizing agents, 227—229
Sanitizing agents, 227—229
Sarcoplasmic protein, 31, 206
Sardines
   freezing, 116
   grading, 78
   minced-type products, 205, 206
   mineral content, 29
   postharvest changes, 64
   resource limitations, 27
   salting, 148
   scombroid fish poisoning, 223
   smoking, color, 167
   storage life, 97
   vitamin content, 47
Sashimi, 97
Saury, 27, 37
Sausage products, 204
Scales
   lipid oxidation and, 118
   removal of, 79—80, 84
Scallops
   chemical composition, 33
   minced-type product, 201
   mineral content, 49, 51
   modified-atmosphere storage, 104
   muscle structure, 30
   octopine, 45
Scampi, 60, 69
Scienidae, 19—20
Scomber japonicus, 37
Scomber scombrus, 36
Scombroid fish, 20
   poisoning, 218
   postharvest changes, 67
   protein quality, 36
   vitamin content, 48
Score sheet evaluation, dried fish, 138, 139
Scorpenidae, 20
Sea mullet, 51
Sea perch, 205
Seasonal cycles
   lipid composition and, 42, 44
   marine habitat, 10, 11
   protein composition and, 34
   quaternary ammonium compounds and, 46
   vitamin content and, 47
Seaweed, 13—14
Sebastodes, 36
Seine nets, 22
Selachii, 20—21
Selenium, 50
Semilogarithmic model, 184—185
Sensory quality, 2
   chilling practices and, 97—98
   dried fish, 137—138
   evaluation, 3, 137—138
   flavor compounds, 44—47
   freezing and, 116—118
   freshness assessment, 69—70
   frozen fish, 113
   gross chemical composition and, 31—32
   in irradiated fish, 105—106
   modified-atmosphere storage and, 104
   postharvest changes, 68—69
   smoked product, 167—168
   sulfur-containing compounds and, 46
Seriola quinqueradiata, 37
Serranidae, 19

SFFFDB, see Salt-free, fat-free dry basis
Shark, 17
    dipeptides, 45
    families of commercial importance, 20—21
    lipids, 41
    minced-type products, 205
    mineral content, 50
    protein quality, 36
    quaternary amines, 45
    vitamin content, 47
Shean, 45
Sheen, dried fish quality, 139
Sheepshead, 205
Shelf life, see also Nutrition; Sensory quality
    dried products, lipid oxidation and, 135
    extending, 101—107
        irradiation, 105—107
        modified atmospheres, 102—104
        preservatives used in, 101—102
    frozen foods, 116, 120—122
    marinades
        cold, 156—158
        cooked, 159
        fried, 161
    smoked product, 177—178
Shellfish
    fishing gear, 21
    flavor compounds, 45
    freezing, 119
    mineral content, 49
    preservatives, 102
    resource limitations, 27
    sanitation problems in developing countries, 223
    toxins, 222
Shewanella, 67
Shigellosis, 218
Ships, see Fishing vessels
Shrimp
    canning, 195
    creatine in, 45
    fluoride in, 52
    freezing, 119, 120
    irradiated, 107
    minced-type product, 201, 205
    mineral content, 49
    modified-atmosphere storage and, 104
    postharvest changes, 64, 67—69
    preservatives, 102
    quaternary amines, 45
    resource limitations, 27
    species of commercial importance, 15, 16
    vitamin content, 48
Silago schomburgkii, 51
Size, chilling and, 99
Skeleton, 17
Skin
    amino acid composition, 35
    collagen sugars, 40
    fluoride in, 52
    freezing and, 118
    microflora, species of, 66
    postharvest changes, 64, 69
    salting and, 150—151
    vitamin content, 47
Skinning
    operations, 86—87, 90, 91
    shelf life of frozen product and, 120
Skipjack, 36, 38, 45, 116
Slant cut, deheading, 80
Smelt, 27, 36
Smoking
    botulism and, 220
    collagen and, 39
    dried fish quality, 139
    equipment, 175—176
    families of commercial importance, 19, 20
    lipid oxidation and, 135
    methods and equipment, 169—170
    process, 172—175
    production of smoke flavorings, 170—172
    quality, product, 176
    salted products, 148, 154—155
    shelf life, product, 177—178
    wood smoke, 164—169
        generation and chemical composition, 164—166
        preserving action, 168—169
        sensory properties and, 167—168
Smoldering method of smoke production, 169
Snails, 49
Snapper, 19
    chilling, 98, 99, 101, 104
    postharvest changes, 66
    salt uptake in refrigerated sea water, 101
    storage life, 97
Snoek, 27
Sodium bicarbonate, 206
Sodium chloride, see Salting
Sodium content, 49
Sodium metabisulfite, 102, 200
Sodium nitrite, 174, see also Nitrites
Solar drying, 127, 128
Sole, 20, 27, 36
Soleidae, 20
Sorbate, 102, 157
Sorbitol, 204, 207
Sorption isotherms, 131—133
Soy protein isolate, 203
Sparidae, 19
Spicy preserves, 153
Spiking, brain, 62
Spiny lobster, 40, 119, see also Lobster
Spissula solidissima, 36
Spoilage, 2
    chilling and, see Chilling
    dried fish quality, 138—139
    drying and, 134—137
    fish protein concentrate preparation, 140
    marinades, fried, 161
    postharvest changes
        bacteria and, 68
        freshness assessment, 69—72
        microbial activity, 67

texture, 69
sulfur-containing compounds and, 46
Spore-forming microbes, 66
   canning and, 182, 183, 186
   freezing effects, 112
   ionizing radiation effects, 105, 106
   normal microflora, 66
Sporondonema, 136
Sprat, 19
   canning, 184
   deheading, 80
   grading, 78
   gutting, 83
   mineral content, 49, 51
   postharvest changes, 64
   preparation for freezing, 119
   smoking, 167, 176
Squalidus, 21
Squid
   collagen, 39, 40
   fermented products, 137
   freezing, 117, 119
   lipid composition, 42
   minced-type products, 202, 205
   mineral content, 49
   muscle structure, 30—31
   myofibrillar proteins, 38
   octopine, 45
   preprocessed, major forms, 80
   protein quality, 36
   quaternary amines, 45
   species of commercial importance, 14
   toxins, 222
Standards
   regulation of, 7—8
   hygiene, 224
Staphylococcal food poisoning, 218, 220
Staphylococcus, irradiation and, 105, 107
Staphylococcus aureus, 105
Staphylococcus xylosus, 135
Starch additives, 203
Steam
   canning, 190—191
   sanitizing with, 228—229
Sterilization, collagen and, 39
Sterilization value of heat process, 186
Sterols, 41
Storage
   bacterial growth and, 67
   canned product, 194
   chilling and, 96—97
   dried fish, 136, 137
   food-borne diseases and, 225
   frozen product, 116, 118
   marinades, 156, 158—161
   modified atmosphere, 102—104
   on-board stowage, 96
   postharvest changes, protein hydration, 68
   salted product, 148—149, 153—156
   shelf life, see Shelf life
Stowage, 96

Streptococcal infections, 218
Streptococcus faecium, 105
Stress, fish, 44, 56
Stroma, 39—40
Sturgeon, 26, 152, 155
Suction gutting, 83, 88
Sugars
   canning and, 196
   collagen composition, 40
   minced-type product additives, 203, 204
Sulfhydryl groups
   canning and, 196
   freezing and, 115, 116
   minced-type product, 200
   myofibrillar proteins, 38
   postharvest changes, 68
Sulfiting agents, 102, 200
Sulfolipids, 41
Sulfur, mineral content, 49
Sulfur compounds, 46, 69, 72
Sun drying, 126, 127
Superchilling processes, 98—100
Surimi, 200, 206, see also Minced-type products
Survivor curve, 184
Swordfish, 36, 50, 104
Synthetic smoke flavorings, 171—172

T

Tapeworm, 221
Taste, see Flavor; Sensory quality
Taurine, 45
Temperature
   bacterial growth and, 66, 67
   body, 18
   canning, see Canning
   chilling, see Chilling
   Clostridium perfringens inactivation, 219
   collagen and, 39—40
   dried product spoilage, 135
   drying and, 132—133
   environment, 18, 42, 44
   food-borne diseases and, 225
   freezing
      chemical reaction rates, 112—113
      ice crystal formation, 112, 113
      points, 112
      product storage, 116, 121, 122
   insect larvae removal, 137
   irradiated fish, 106
   marinades, 157, 160, 161
   marine habitat, 11—12
   minced-type products, 202
   postharvest changes and, 60
      enzymatic protein degradation, 64
      microbial spoilage, 67
      pH, 60
      rigor mortis, 62
   salted product, 151, 153—156
   smoked product shelf life, 178
   smoke generation, 170

smoking process, 172, 173
  drying and heat processing, 174—175
  smoke constituents and, 165—166
Tetraodon poisoning, 223
Texture
  dried fish quality, 139
  freezing and, 114
  minced-type product, 200—201, 206—208
  postharvest changes, 69
  salted products, 151, 152, 156
  smoking and, 168
Thermal death time, 183, 185—187
Thermal resistance curves, 183, 185—187
Thialdine, 46
Thunnus orientalis, 37
Thunnus thynnus, 33
Tilapia, 62, 205
Time temperature tolerance (TTT), 121—122
Tissue fluids, see Water
Titin, 38—39
TMA, see Trimethylamine/trimethylamine oxide
TMAO, see Trimethylamine/trimethylamine oxide
Todarodes pacificus, 14
Torry freshness meter, 72
Torsk, 36
Torulopsis, 66
Total volatile bases, 71
Toxins, 222—223
  aflatoxin, 136
  bacterial, 220
  botulinus, see Botulinus toxin
  food-borne diseases, 222—223
  mineral, 49—51
  modified atmospheres and, 103
  pathogenic microflora, 66
  preservatives and, 102
  sources of contamination, 218
Traps, fishing, 22, 23
Trawlers, 25
Trawls, 22, 24
Trematodes, 222
Triacylglycerols, 41, 44
  frozen fish, 117
  lipolysis and oxidation interactions, 118
  postharvest changes, 65
Trimethylamine (TMA)/trimethylamine oxide (TMAO)
  composition, 34
  content, 45—46
  dried fish, 138
  freezing and, 114—116
  freshness assessment, 70
  modified-atmosphere storage and, 104
  postharvest changes, 63—64, 67, 71
  preservatives and, 102
  shark meat, 21
Trimethylarsine, 46
Trithiolane, 46
Tropical species
  chilling, 99
  crustaceans, 15—16
  dried, 136, 137
  families of commercial importance, 19, 20
  insect spoilage, 137
  microflora, species of, 66
  rigor mortis in, 62
  storage life, 97
Tropomyosin, 38
Troponins, 38
Trout
  aquaculture, 2
  chemical composition, 33
  dipeptides, 45
  minced-type products, 205
  protein quality, 36
  resource limitations, 27
TTT, see Time temperature tolerance
Tuna, 17
  aquaculture, 2
  body temperature, 18
  canning, 195
  chemical composition, 33
  chromoproteins, 37
  clippers, 24—25
  collagen sugars, 40
  dipeptides, 45
  families of commercial importance, 20
  fishing gear, 21, 22
  fishing methods, 24—25
  flavor compounds, 45
  freezing, 119
  lipids, 41
  minced-type products, 204, 205
  mineral content, 49, 50
  myofibrillar proteins, 38
  postharvest changes, 60
  protein quality, 36
  resource limitations, 27
  scombroid fish poisoning, 223
  vitamin content, 47, 48
Turbot, 20, 36, 47
TVN, 104
Typhoid fever, 218
Tyrosine, color changes, 68—69

U

Umami, 45
Unit operations, see Operations
Urea, 21, 57

V

V-cut for deheading, 80, 85
V-cut fillet, 86
Vertical axis drum washer, 79, 83
Vessels, fishing, see Fishing vessels
Vibrio, 66
Vibrio cholerae, 218
Vibrio parahemolyticus, 67, 102, 218, 219
Vibrio vulnificus, 218
Viral diseases, 66, 218, 220

Viscera, 18, see also Digestive tract; Gutting
  mineral content, 51
  postharvest changes, 64
  salted products, 151
Vitamins
  composition, 31—32, 47—49
  dried fish quality, 139
  fat-soluble, 47, 117
  frozen fish, 117
  water-soluble, 47, 48, 196, 197
VNIIMP-1, 172

W

Wallemia sebi, 136
Washing
  canning process, 193
  for marinades, 157, 158, 160
  minced-type products, 201—202, 206, 207
  on-board processing, 95
  operations, 78, 79, 83, 84
Water, see also Washing
  activity, 133—134
    dried fish products, 137
    insect spoilage and, 137
    lipid oxidation and, 135
    marinades, cold, 157
    microbial spoilage and, 135—136
  canning, sterilization in, 190
  food-borne diseases and, 225
  sanitation, 215—218
    fishing vessel, 213
    manufacturing plants, 216
    steam sanitizing, 228—229
  tissue fluids
    composition of major groups of marine organisms, 31, 33—34
    drying, sorption isotherms and, 131—132
    frozen product, dessication of, 121
    marinades, fried, 160
    minced-type products, 200—201
    postharvest changes, protein hydration, 68
    salting-in process, 150—151
  smoked product, 167
  smoke partitioning, 166
  smoking and, 174, 175
Water-soluble vitamins, see Vitamins
Wax esters, 41, 65
Whales, 45
Whitefish
  minced-type products, 205
  postharvest changes, 64
  protein quality, 36
White muscle
  connectin, 38—39
  lipid distribution, 44
  postharvest changes, enzymatic protein degradation, 64
  protein composition, 36, 37
Whiting, 51
Wholesomeness, 2
WHO standards, hygiene, 224
Wood smoke, 164—169
World catch, 26, 27
Wounding gear, 21—22

X

Xanthan gums, 203
Xanthomonas, 66
Xenoma, 222

Y

Yeasts and molds
  associations of, 66
  dried fish, 136, 138, 139
  freezing effects, 112
  marinades, cooked, 159
  smoking and, 169
  sorbates and, 102
Yellowtail, 37, 39, 117

Z

Zooplankton, 12, 13, 42, see also Krill